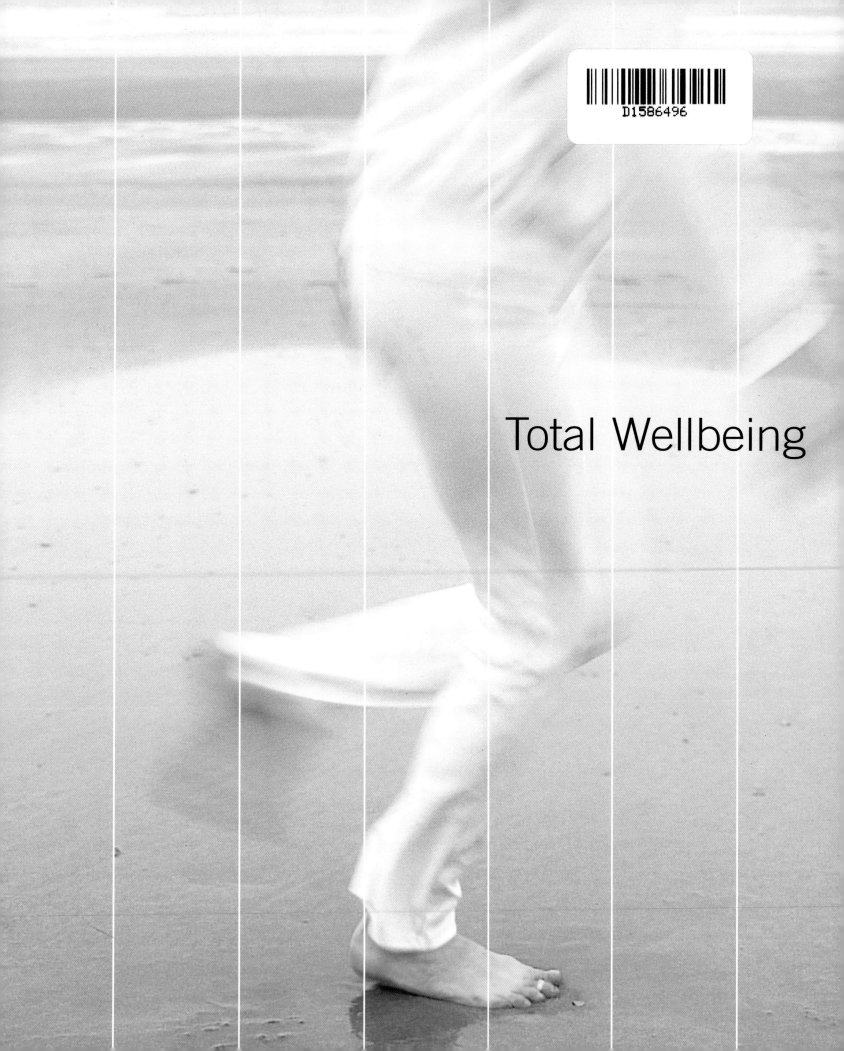

Total Wellbeing

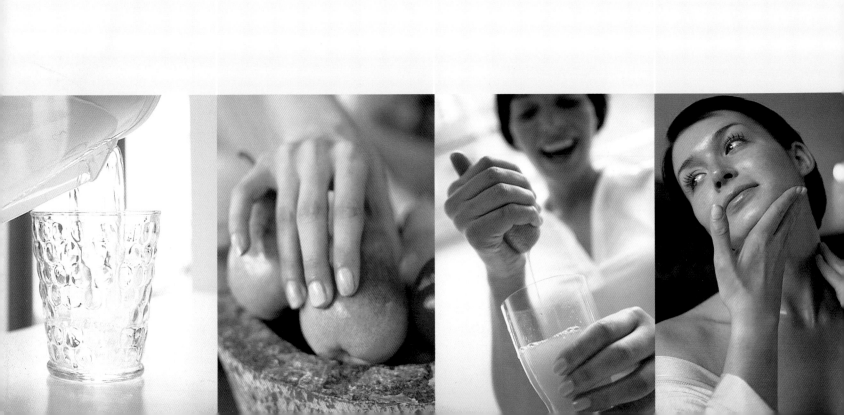

hamlyn

Total Wellbeing

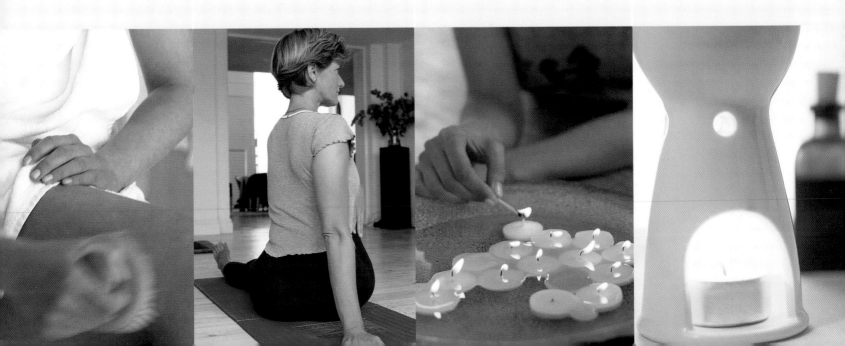

Introduction
6

Foodwise
10

Detoxifying your body
88

Face and hair
110

First published in Great Britain in 2002 by Hamlyn, a division of Octopus Publishing Group Ltd 2–4 Heron Quays, London E14 4JP

This paperback edition first published 2003

Copyright © Octopus Publishing Group Ltd 2002, 2003

ISBN 0 600 60796 8

A CIP catalogue record for this book is available from the British Library

Printed and bound in China

10 9 8 7 6 5 4 3 2

SAFETY NOTE

It is advisable to check with your doctor before embarking on any exercise, massage, diet or detox programme. *Total Wellbeing* should not be considered a replacement for professional medical treatment; a physician should be consulted in all matters relating to health and particularly in respect of pregnancy and any symptoms which may require diagnosis or medical attention. While the advice and information in this book is believed to be accurate and the step-by-step instructions have been devised to avoid strain, the publisher cannot accept legal responsibility for any injury or illness sustained while following the exercises and diet plan.

Some of the material in this book has appeared in titles previously published by Hamlyn.

4

Pampering your body

148

5

Posture and exercise

180

6

Rest and relaxation

228

7

Therapies and treatments

274

RECIPE NOTES

1 Standard level spoon measurements are used in all recipes.
 1 tablespoon = one 15 ml spoon
 1 teaspoon = one 5 ml spoon

2 Both metric and imperial measurements are given for the recipes. Use one set of measurements only, not a mixture of both.

3 Measurements for canned food are given as a standard metric equivalent.

4 Eggs should be large unless otherwise stated. The Department of Health advises that eggs should not be consumed raw. This book contains some dishes made with raw or lightly cooked eggs. It is prudent for more vulnerable people, such as pregnant and nursing mothers, invalids, the elderly, babies and young children, to avoid dishes made with uncooked or lightly cooked eggs. Once prepared, these dishes should be kept refrigerated and used promptly.

5 Milk should be full-fat unless otherwise stated.

6 Fresh herbs should be used unless otherwise stated. If unavailable, use dried herbs as an alternative but halve the quantities stated.

7 Pepper should be freshly ground black pepper unless otherwise stated.

8 Ovens should be preheated to the specified temperature. If using a fan-assisted oven, follow the manufacturer's instructions for adjusting the time and temperature. Grills should also be preheated.

9 This book includes dishes made with nuts and nut derivatives. It is advisable for readers with known allergic reactions to nuts and nut derivatives and those who may be potentially vulnerable to these allergies, such as pregnant and nursing mothers, invalids, the elderly, babies, and children, to avoid dishes made with nuts and nut oils. It is also prudent to check the labels of pre-prepared ingredients for the possible inclusion of nut derivatives.

10 Vegetarians should look for the 'V' symbol on cheese to ensure that it is made with vegetarian rennet. There are vegetarian forms of Parmesan, feta, Cheddar, Cheshire, Red Leicester, dolcelatte and many goat's cheeses, among others.

11 The nutritional values given in each recipe refer to one serving of.the dish.

Introduction

How often do you spend some time on yourself? In our busy lives, we pack so much in that we have no time left for the basics in life: to prepare a proper meal, take a little gentle exercise or simply to relax and allow the stresses of the day to drain away. We start to feel tired, we become pallid, our waistlines fill out and we suffer from nagging symptoms such as headaches and digestive problems. Taking some time out to pamper yourself and improve your overall health will boost your general wellbeing and make you feel more energized. You will have a better outlook on life and more self confidence to face the world. You don't have to spend a lot of time in order to make a difference. A little effort goes a long way to reducing stress and invigorating your emotional, physical and spiritual wellbeing.

As an added bonus, if you take steps to improve your health you will not only feel better, but look better too. Good health on the inside really shines through on the outside in the form of a better complexion, glossy hair, a more upright posture and toned figure.

Though it may sound strange, devoting time to yourself can actually improve your relationships with others. Most of us feel pulled in many different directions at once, with demands from our partners, work, children and the home. It is only natural to begin to resent the time you have to spend on others when there is none left over at the end of the day. If you take a little time out for yourself, you will feel happier and more generous with the rest of your time. You owe it to those around you as much as you do to yourself.

Making time

You can invest as little or as much time as you can spare. Even a few minutes a day or an hour a week will give you a boost, whether it's a regular fixture or a one-off session. For example, with just a few minutes to spend before work each day you can do a regular facial massage to tone your skin and improve your complexion. With a free hour two or three times a week you could practise yoga or body toning exercises, or some relaxation techniques before bed. And when you have an evening free, indulge in an aromatherapy bath or skin brushing session. When you have more time to yourself and you feel like really making an effort, take on a 7-day detox diet or a detoxing weekend home health spa, to revitalize body and soul.

However much time you are able to invest, make sure it is at a time when you will not be interrupted. Take the telephone off the hook so you can really relax and make sure you don't have to cut the session short. To gain maximum benefit, you really need to feel that you are indulging yourself and spending time and effort just for you. If you are planning regular sessions, set aside the same slot each day or week and stick to it. You will soon get into the habit and it will become part of your routine so you won't even have to think about it. You are much more likely to keep it up if you aren't constantly worrying about when you are going to fit it in each day – more stress is what you don't need.

What to concentrate on

Take a look at yourself and your lifestyle and decide which area of your life needs most attention. Most of us have niggling feelings about what we could improve on, or an aspect of our lives we feel guilty about. We usually put these feelings to the backs of our minds, with the misguided notion that we will deal with them when we have more time. Just by facing up to possible problems and tackling them head on, even for just a few minutes a day, you will feel more positive about yourself and your life in general. Ask yourself whether you most need to concentrate on:

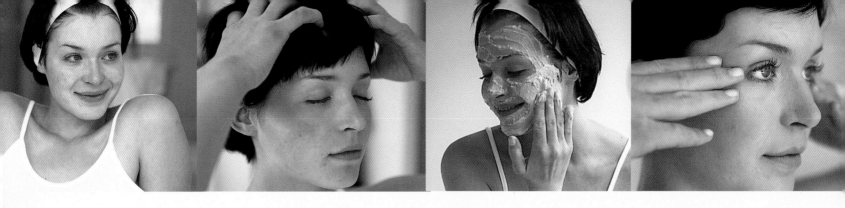

- fitness
- diet
- face, skin and hair
- posture and exercise
- rest and relaxation

If you are having trouble deciding, try completing the questionnaries on pages 13, 91, 113 and 231 to show you where there is most room for improvement. If the results reveal you need to work on more than one area, then choose the one you feel would make the biggest difference to your life – half the battle is in the motivation.

Concentrate on one area at a time and work it into your routine, then build up to more when you think you have the time. There's no point in trying to tackle everything at once as you are much more likely to let it all slip. Introduce it gradually and you will succeed.

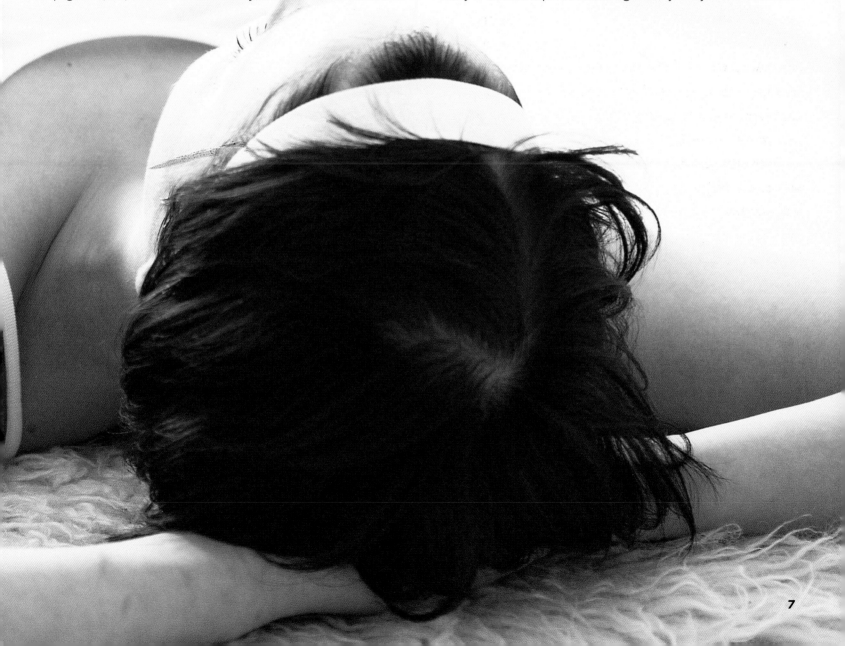

About this book

This hands-on guide takes you through all aspects of improving your wellbeing, showing you quick and simple ways to make you feel great and look even better, from diet and exercise to skincare, body pampering and relaxation techniques. Most of it can be done at home, but there are also details of professional treatments, such as aromatherapy massage, herbal healing and Reiki.

There are many exercise, toning and massage routines to try out, clearly illustrated with step-by-step photographs. Over 35 delicious recipes are included for nutritious and healthy dishes to add to your repertoire, plus recipes for homemade natural beauty products to give you a healthy glow.

Cross-references at the end of each section guide you around the book, and suggest related topics. The book has the following chapters:

Foodwise

This section tackles food and drink and shows how to achieve a balanced and nutritious diet for optimum health. It explains the major food groups – proteins, fats, carbohydrates, vitamins and minerals – and tells you which foods contain which nutrients. It then highlights the top foods for health, the ones bursting with beneficial nutrients. Food allergies and intolerances are tackled, and clear advice is given on buying organic produce. A recipe section gives flavoursome dishes packed with natural, healthy ingredients, suitable for all occasions.

Detoxifying your body

A modern lifestyle exposes us to unavoidable and potentially harmful atmospheric pollution, food additives and other chemicals. Their effects can build up over time, making us feel generally unwell, or causing more serious symptoms. A questionnaire helps you decide whether you are at risk, then offers ways to reduce the build-up of chemicals in your body and detoxify your system to bring you back to good health. Choose from a 7-day detox diet to follow when you need a boost, and a weekend home health spa programme to cleanse and restore body and mind when you have a few days to spare.

Face and hair

Of all body parts, your face is most at risk from the effects of dirt, atmospheric pollution, make-up, lack of sleep and stress. Yet it is also

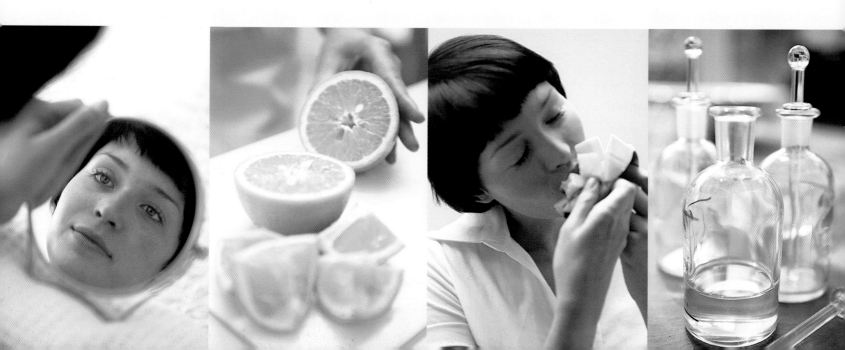

the part with which you greet the world, so you want it to look its best. This chapter discusses ways to improve your complexion and muscle tone by means of facial exercises and facial massage routines, clearly illustrated in step-by-step photographs. The section ends with haircare essentials: advice on how to achieve naturally healthy hair.

Pampering your body

What better way than body pampering to relax and feel good about yourself? This chapter covers all aspects of looking after your skin, including your hands, nails and feet. It offers advice on bathing and showering for maximum benefit to your skin, then looks at sun safety and how to reduce cellulite. Step-by-step photographs show basic massage strokes, a full body massage routine, plus foot massage. Treatments to make your skin feel toned and refreshed, such as salt scrubbing, skin brushing and hydrotherapy, are covered, too.

Posture and exercise

Exercise doesn't have to leave you gasping: there are many gentle, relaxing ways to improve your posture and muscle tone. By means of carefully illustrated exercises, this section gives ways to work on posture; a selection of Pilates exercises; and body shaping and toning exercises, showing you how to achieve a flatter stomach, a beautiful bottom and trimmer thighs. The chapter ends with a discussion of different types of aerobic exercise to improve fitness.

Rest and relaxation

Being able to wind down is one of the keys to total wellbeing. This section offers advice on reducing and dealing with stress. It includes many ways to unwind, through yoga, meditation, visualization, autogenic training and *feng shui*, and ends by showing you how to indulge yourself with a full-blown relaxing weekend home health spa.

Therapies and treatments

Many therapies and treatments can alleviate nagging symptoms brought about by a hectic lifestyle, or simply help you unwind and lift your spirits. Try aromatherapy, reflexology, acupressure, herbal healing, chi kung or Reiki. Each treatment has something to offer and is explained in full. Some you can even do for yourself at home.

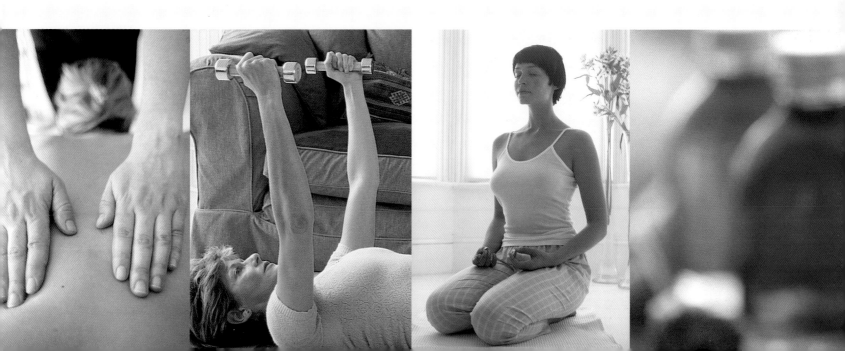

Foodwise

We are what we eat, and any deficiency of specific nutrients in the diet has far-reaching consequences on all of the body's systems. Our bodies need a balanced diet that provides all of the necessary vitamins, minerals, protein, carbohydrates, fibre and fats to maintain our health and wellbeing. Whatever your lifestyle, try to ensure that the food you eat is conducive to good health. Instead of relying on processed convenience foods with all their chemical additives, extra salt, fat and sugar, consider doing more home cooking using simple unprocessed ingredients, making your own fresh fruit and vegetable juices and drinking herbal teas.

Health from within

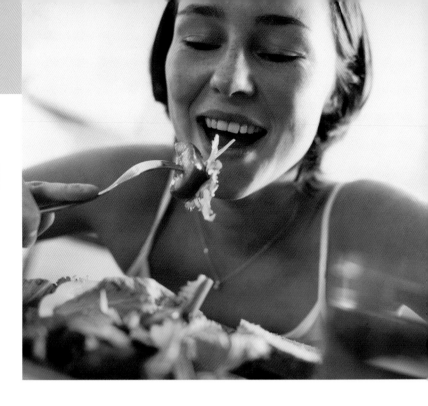

As well as offering protection against colds or more serious illnesses, eating a healthy diet has other beneficial effects. It can make you feel good from within and generally more optimistic about life. It should also give you more energy, and take away that sluggish, lacklustre feeling caused by eating too much junk food.

Healthy eating will make you look better, too. A regular intake of all the necessary nutrients will greatly improve the appearance of your skin and your complexion, giving you a healthy radiance. Your hair will shine, and your teeth and nails will also be stronger.

How to think about food

Food should be one of life's great pleasures. Make an effort with what you eat and take the time to pamper yourself with healthy luxuries – it's a cheap and easy way to treat yourself as healthy eating doesn't have to rely on limp, dull salads and plain brown rice. Just think how delicious a simple slice of luscious ripe melon can be or a plate of sumptuous asparagus tips. Consider fragrant exotic fruits, fresh salad leaves, healthy and delicious sushi, sweet ripe tomatoes, good quality Italian pasta, smooth homemade guacamole, a succulent organic chicken breast grilled with lemon and herbs, cold poached organic salmon, or a bowl of live, low-fat natural yogurt with a drizzle of honey and some toasted almonds. When starting to eat more healthily, you don't have to give up all treats, as an occasional chocolate or ice cream won't hurt.

Shopping for food

Regular shopping to maintain a supply of fresh ingredients is important for healthy eating, so shop little and often. This gives you the opportunity to buy and cook what you fancy when you fancy it. If you have a good supply of fresh ingredients in the house, you are more likely to cook a proper meal rather than ordering a take away.

If you don't get home until late, buy natural convenience foods which cook quickly or don't need cooking at all. Create delicious meals in minutes from salad ingredients, pesto for instant pasta sauces, baby new potatoes, sweet peppers, pitta breads, fresh herbs, tinned fish, meat or fish for grilling, and fresh vegetables.

Cooking methods

Healthy eating is almost as much about how you cook as what you cook. The two main principles are to retain vitamins and reduce oil and fat.

- As a general rule, cook fruits and vegetables as little as possible or not at all
- Add as little oil or fat to foods as possible
- Boil, steam or poach foods rather than frying or roasting with oil
- Grill meat rather than roasting or frying
- Steam vegetables if they need to be cooked
- Tear up leaf vegetables rather than slicing them with a knife
- Remove any visible oil or fat from food before serving

How healthy is your diet?

1 Do you eat breakfast:
- ☐ **A**: Never?
- ☑ **B**: Only at weekends?
- ☑ **C**: Every day?

2 How many portions of fruit, vegetables and salad do you eat each day?
- ☑ **A**: One or two?
- ☐ **B**: Three or four?
- ☐ **C**: Five or more?

3 Would you say your diet is:
- ☐ **A**: Predictable – you eat a relatively small variety of different foods most weeks
- ☑ **B**: Reasonably varied – you try not to stick to old favourites all the time
- ☐ **C**: Very varied – you love experimenting with new recipes and ingredients

4 Do you eat a takeaway:
- ☐ **A**: Most days?
- ☐ **B**: Several times a week?
- ☑ **C**: Occasionally or never?

5 Do you eat high-fat foods (like sausages, pies, burgers, chips, cheese and butter):
- ☐ **A**: More than once every day?
- ☑ **B**: Most days?
- ☐ **C**: Once a week or less?

6 What cooking method do you use most often?
- ☐ **A**: Frying or roasting?
- ☑ **B**: Grilling?
- ☐ **C**: Steaming?

7 Which is your favourite snack?
- ☐ **A**: A chocolate bar?
- ☑ **B**: A cake or biscuits?
- ☐ **C**: Fresh fruit?

8 Do you usually eat:
- ☐ **A**: At your desk or on the move?
- ☑ **B**: In front of the television?
- ☐ **C**: Slowly, sitting at the table?

9 Given the choice, do you drink:
- ☑ **A**: A can of fizzy drink such as a cola or something alcoholic?
- ☐ **B**: Tea or coffee?
- ☐ **C**: Water or herbal tea?

10 Do you have calcium-rich dairy foods, such as milk, cheese, yogurt or crème fraîche:
- ☐ **A**: Now and then?
- ☐ **B**: Several times a week?
- ☑ **C**: At least once a day?

HOW YOU SCORED

MOSTLY As

It's time to clean up: you're unlikely to be eating a sufficiently varied diet, probably overdosing on fats and sugars and you may be missing out on essential nutrients. Your main priorities should be to increase fruit and vegetable consumption to five portions a day, cut down on fats and eat more complex carbohydrates such as wholemeal bread and pasta. You don't have to cut out every single 'baddie' – just regard them as an indulgence to be enjoyed now and again.

MOSTLY Bs

Your diet isn't a disaster but there's room for improvement. You should aim to keep the fat content of your diet down to 30 per cent in calorie terms – if you switch to low-fat dairy foods and spreads, and cut down on 'processed' foods you'll get there fairly easily. Eat a couple of extra portions of fruit and veg every day and try to vary your diet a little more – make a point of trying a new dish every week. Opt for water or herbal teas sometimes instead of caffeine-rich drinks.

MOSTLY Cs

You're eating a healthy diet and providing your body with a good variety of nutrients while steering clear of 'empty calories'. Don't get too earnest though – there's still lots of scope for new tastes and cooking techniques. Remember that a healthy diet isn't just about nutrition – it's important to make meal times a pleasure so that you really enjoy your food.

A balanced diet

A healthy diet is primarily about balance. Our bodies need certain amounts of carbohydrates, proteins, fats, vitamins and minerals in order to function properly and, by eating sensibly, this is easy to achieve. (They also need plenty of water – see page 96.) With busy lifestyles and stressful jobs, it is all too easy to neglect our diets. However, it is well worth taking the time to think about what you eat, since a sensible diet will boost energy and vitality and doesn't necessarily mean hours of preparation and cooking.

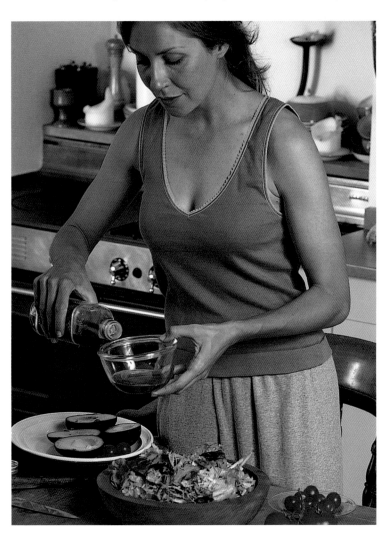

Guidelines for healthy eating

Healthy eating does not mean compromising on enjoyable foods or cutting out treats, it simply means that you should be aware of the food that you eat and follow a few simple guidelines.

Enjoy your food Food should be one of life's pleasures, to be savoured and enjoyed. Don't add stress to your life by worrying unnecessarily about food. Take time to enjoy food with family and friends and be a bit adventurous in trying new recipes and new ways of cooking.

Eat a variety of different foods There is no one food that will provide all the nutrients we need (apart from human milk, which provides for a baby's needs in the first few months of life). For this reason it is important to eat a wide variety of foods, and to make sure we include foods from all of the main food groups (see The food pyramid, page 16).

Maintain a healthy weight Body weight is the result of the balance between energy taken in, usually measured in calories, and the amount used up. Those who consume more calories than they use gain weight.

The more physically active we are, the greater our energy need. Cutting down very strictly on food intake to keep body weight down can mean that not enough of the essential nutrients are eaten. A healthy balance of food and exercise is therefore the best plan.

Eat plenty of foods rich in starch and fibre Most people do not eat enough starchy foods, but they are valuable sources of fibre (see page 19), and can be used in lots of different, interesting ways. For a well-balanced diet you should have plenty of the starchy foods at two, or preferably three, meals daily. At a main meal, most of the space on the plate should be taken up with starchy foods and vegetables, with the amount of meat or fish being quite small in proportion.

Eat plenty of fruit and vegetables Fruit and vegetables are protective foods, because they contain vitamins and minerals which help to keep us healthy (see pages 24–25). They may also protect us from diseases

Top tips for a healthy lifestyle

- Eat a variety of foods
- Maintain a healthy weight
- Always refuse second helpings if you need to watch your weight
- Eat slowly and not in front of the television or while otherwise distracted from the food on your plate
- Eat plenty of fruit and vegetables and foods rich in starch and fibre
- Choose foods that are low in fat and the unhealthy form of cholesterol

- Restrict your use of salt and sugar
- Opt for 'grazing', which means eating small meals and healthy snacks throughout the day, rather than eating two or three large meals
- Eat only when you are hungry
- Never go food shopping when you are hungry
- Don't buy the foods you find hard to resist. That way there will be no temptation in the cupboards at home
- Drink alcohol only in moderation

such as coronary heart disease, and some forms of cancer. Aim to eat at least five portions of fruit and vegetables a day, excluding potatoes.

Cut down on foods containing a lot of fat There are several different kinds of fat and they have different effects on the cholesterol level of our blood. Fat helps to make our diets more palatable and interesting and some fats are good sources of important vitamins, so a certain amount of fat is essential in our diets. In particular we need small amounts of the so-called 'essential fatty acids' (EFAs), which our bodies cannot manufacture themselves (see Fats, page 22).

Evidence shows that too high a proportion of certain fat in the diet leads to coronary heart disease – another reason to limit the amount of fat we eat. The important thing is to reduce the total amount of fat in the diet and then decide what kind of fat to use within the reduced amount.

Restrict your use of salt Salt affects the balance of fluid in the body and raises blood pressure. It draws water out of body cells, drying tissues including the skin. Therefore limit your intake of sodium by not adding salt to foods and by eating foods that are already salted only sparingly.

Limit your consumption of sugary foods and drinks Most of us enjoy the taste of sweet things. Sugar (white and brown sugar, honey and syrup) provides energy in the form of calories but very little in the way of other nutrients, and it upsets your body's blood sugar levels (see Carbohydrates, page 18). It is therefore sensible to cut right down on your intake of sugar and sugary foods, to maintain long term health.

If you drink alcohol, drink sensibly For many people alcohol is something to be enjoyed and it can enhance the enjoyment of a meal or social occasion. Research has shown that a certain amount of alcohol may improve some aspects of our health. However, moderation is the important aspect to remember, as there are also a number of risks associated with drinking alcohol; it is sensible to know what the recommended limits are and not to exceed these (see Everyday toxins, page 94).

SEE ALSO:

→ Carbohydrates, page 18
→ Proteins, page 20
→ Fats, page 22
→ Vitamins, page 24
→ Minerals, page 26

→ Top foods for health, pages 28–35
→ Making juices, page 40
→ Water, page 96
→ Aerobic exercise, page 224

The food pyramid

The food pyramid is all about eating a wide variety of foods, from each of the major food groups. The pyramid below is made up of these groups. Eating foods from each section of the pyramid every day, in the proportions shown, will provide a balance of the necessary nutrients. Good nutrition entails thinking in terms of both quality and quantity. The amount we eat of certain foods, and how often we eat them, is very important for a healthy diet. See the box on the right for recommended daily quantities.

Level 1 Sugars and fats

Foods containing sugars and fats are at the top of the pyramid. These include butter, cooking oils, oil-based dressings, ice cream, pastries, confectionery and certain soft drinks, and should be eaten sparingly as they are high in fat or refined carbohydrate such as sugar and honey. Although they make food taste good, too much fat raises blood cholesterol levels. Sugars provide calories yet few nutrients, and too much sugar can result in weight gain and tooth decay.

Level 2 Protein and dairy foods

The next step of the pyramid contains protein and dairy foods. Protein can come from animal sources (meat, fish and eggs, milk, cheese and yogurt); or vegetable sources such as beans and lentils (see page 34), and seeds (see page 34). Meat, fish and alternatives provide protein, iron, zinc, magnesium and some B vitamins, especially B12. Milk and dairy foods supply our bodies with protein, calcium and zinc, and vitamins B12, B2, A and D. Try to choose lean cuts of meat and low-fat dairy products to avoid too high an intake of fat. Similarly, certain nuts and seeds are high in saturated fat so eat them in moderation.

Level 3 Fruit and vegetables

Fruits and vegetables form the next step of the pyramid. These provide fibre and some carbohydrates, as well as many of the vitamins and minerals that are essential for our bodies to function efficiently. In terms of their nutritional value, it is best to eat fruits and vegetables when fresh, although certain varieties are fine frozen, too. Canned produce and dried fruit do also provide some of the nutrients needed.

Level 4 Starchy foods

The large base section of the pyramid contains the staple, starchy, carbohydrate foods that should provide the major source of energy in the diet. These include cereals (such as wheat, rye, oats, barley, millet), rice and products made from them, such as bread, pasta, noodles, cornmeal and breakfast cereals. Other staple carbohydrate foods in this group include potatoes, yams and other starchy vegetables. All the foods in this group are rich in nutrients – supplying fibre, B vitamins and some calcium and iron as well as carbohydrates (see page 18).

Quantities of foods required

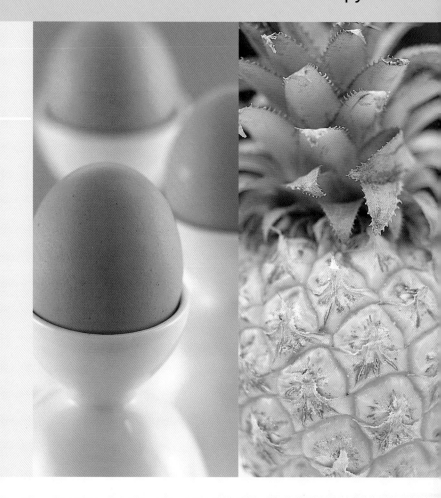

For a balanced diet, aim to have the following daily:

1	SUGARS AND FATS	1 serving
2	PROTEIN AND DAIRY FOODS	2–3 servings
3	FRUIT AND VEGETABLES	5 servings
4	STARCHY FOODS	4–5 servings

SUGARS AND FATS 1 SERVING:

One serving could include a small amount of spreading or cooking fat, and/or a small amount of sugary food. Sugar is best included in a starchy item, such as a cake or biscuit, rather than on its own.

PROTEIN AND DAIRY FOODS
1 SERVING:

1 small portion of meat (50–75 g/2–3 oz)

1 portion of fish (125–150 g/4–5 oz)

1 egg

25 g (1 oz) hard cheese

600 ml (1 pint) milk or yogurt

1 portion of cooked lentils, beans or peas
  (175–200 g/6–7 oz)

FRUIT AND VEGETABLES 1 SERVING:

apple, orange, peach, banana or pear

1 slice of large fruit (melon, pineapple,
  mango)

1 handful of berries or soft fruit

1 dessert bowl of salad

1 portion fresh or frozen vegetables
  (about 75 g/3 oz)

1 side salad

1 small bowl of canned fruit in fruit juice

1 glass of fresh fruit juice

STARCHY FOODS 1 SERVING:

1 large slice of bread

1 medium bowl of pasta or rice

1 bowl of breakfast cereal

2 medium potatoes or equivalent in yams, etc

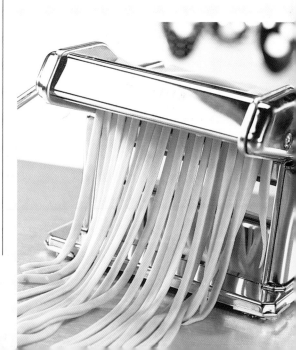

Carbohydrates

Carbohydrate foods provide the fuel the body needs to function in an efficient manner. Typical sources of carbohydrates include grains, vegetables, fruits and legumes.

Until recently, carbohydrates were classed as either 'simple' or 'complex'. Simple carbohydrates comprise simple sugars – found in milk, fruits and some vegetables. Complex carbohydrates are starchy foods, found in grains or foods made from wholegrains, such as bread, pasta and breakfast cereal. Potatoes, peas and beans are also high in starch.

Certain complex carbohydrates that are high in fibre, such as vegetables, legumes and unrefined wholegrain foods that have lost nothing in their processing, are particularly good for you. This is because high-fibre carbohydrates are digested more slowly. As a result the blood sugar level in the body doesn't rise as quickly, whereas low-fibre carbohydrates are digested faster and consequently raise blood sugar rapidly. Rapid rises in blood sugar are undesirable since they cause the body to produce higher levels of insulin, the hormone that helps regulate blood sugar levels. Over time, this can result in health problems.

Increasing your intake of high-fibre carbohydrates

- Replace refined low-fibre carbohydrates (for example white bread, white rice, sugary breakfast cereal) with unrefined carbohydrates (for example **wholemeal bread**, **brown rice**, **porridge oats**, **bran flakes**, **wholewheat pasta**)
- Snack on **dried fruit**
- Use **legumes** as a base for hearty soups and stews

Starches

In addition to the fact that starchy foods are very important as they make the blood sugar level rise quite slowly (especially important for diabetics), their bulkiness gives a feeling of fullness when they are eaten and the slow release of their carbohydrate helps to sustain energy over a long period of time. Indeed, for some forms of athletics, such as long-distance running, a very starchy meal eaten some hours before a race has been proved to be an extremely effective way of storing energy for slow release during a long, gruelling race.

Encompassing the staple foods common to every culture, starchy foods include bread, rice, pasta, couscous, all sorts of grains such as oats, rye, buckwheat, millet, and the starchy vegetables such as potatoes, yams and plantain. Many of these foods, particularly the wholegrain cereals, are good sources of important vitamins and minerals and many of them also contribute to the protein content of the diet. Some vitamins are lost in the milling process, for example rice loses its B vitamins in the polishing process, when it is changed from brown to white rice.

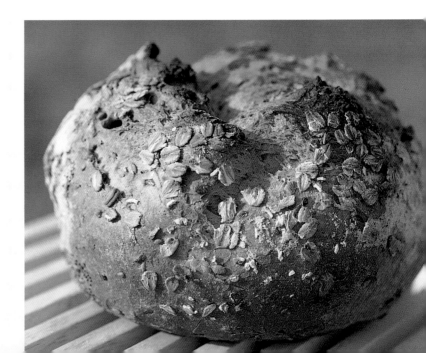

Fibre

We require plenty of fibre in our diets for fitness and wellbeing. The best sources are the wholegrain cereal foods, such as wholemeal bread, wholewheat pasta and brown rice. Vegetables and legumes (chickpeas, beans and lentils) are also very good sources of fibre, as are seeds and fruit (especially pears, prunes, figs and raspberries).

Dietary fibre (also called roughage) is formed from the cell walls of plants and occurs in two forms, insoluble and soluble, both of which are needed for good health. The fibre in wheat is mainly insoluble, whereas in other cereals a higher proportion of the fibre is soluble. In fruit and vegetables the proportion of soluble to insoluble fibre is about equal.

Dietary fibre is important for slowing the release of sugars into the bloodstream; it also keeps the bowel healthily active. A low-fibre diet causes constipation and over a period of time the bowel can lose its natural strength and elasticity. If there is too little fibre in the diet, the transit time of food residue is slowed, resulting in possible damage such as diverticulosis – the formation of small pockets in the lining of the gut. Too little fibre may also be a factor in the development of some forms of cancer. Fibre may also help to keep levels of blood cholesterol down.

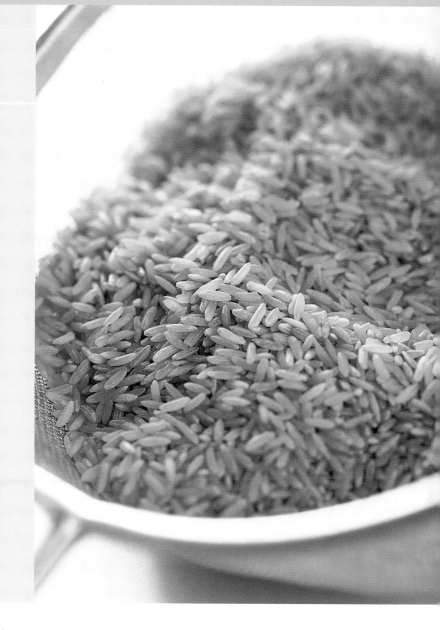

The great variety of starchy food now available to us from all over the world can be used to add interest and variety to the diet, so that the humble starchy staple food can be quite glamorous, as well as being a very important basis for good nutrition and a healthy balanced diet.

Quantities

Nutritionists recommend that a high percentage (40–50 per cent) of the calories consumed daily should be taken in the form of unrefined carbohydrates. By eating large portions of starchy foods, cooked and served with little or no fat, we can satisfy our hunger, making it easier to restrict the quantity of high-fat foods we eat. A diet high in unrefined carbohydrates and fruit and vegetables, and low in fatty foods, may have a protective effect against a number of diseases such as coronary heart disease and some forms of cancer.

SEE ALSO:

→ The food pyramid, page 16

→ Oats, page 33

→ Beans and lentils, page 34

Proteins

Proteins are the basic building blocks that are found in all cells in our bodies. They make up the structure of the cells as well as the elements inside, including enzymes and hormones. These structural elements are constantly being worn out so they need to be replaced by new proteins from the food we eat.

What are proteins?

Proteins, found mainly in meats, eggs, dairy products, cereals, beans, peas and lentils, are made up of chains of amino acids. There are about 20 different amino acids and the order in which they are linked in the chain depends on the type of protein they are making, whether it is a grain of wheat or muscle tissue in a cow. When we digest and absorb these foods, the chains are broken down into the individual amino acids. The body then builds up new chains with the amino acids in the right order to form different parts of the human body, such as hair, muscle, or a hormone.

It used to be thought that proteins from vegetable sources, such as grains and beans, were of a lower quality than those from animal sources such as meat and eggs, but it has since been shown that this

Dairy products

Products such as milk, yogurt and cheese are good sources of protein and also provide essential minerals and vitamins. Milk is a very important source of calcium and also of the B vitamin, riboflavin. If you use low-fat dairy products you will lose much of the content of fat-soluble vitamins (A, D, E), but the essential minerals such as calcium will still be available.

Good sources of protein

- Meat
- Offal
- Milk
- Cheese
- Yogurt
- Corn
- Wheat
- Bread
- Pasta
- Rice
- Potatoes
- Couscous
- Nuts
- Beans
- Peas
- Lentils
- Eggs

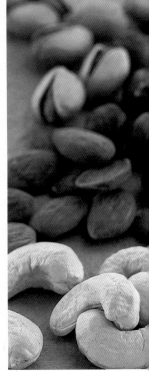

is not true. They do have less protein per unit weight than meat products but the quality is the same. Research has shown that just about all diets around the world have a more than adequate supply of protein and that the protein quality varies little, whatever the percentage of meat to vegetables in the diet. Even diets based almost solely on one source of vegetable protein, such as rice, contain adequate protein for healthy growth.

In fact, in Western countries today there is a general move towards sources of vegetable protein such as bread, pasta, beans and lentils to replace meat products. Vegetables and grains contain a lot less fat than animal protein foods such as meat, cheese and milk, as well as more fibre, so they are much healthier.

Why do we need proteins?

Every cell in our bodies is partly composed of protein. We need to have adequate supplies of protein to build cells, and for the existing cells to go through their continuous process of growing and replacing themselves. As well as their role as building blocks, proteins like carbohydrates also supply us with energy to fuel our bodies.

What provides 60 g (2½ oz) of protein?

To compare, 1 g of protein supplies 4 calories, whereas 1 g of carbohydrate supplies 3.5 calories and 1 g of fat supplies 9 calories. If we are low on energy, our bodies will use proteins for fuel first but this is rather like fuelling a furnace with paper money, as unlike fats and carbohydrates, proteins have a much more important structural role, too.

How much do we need?

In most diets around the world, 10–15 per cent of the total energy (calories) consumed is provided by proteins, though the recommended intake is about 10 per cent. This works out at about 60 g (2½ oz) of protein per day for an average person. In Western societies, protein deficiency is extremely rare; in fact there is more concern about eating too much protein as research suggests an association between red meat consumption and heart attack, stroke and bowel cancer.

(all uncooked weights)

- 1.8 litres (3 pints) milk
- 2.8 kg (4½ lb) potatoes
- 240 g (7¾ oz) dried lentils
- 230 g (7½ oz) peanuts
- 460 g (14½ oz) dried pasta
- 800 g (1lb 10 oz) brown rice
- 19 slices of wholemeal bread
- 340 g (11½ oz) rump steak
- 240 g (7¾ oz) Cheddar cheese
- 300 g (10 oz) chicken
- 400 g (13 oz) lamb chops
- 660 g (1 lb 5½ oz) sausages
- 325 g (11 oz) haddock
- 16 fish fingers

Proteins for vegetarians and vegans

Like meat-eaters, vegetarians and vegans must ensure their diet contains adequate protein and calories for energy and for rebuilding the tissues of the body. This is not usually a problem as it is easy to substitute cereals, beans, nuts and vegetables for meat. If a variety of these protein foods is eaten in sufficient quantity to provide enough calories, then it is unlikely that a vegetarian or vegan will not get enough protein.

It is a mistake to replace meat with just cheese, eggs and milk as these foods are relatively high in fat and large quantities will lead to obesity.

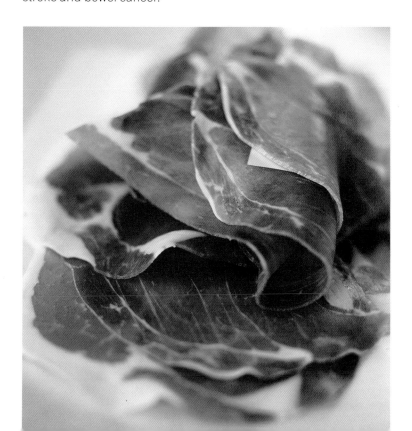

SEE ALSO:

→ The food pyramid, page 16

→ Fats, page 22

→ Beans and lentils, page 34

→ Nuts and seeds, page 34

→ Soya and tofu, page 35

→ Yogurt, page 35

Fats

Fat adds richness and moistness to food and improves the taste. We need some fat in the diet for energy and to provide fat-soluble vitamins. The body can make the fatty acids it requires except for the essential fatty acids (EFAs), which must be supplied in the diet. However, all fats are very concentrated sources of calories and excess consumption causes weight gain. A high concentration of saturated fat in the diet may also increase the risk of coronary heart disease and some forms of cancer. It is advisable to restrict the total amount of fat in the diet (see box opposite), to maintain a healthy weight and control the level of cholesterol in the blood.

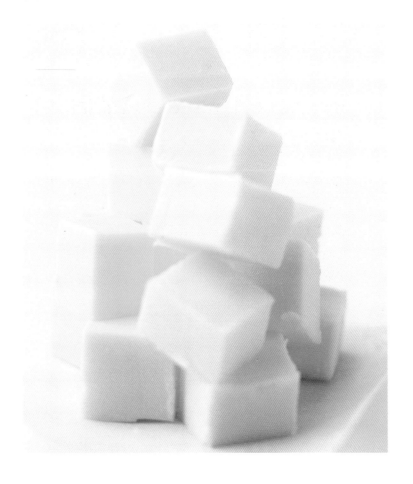

Cholesterol

This is a natural and necessary form of fat manufactured in the body from dietary fats. There are two types: 'good' cholesterol (high-density lipoprotein, HDL) and 'bad' cholesterol (low-density lipoprotein, LDL). The former is necessary to make oestrogen and testosterone among other vital bodily functions, but too much LDL cholesterol can clog the arteries, leading to coronary heart disease and strokes. High levels of cholesterol may be reduced by restricting fat in the diet, and changing the type of fat that is eaten.

What kind of fat?

The chief sources of fat in the diet are dairy products, meat, oils and fried foods. Oily fish such as mackerel contain the EFAs necessary for good health (see Polyunsaturated fats, opposite). Some foods may be high sources of hidden fats, for example biscuits, cakes and pastries. Fats can be divided into saturated, monounsaturated or polyunsaturated fats.

Saturated fats These are usually solid at room temperature and tend to come from animal sources – the fat on meat, butter, lard and cheese. Vegetable sources of saturated fat are coconut butter and palm oil. The process of hardening vegetable oil to make margarine is called hydrogenation and changes the fat content to a higher proportion of saturated fat. A high intake of saturated fat raises blood cholesterol, particularly the fraction of cholesterol that is thought to be the most harmful, the low-density lipoproteins (LDL). High quantities of saturated fats are found in many fast and processed foods.

Monounsaturated fats Olive oil is our main source of monounsaturated fat. It has been observed that populations who use olive oil regularly have a much better health record than those who rely on animal fats. Monounsaturated fats help to lower LDL

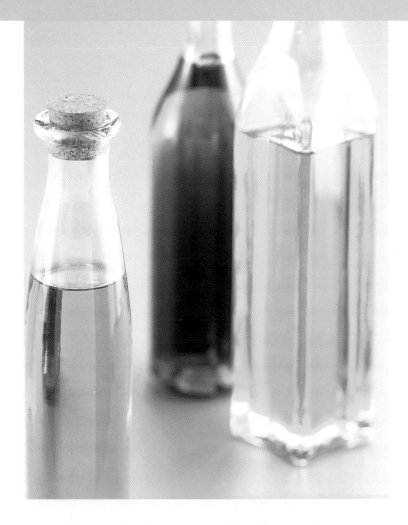

cholesterol in the blood and maintain the important HDL levels, and are therefore thought to protect against coronary heart disease. Other good sources of monounsaturated fat are rapeseed oil, many kinds of nuts and avocados.

Polyunsaturated fats These contain the essential fatty acids that our bodies need from our diet. They help decrease the LDL cholesterol level in blood. Good sources are fresh nuts and seeds and their oils (such as sunflower, safflower, walnut and corn oils), leafy green vegetables, seafood and oily fish (herring, kippers, mackerel, tuna, salmon, sardines, whitebait and anchovies). Ideally, EFAs should account for at least 15 per cent of our calorie intake.

Everyday fats

Butter and margarine have the same calorie content, whether or not the margarine is marked 'polyunsaturated'. Butter is a good source of the fat-soluble vitamins A and D, and these vitamins are added to margarine.

Low-fat spreads all have a high water content and therefore a lower calorie content than margarine or butter. Low-fat spreads usually have added fat-soluble vitamins.

Most cheeses have a high fat content; however, lower-fat varieties of some hard cheeses are available. Many soft cheeses can be bought in low-fat varieties. Quark is very low in fat, and low-fat ricotta or fromage frais are also good. Double cream, however, is a wopping 50 per cent fat.

Reducing the total amount of fat in the diet

- Choose lower-fat versions of dairy products, e.g. **skimmed** and **semi-skimmed milk** and **reduced-fat cheese**
- Use less fat in cooking. **Grill** and **bake** instead of frying and roasting
- Opt for **low-fat spreads** for bread
- Use **lean cuts** of meat and **remove skin** from poultry

SEE ALSO:

→ The food pyramid, page 16   → Oily fish, page 33

→ Proteins, page 20   → Nuts and seeds, page 34

Vitamins

If you eat a wide variety of food and a balanced diet you should get all the vitamins you require, with no need for supplements. If you do take a supplement, it is sensible not to exceed the recommended dose. There are two main types of vitamins – fat-soluble and water-soluble ones. The fat-soluble vitamins, A, D, E and K, are stored in the body and taking excessive amounts of them could be harmful. The water-soluble vitamins, vitamin C and the B complex vitamins, are not stored in the body and any excess amounts are excreted in the urine. A good mixed diet should contain adequate amounts of all these vitamins.

Vitamin A (retinol)

Vitamin A is essential for vision in dim light and for the maintenance of healthy skin and surface tissues of the body. It is stored in the liver and is toxic in very excessive amounts. Vitamin A is found in natural fats such as whole milk and butter, and liver has a very high content. It can also be made in the body from beta-carotene, which is found in leafy green vegetables and in orange-coloured fruit and vegetables such as carrots, apricots, mangoes, pumpkin, tomatoes and peppers.

Vitamin D (cholecalciferol)

Vitamin D is essential for maintaining calcium and phosphorus levels in the blood and for building healthy bones and teeth. Deficiency causes rickets in children and osteomalacia (bone thinning) in adults.

The best source of vitamin D is the action of sunlight on the skin. Dietary sources are less important, except for people who cannot go out or who do not expose their skin to light. Sources include oily fish, milk, butter and egg yolks. Vitamin D is added to margarine, and some manufacturers add vitamin D to breakfast cereals and some types of yogurt.

Vitamin E (tocopherol)

One of the top antioxidants, Vitamin E fights free radicals (see page 28) and helps your skin stay healthy. It is found in poultry, fish, vegetables, vegetable oils, nuts and seeds.

Vitamin K

Vitamin K helps the body make a number of proteins, one of which is necessary for blood clotting. It is found in leafy green vegetables, soya oil and margarine.

Vitamin B

The vitamin B complex includes thiamine (B1), riboflavin (B2), niacin (B3), vitamins B5, B6, B12, biotin and folate. Thiamine, riboflavin and niacin are essential for the release of energy from the food we eat, particularly from carbohydrates. These vitamins are widely distributed in foods, including milk, offal, eggs, vegetables, fruit and wholegrain cereals. Many breakfast cereals are fortified with B vitamins.

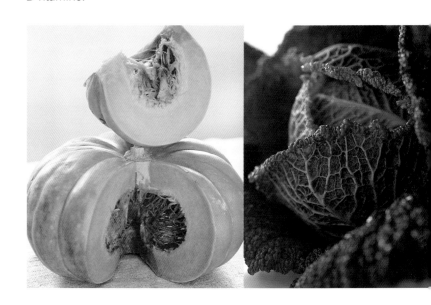

Vitamin B5 (pantothenic acid) This helps break down carbohydrates, proteins and fats, and encourages the growth and maintenance of body tissues. It is found in meat, especially offal, fish, egg yolks and beans.

Vitamin B6 (pyridoxine) This is involved in the metabolism of amino acids (the breakdown products of protein), and is necessary for the formation of haemoglobin. Deficiency of vitamin B6 is rare, and very high intakes could be dangerous. It occurs widely in food, especially in meat, fish, eggs, wholegrain cereals and some vegetables.

Vitamin B12 (cobalamine) A mixture of compounds, B12 is necessary (with folate) for the development and maintenance of cells in the blood. It occurs mainly in animal products, particularly liver, eggs, cheese, milk, meat and fish. It is also available from yeast extracts, and is added to some breakfast cereals. Deficiency leads to a form of anaemia.

Biotin Like pantothenic acid, biotin helps break down carbohydrates, proteins and fats. It is found in meat, milk, eggs, beans, nuts and wholegrains.

Folate (folic acid) Folate has a number of functions, but is important for the development of rapidly dividing cells. Folate deficiency can arise from poor diet, and also when there are increased needs for the synthesis of red blood cells, for example in pregnancy. There is some evidence that adequate folate in the diet in the very early stages of pregnancy can protect against the development of spina bifida in the fetus. The best dietary sources of folate are offal and leafy green vegetables. Folate is easily destroyed by cooking vegetables, as it is lost in the water used for cooking. Avoid boiling leafy green vegetables – choose steaming, stir-frying or wilting in a little oil instead, or eat them raw if at all possible.

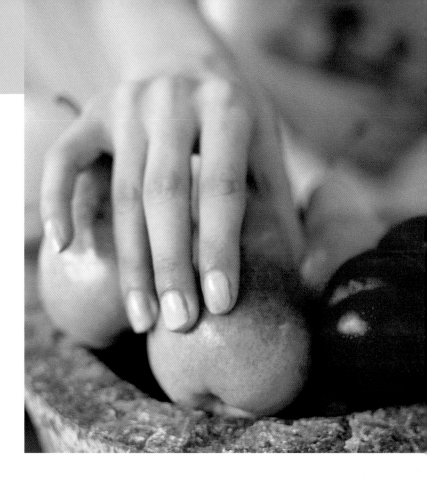

Vitamin C (ascorbic acid)

Vitamin C is necessary for growth and the maintenance of healthy connective tissue in the body. It also helps in the absorption of iron. Lack of vitamin C leads to gum bleeding, bruising and poor wound healing. Only humans and guinea pigs need to get vitamin C from their diet. All other animals can make the vitamin within their bodies.

The best sources of vitamin C are vegetables and fruit. Potatoes are a good source of the vitamin because of the large amounts generally eaten. Blackcurrants are very high in the vitamin and citrus fruits and strawberries are good sources, too. Green salads and vegetables are also useful.

The amount of vitamin C in fruits and vegetables diminishes with storing and cooking. Frozen vegetables may therefore sometimes have a higher vitamin C content than fresh vegetables that have been stored for some time.

SEE ALSO:

→ A balanced diet, page 14   → Top foods for health, page 28

→ Minerals, page 26   → Making juices, page 40

Minerals

Our bodies need to take a number of minerals from our diets in order to stay healthy – for the growth and the maintenance of bones, cells and tissues. Some are needed in only very small quantities and are called trace minerals. Examples of these include zinc, selenium, iron, iodine and chromium. Other minerals, for example calcium, phosphorus and magnesium, are required in much larger amounts. By eating a healthy, mixed diet it is possible to get all the minerals needed every day. The most important dietary minerals are calcium, iron and zinc. Phosphorus and magnesium are also important, but a diet that provides sufficient calcium will also provide adequate phosphorus and magnesium.

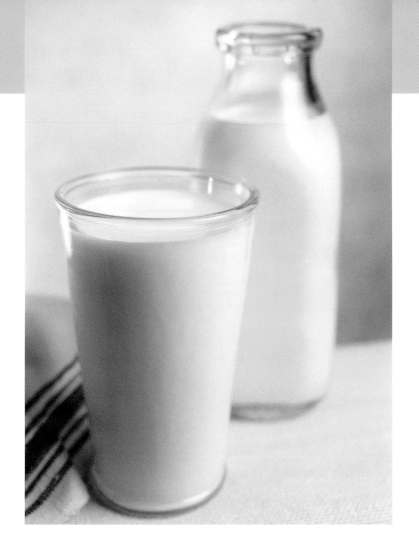

Calcium

Calcium and phosphorus together form the framework of our skeleton, giving strength to bones and teeth. A deficiency of calcium in some elderly people may result in osteoporosis, where calcium is lost from the bone, making it painful to bear weight. In order to prevent osteoporosis, it is important to build strong bones early in life, when the bones are growing actively, through weight-bearing exercise and adequate dietary calcium. The best sources of dietary calcium are milk, cheese and other milk products such as yogurt. The calcium in milk is in the watery part of the liquids, so using skimmed or semi-skimmed milk, or low-fat yogurts and cheeses, will not lower your calcium intake.

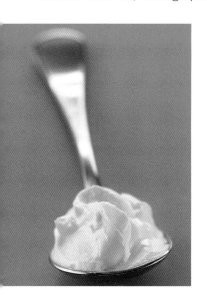

Butter and cream contain very little calcium. For people who do not take milk, calcium is available in some vegetables and seeds. Some kinds of soya milk have added calcium, and it is often added to white bread and soya curd products such as tofu (see page 35). In addition to strengthening bones and teeth, calcium acts as a natural tranquillizer, soothing irritability and aiding insomnia.

Iron

Iron is particularly important for the formation of haemoglobin, the red pigment in blood. In theory we are born with enough iron to last through life, but if we do not eat enough dietary iron to restore any losses, anaemia can result. The amount of iron we absorb from food is quite low, but it is increased if the body's stores are depleted or when there is a need, such as with growing children or pregnant women. The best sources of iron in the diet are red meat and liver because this iron is most easily absorbed. The iron in eggs is also well absorbed but the iron in vegetables or added to

Other dietary minerals

- **Chromium** A trace mineral that works with insulin to balance blood sugar levels and helps lower cholesterol levels. Found in chicken, shellfish, brown rice and certain fruits and vegetables
- **Copper** A trace mineral that helps the body to use iron properly. Found in fish and green vegetables
- **Fluoride** A trace mineral that helps protect teeth. Naturally present in tea and fish
- **Iodine** A trace mineral that helps to control metabolic activity. Found in milk, seaweed and seafood
- **Magnesium** Helps cells and muscles work efficiently. Widely found, especially in leafy green vegetables, wholegrain cereals, nuts and peas
- **Manganese** A trace mineral that is important for bone structure. Found in nuts, leafy green vegetables, beetroot and egg yolks
- **Phosphorus** Required for healthy cells, bones and teeth. Found in meat, fish, dairy foods and eggs

- **Potassium** Helps in cellular growth and controlling blood pressure. Also good for the nervous system and for regulating bodily fluids and the acid-alkali balance in the body. Found in all foods (except sugars, fats and oils), especially bananas
- **Selenium** An antioxidant (see page 28) trace mineral found in cereals, meat, offal, fish, cheese, eggs and brazil nuts
- **Sodium** Helps regulate the body's water content and enables the nerves to function effectively. Most raw foods contain small amounts of sodium chloride (salt)

flour is less well absorbed. A source of vitamin C, such as orange juice or salad, included in a meal containing iron-rich vegetables helps in the absorption of the iron. Tea inhibits absorption of iron, so avoid it around meal times.

Zinc

Zinc helps in the healing of wounds and is involved in enzyme activity. It is present in a variety of foods, but may be deficient in some diets. Zinc is associated with protein, so meat and dairy foods are good sources, as are nuts, wholegrains and seeds.

SEE ALSO:

→ A balanced diet, page 14

→ Vitamins, page 24

→ Top foods for health, page 28

Top foods for health

Since it is the food that we eat that provides our bodies with the necessary fuel with which to function efficiently, fight off infection, grow, repair and regenerate cells, it makes sense to choose the best foods possible for the purpose. The nutrient-rich foods that constitute the best possible raw materials could be termed 'miracle foods' and a selection of the best of them appear on the following pages.

When buying any fresh produce, look for good-quality healthy-looking specimens. Any produce past its best should be avoided as it will have lost much of its nutritional value – vitamin C in particular disappears very quickly. Similarly, cooking can reduce many of the key vitamins and minerals, so cook vegetables lightly where possible, or not at all.

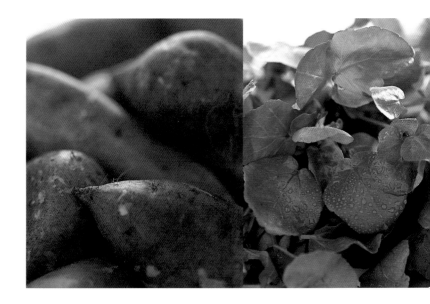

Antioxidant foods

Antioxidants are nutrients that slow the oxidative process in the body caused by the action of free radicals. Free radicals are electrochemically unbalanced molecules, generated within our bodies by such things as pollution, cigarettes, certain foods and

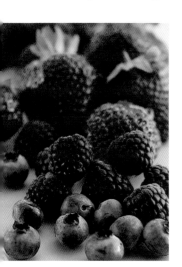

stress. They react with other, healthy molecules to make them unstable, too, and a chain reaction can start up, which leads to a process of cellular destruction and disease.

Antioxidants protect us against minor infections, serious degenerative diseases such as cancer and heart disease, as well as conditions that come with premature ageing – for example they help protect the brain

and preserve the memory. The key antioxidants are vitamins A, C and E. The minerals selenium, manganese and zinc, some of the B complex vitamins and certain enzymes and amino acids also have antioxidant properties. Vitamins C and E actually work together to make each other more effective – vitamin C recycles vitamin E, allowing it to carry on working longer. A group of flavonoids called anthocyanidins are another group of very powerful oxidants – thought to be 50 times more powerful than vitamin E – and found in abundance in certain fruits and berries. Anthocyanidins provide protection from a wide variety of toxins and free radicals in both watery and fatty parts of the body. Red, purple and blue fruits (especially berries) are rich in anthocyanidins.

Uncooked fresh fruit and vegetables are the best places to find antioxidants. Prunes, raisins, cherries, berries (strawberries, raspberries, blackberries, blackcurrants, redcurrants), black grapes, bananas, carrots, sweet potatoes, peas, chestnuts, brazils and hazelnuts are particularly good sources.

Foods for specific ailments

Eat more of the suggested foods if you suffer from the complaints shown here.

Anxiety/depression Bananas, broccoli, oats

Cancer (These foods protect against the risk of cancer) Bananas, beans and lentils, broccoli, cabbage, oats, oily fish, olive oil, papayas and mangoes, peppers, seeds, soya and tofu, spinach, sweet potatoes, tomatoes, watercress

Cholesterol (To reduce) Apples, bananas, beans and lentils, garlic, nuts, oats, oily fish, olive oil, soya and tofu, watercress, yogurt

Circulatory problems and anaemia Beetroot, blackberries, blackcurrants, blueberries, redcurrants, cabbage, carrots, game, garlic, honey, nuts, oats, papayas, mangoes, spinach, sweet potatoes, tomatoes, watercress

Detoxifying (These foods help prevent a build-up of toxins) Apples and pears, beans and lentils, broccoli, carrots, spinach, sweet potatoes, watercress

Digestive problems Apples and pears, bananas, beans and lentils, broccoli, cabbage, carrots, garlic, honey, linseeds, oats, olive oil, papayas and mangoes, raspberries, seeds, soya and tofu, spinach, sweet potatoes, tomatoes, watercress, yogurt

Energy deficiency Apples and pears, bananas, blackberries, broccoli, honey, nuts, papayas and mangoes, peppers, spinach, sweet potatoes and yams, watercress

Eyesight Carrots, spinach, sunflower seeds

Heart disease and stroke/high blood pressure (These foods lower the risk of heart disease and stroke and help reduce high blood pressure) Bananas, broccoli, carrots, garlic, nuts, oily fish, olive oil, peppers, seaweed and sea vegetables, seeds, soya and tofu, spinach, sweet potatoes, tomatoes, watercress

Immune system deficiency Apples and pears, beetroot, broccoli, cabbage, carrots, game, garlic, honey, oily fish, papayas and mangoes, peppers, seaweed and sea vegetables, seeds, spinach, sweet potatoes, tomatoes, watercress

Kidney, liver, bladder and urinary infections Beans and lentils, beetroot, blackcurrants, broccoli, cabbage, carrots, chickpeas, cranberries, garlic, honey, sweet potatoes, tomatoes, watercress, yogurt

PMS/Menstrual problems Bananas, beans and lentils, beetroot, berries, carrots, linseeds, nuts, oats, oily fish, soya and tofu, yams

Nervous system Bananas, broccoli, cabbage, game, nuts, oats, seaweed and sea vegetables, seeds, spinach, sweet potatoes, watercress

Respiratory problems/coughs and colds Apples, blackberries, broccoli, cabbage, carrots, cranberries, garlic, honey, olive oil

Rheumatism and rheumatoid arthritis Apples, beans and lentils, honey, nuts, oily fish (especially tuna), seeds, strawberries

Skin conditions Apples and pears, broccoli, cabbage, carrots, nuts, oily fish, olive oil, papayas and mangoes, strawberries, sweet potatoes, watercress

Sleeping problems Bananas

Strong teeth, bones, connective tissue (To build strong teeth, bones and tissue) Carrots, oats, oily fish, papayas, mangoes, soya and tofu, spinach, sweet potatoes, watercress

Thyroid problems Cabbage, oats, pears, seaweed and sea vegetables, watercress

Top foods for health

Berries

Berries are important for immune health, being rich in the antioxidant vitamins – vitamins C, E and beta-carotene, which converts within the body to vitamin A. These provide **protection against infection and disease** by neutralizing the free radicals responsible for cellular damage in our bodies (see page 28). Blackberries, blueberries, cranberries, blackcurrants and black grapes are also rich in anthocyanidins, another group of powerful antioxidants (see page 28). Anthocyanidins have an important role to play in **anti-ageing** – for example they have been found to prevent collagen from breaking down. They are robust nutrients and survive various food processes, so when fresh berries are not available, canned and frozen berries remain nutritious alternatives. Berries also have high levels of phytoestrogen (plant oestrogens), which have a **stabilizing effect on the menstrual cycle**, as well as high levels of minerals, especially calcium, magnesium and potassium (see pages 26–27).

Strawberries are believed to **soothe arthritic inflammation**; raspberries are good for **indigestion** and **menstrual problems**. Blackberries are very **energizing** and make excellent **blood cleansers**, as do blackcurrants, redcurrants and blueberries. Blackberries and cranberries are useful for **clearing congestion** in the respiratory tract and **soothing sore throats**. Cranberries and blackcurrants are beneficial for **kidney** and **urinary tract infections**.

Bananas

A surprisingly rich source of protein and a good source of fibre, bananas also have potent **energizing qualities**, making them an ideal snack when you feel low on energy. They are also a healthy option for fulfilling a craving for something sweet. The amino acid tryptophan found in bananas has a **mildly sedative effect** so makes them a good snack to have at bedtime; tryptophan also has uplifting qualities and can help **alleviate the symptoms of depression**, **anxiety** and **PMS**.

Bananas are high in antioxidants (see page 28) – vitamin C and beta-carotene, the precursor of vitamin A – and in potassium (see page 27). They also contain vitamin B6, which helps **protect against heart disease** and **regulates the nervous system**. Being generally easy to digest, bananas make particularly good food for convalescents or those with appetite-related conditions.

Broccoli

An ideal food, broccoli is packed with vitamins and minerals – vitamins A and C (a cup of cooked broccoli contains more vitamin C than two oranges), beta-carotene, B2, B5 and folate, zinc and iron. It comprises 90 per cent water and contains very few calories. Broccoli is another free radical-fighting food, **protecting cells** in the brain and body **from oxidative damage**. It provides **protection against heart disease** and a range of infections, particularly respiratory ones, and is thought to be a major force in **fighting bowel cancer**, thanks to the sulphuraphane it contains, a substance that detoxifies and excretes the carcinogens encountered in daily life.

Its detoxifying properties mean that broccoli can **prevent a build-up of harmful toxins** within the body, allowing the liver and digestive system to function more effectively, and ultimately **improving skin condition**. In addition, the folate found in broccoli promotes the production of the mood-lifting chemical serotonin, beneficial for those suffering from **depression**.

Carrots

Carrots are a powerful **detoxifying** food and are especially effective taken as a juice with apple (see page 40). Their rich orange colour indicate that they are loaded with beta-carotene. This carotenoid pigment converts to vitamin A in the body when needed and is a powerful force in the fight against free radicals. In addition, beta-carotene has a **healing effect on the skin**, especially in cases of **eczema**, **dermatitis** and **acne**, and is believed to result in **healthy eyes** and **good night vision**.

In addition to beta-carotene, carrots contain vitamin C. These two antioxidants mean that carrots are valuable for **boosting the immune system** and restoring health to convalescents. Carrots are believed to offer **protection against various cancers** and **heart disease** and to help **lower cholesterol levels** if eaten daily.

Top foods for health

Spinach

Spinach is just one example of the leafy green vegetables rich in calcium and magnesium. Half a cup of cooked spinach contains more calcium, magnesium and iron than half a cup of milk. The calcium and magnesium in spinach work together to ensure **efficient nerve transmissions**. Calcium also **strengthens bones**, **teeth** and **gums**, while magnesium and vitamin K build **healthy red blood cells**; the iron in spinach **strengthens the blood** and the potassium **regulates high blood pressure**. Leafy greens are particularly rich in antioxidants, too, and therefore important for **strengthening the body's immune system**. The antioxidants in spinach are believed to **reduce the risk of** both **heart disease** and **stroke** and **lower the risk of skin** and **stomach cancer**. Spinach is another energizing food, and is most effective in combating **long-term fatigue**.

NOTE:Spinach contains oxalic acid, which can exacerbate kidney or bladder stones and can also interfere with the absorption of calcium by preventing it from dissolving into a usable form. The goodness of spinach is therefore diminished when it is served with calcium-rich dairy products. So eat this combination in moderation, or eat spinach on its own to benefit fully from its nutrients.

Garlic

A perfect food, garlic has many properties beneficial to health. Taken regularly, it helps build up high levels of resistance to infection within the immune system. It is antiviral, antibiotic, antibacterial and antiseptic. Garlic contains the antioxidants, selenium and vitamin C, which help to fight free radicals. It is a good **detoxifying agent**, **cleanses** and **tones the liver** and its decongestant properties make it excellent for **clearing respiratory ailments**. Renowned for its beneficial effects on the **heart** and the **circulation**, garlic can **reduce high blood pressure** and **lower cholesterol levels**. It contains a substance called allicin, which dilates the blood vessels and reduces clotting; it also contains sulphur, which is believed to **inhibit the growth of tumours**.

Oily fish

All oily fish (for example herring, kippers, mackerel, tuna, salmon, sardines, whitebait and anchovies) contain omega-3 essential fatty acids (EFAs). They are called essential because they cannot be made within the body and must be obtained from the diet. Omega-3 oils provide a range of health benefits. They are crucial for protecting the parts of our brain that send messages to the body, and improving memory. They also **strengthen cardiovascular health** – providing **protection against heart disease**, helping **prevent blood clots**, and **lowering cholesterol levels** and **high blood pressure**. Fish oils also have a beneficial effect on **rheumatoid arthritis**, **swollen joints**, **dry skin** and **inflammatory skin conditions**. Another health benefit of taking fish oils is a reduction of the symptoms of **PMS**.

Besides containing EFAs, fish are a good source of the antioxidant selenium. This mineral helps **protect against** the development of **cancer** by detoxifying the body, removing heavy metals such as mercury from the body and mopping up free radicals. Selenium also **protects against heart disease** so oily fish are an excellent inclusion in the diet. Vitamin E is another antioxidant found in many oily fish.

Oats

The oat grain is very like a kernel of wheat in structure. However, unlike wheat, the nutritious bran and germ are not removed in the normal processing because oats are not refined. Oats can often be eaten by those intolerant of wheat (see page 36). Very nutritious, they are full of protein and minerals – they contain high levels of calcium, phosphorus and iron. Oats also contain antioxidants and high levels of the mood-lifting amino acid tryptophan, which accounts for their **tranquillizing** and **uplifting effects**.

Besides providing dietary bulk and improving the digestive process in general, the soluble fibre found in oats helps to **lower cholesterol** and **boost cardiovascular health** generally. In addition, because oats are digested slowly they help to maintain an even supply of energy to the brain by sustaining steady blood sugar levels. This is **beneficial for diabetics** and can help **reduce mood swings**, particularly those associated with **PMS**.

Top foods for health

Beans and lentils

Beans, lentils, peas and chickpeas are the seeds of various plants belonging to the legume family. They are a valuable source of protein, especially for vegetarians, as vegetable proteins are no longer considered to be inferior to those from animal origins.

Beans and lentils are a good source of carbohydrates and the slow release of their sugars helps to **sustain energy** over a long period of time. The phytoestrogens (plant oestrogens) found in these foods have a **stabilizing effect on the menstrual cycle**, are increasingly used as an alternative to hormone replacement therapy (HRT), and are believed to **protect against breast cancer.** Most beans and lentils are high in minerals, supplying potassium, calcium, selenium, magnesium, phosphorus, iron, zinc and manganese. They can improve **intestinal health**, have useful **detoxifying properties** and help **lower cholesterol.**

Fresh beans contain vitamin C but this starts to decline soon after harvesting. Canned beans retain about half their vitamin C, while frozen beans keep only one-quarter. However, the other vitamins, the minerals, protein and carbohydrate found in beans are more robust, and canned, frozen and even dried beans are useful in the diet.

NOTE: It is not safe to eat raw or undercooked kidney and soya beans. There is no need to avoid them as long as they are thoroughly soaked and cooked.

Nuts and seeds

Crammed with lots of smart nutrients, nuts and seeds are important rich sources of omega-6 fats, one of the two groups of essential fatty acids (EFAs) required by the body. Nuts also contain the antioxidant vitamins essential for **immune health** and are high in both protein and carbohydrates, which makes them an **energizing food**.

Since each nut and seed has its own unique combination of nutrients, try to eat a mixture for maximum benefit. Almonds are the best choice of nuts – low in saturated fat, rich in omega-6 oils, particularly rich in calcium (50 g/2 oz almonds contain more calcium than half a cup of milk), with plenty of protein and vitamin E. Hazelnuts are another good choice – they have less omega-6 oils than almonds but double the amount of manganese of any other nuts.

Peanuts, brazils and cashew nuts are very high in saturated fats and should be eaten more sparingly. Walnuts and pumpkin seeds unusually contain both omega-6 and omega-3 oils (usually found only in oily fish). Sesame seeds contain plenty of zinc, while sunflower seeds are rich in the mineral magnesium and vitamin E.

WARNING: Some people are very allergic to nuts and seeds. Take great care with nuts or products containing nuts if you suspect someone has an allergy to them.

Soya and tofu

An excellent source of protein, slow-releasing carbohydrates, vitamins, minerals and fibre, the soya bean is the most nutritious of all beans. Soya beans contain the essential omega-3 fatty acids and have a high content of phytoestrogens, the naturally occurring plant oestrogens thought to **protect against hormone-related cancers**, including breast, cervical, ovarian and prostate cancers. The protein found in soya beans helps to **reduce blood pressure** and **cholesterol levels**. Its minerals include a high content of iron, as well as potassium, magnesium and phosphorus.

Made from coagulated soya milk, tofu provides an excellent alternative to meat for people who avoid all animal products including eggs and dairy foods. Silken tofu is smooth and creamy, while the denser, firmer-textured varieties are often smoked or marinated. Tofu is already cooked and can be eaten straight from the packet or used in cooking. Other soya bean products include miso, a fermented bean paste useful for soups and flavourings, and tempeh, made from soya beans that have been cooked, fermented and mashed into blocks.

Yogurt

A living food, yogurt is produced by the action of friendly bacteria on the sugars in milk. The *Lactobacillus acidophilus* bacteria found in live, or 'bio', yogurt are particularly helpful and aid in **digestion** and **absorption** and help maintain an overall **healthy digestive tract**. Live yogurt is especially beneficial for recovery after taking a course of antibiotics or after a yeast infection such as *Candida albicans*.

Besides helping the digestive system, yogurt also supports the **immune system**. It **protects against urinary tract infections** and **peptic ulcers**; it is thought to offer some **protection against heart disease** and **reduce cholesterol levels**, too.

Yogurt is rich in protein, contains the B complex vitamins and has a higher percentage of vitamins A and D than does milk. Its high calcium levels ensure **strong bones** and **teeth**; calcium also acts as a **natural tranquillizer** and helps with **insomnia**. The motivating amino acid tyrosine is found in yogurt, too.

Avoid flavoured yogurts sweetened with lots of sugar. Instead choose low-fat natural varieties for maximum protein with minimum fat and sugar.

Food allergies and intolerances

Many people have a sensitivity to certain foods, which produce a mild stomach upset when eaten. For others the intolerance is more serious and has a greater impact on everyday life, especially if the offending food is a common ingredient, such as wheat. However, in some cases people are actually allergic to certain foods and this can have far more serious consequences.

Food allergies

These occur when your immune system, your body's defence against bacteria and viruses, responds inappropriately to substances found in certain foods. It fails to realize that they are harmless and mounts a full-scale defence against them, causing swelling of the mouth and lips, difficulty breathing and in extreme circumstances, anaphylactic shock, which can be fatal. Peanuts are perhaps the best known foods to cause allergies, but there are many other foods which can have a similar effect.

In some people, certain foods are known to trigger other allergic diseases such as asthma and rhinitis. This is not a food allergy as such and the symptoms often start off mild, but they can get progressively worse with each exposure to the food, until they become life threatening. Wheat, dairy products and some food preservatives and flavourings are among the most common culprits.

Food intolerances

The symptoms of the classic food allergy, which occur straight after eating the food, are easy to recognize but in some people they do not happen straight away and the symptoms are more ambiguous. This makes it difficult to diagnose and to pinpoint which food is causing the reaction. This is known as a food intolerance or sensitivity and is also likely to cause stomach pain and diarrhoea. Usually, the offending food is one the person likes or eats often and although most foods can have ill effects, the most common culprits are wheat, milk, eggs, fish and shellfish.

Do allergies run in families?

In some families, there is an inherited tendency to develop an allergy. If one or both parents have an allergic condition – a food allergy, asthma, eczema or hay fever – their child is more likely (but not certain) to develop an allergy of one sort or another. If you think your baby is susceptible, there are measures that will reduce the likelihood of an allergy. Breastfeeding the child for at least six months before giving solid food will decrease the risk. Avoid eating any of the potential allergy triggers while you are breastfeeding, such as eggs, fish, milk and dairy products, nuts, wheat and oranges. However, take medical advice to ensure you get a balanced diet. When you start to introduce new foods to your baby, do so one by one and leave plenty of time between each to give the child time to adapt and for you to recognize any reaction that may take place.

The symptoms of food allergies

Usually, symptoms start off mild, but become more severe each time the food is eaten, though they may start severe. If any of these symptoms occur inexplicably in you or your child, consult a doctor as next time they may be worse, even resulting in anaphylactic shock (see right). Be aware that the symptoms of food allergy can be set off by merely breathing in tiny particles of the food.

- Tingling and swelling of the mouth and lips
- Breathless feeling
- Skin rashes and blotches
- Vomiting

The most common triggers

- Oranges
- Eggs
- Nuts
- Fish
- Shellfish
- Wheat and other cereals
- Yeast
- Cows' milk

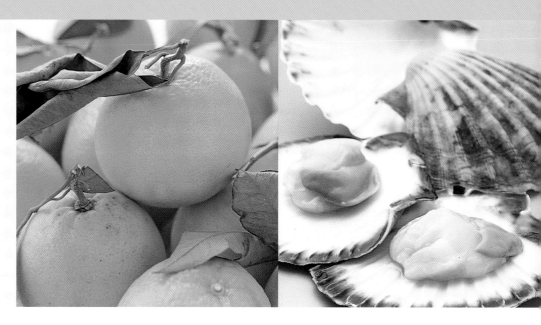

Are you allergic?

If you have suffered from any symptoms of a food allergy, consult your doctor without delay: next time, the reaction could be worse.

The following methods may be used to establish whether in fact you do have an allergy:

Skin prick testing – A small drop of a diluted allergen is applied to the skin, and a tiny hole is made in the skin below it. A red spot will occur at the site if you are allergic to the allergen. This test may not always be reliable.

Blood tests – These are designed to identify specific substances in the blood which have triggered an allergic response. These tests are expensive and not always necessary.

Elimination diets – The principle is to eliminate all suspect foods from your diet, then re-introduce them one by one to see if any of them trigger a reaction. Elimination diets are often slow and painstaking processes which are best performed under the guidance of a qualified dietician who can ensure you maintain a balanced diet and are not inadvertently eating any of the suspect foods.

Food diaries – One of the easiest methods to pinpoint the offending food is to keep a diary of exactly what you have eaten and when, then compare it with details of the symptoms you experience at what times. In some cases, it will be obvious what the culprit is, but other cases can be much more confused.

Anaphylactic shock

This a very severe allergic reaction which can be fatal if not treated swiftly and correctly. It is usually caused by eating a food to which the patient is allergic. Peanuts are perhaps the most common culprits, partly because peanut oil and traces of nuts can appear in otherwise 'safe' foods so the person is unaware that they are eating them. Symptoms appear anything up to two hours after contact with the food. If you experience any of the symptoms below and can't explain what caused them, get medical help immediately.

- **Dizziness or faintness accompanied by a fast pulse**
- **Disorientation and speech slurring**
- **Pale, itchy skin**
- **Diarrhoea, stomach pains or incontinence**
- **Unexplained anxiety**

SEE ALSO:

→ 7-stage detox diet, page 98

Organic foods

Many conventionally grown fruits, vegetables and cereals contain chemicals added in the form of weedkillers, pesticides or fertilizers to increase food productivity. The effects of long-term exposure to these chemicals in humans is not yet understood, but recent research suggests there may be a relationship between these chemicals and depression, memory loss and mood swings.

We know that pesticide residues can cause anxiety, hyperactivity, dizziness, sight problems and muscle weakness. Pesticides can also increase the risk of respiratory and digestive problems. Children are most at risk as they are still growing, and many people attribute hyperactivity in children to these pesticides.

Meat is a worry too, as animals are regularly injected with hormones and antibiotics. Most poultry and livestock is farmed in intensive conditions, making the animals prone to diseases and pests. Farmers treat diseases with antibiotics, but it is thought in many cases they also inject antibiotics just to prevent disease. This overuse leads to the development of resistant strains of diseases, which is a worrying scenario.

Organic standards

'Organic' is a term defined by law and can only be used by farmers and producers who have an organic license. They follow strict guidelines detailing how they must produce food, what ingredients and chemicals they can use, and how the food must be processed, packaged and distributed. The rules and regulations are stringent and the producers are inspected regularly, ensuring a reliable and traceable food line.

Animal feeds are usually made from intensively grown crops, treated with chemical pesticides. The feed then has preservative added to it, and some of these chemicals may end up on our plates.

The best way to avoid these potentially harmful chemicals is to choose organic foods, which are are virtually free from pesticides and contain more nutrients than conventionally farmed produce.

What is organic food?

The term 'organic' refers to the way foods are produced. It is based on a sustainable system of farming which replenishes nutrients in the soil to keep crops healthy without the use of systemic and persistent chemicals, and rears animals in natural conditions, without regular hormone or antibiotic injections. Organic foods receive the minimum of processing so they retain their nutrients, and have no artificial ingredients or preservatives.

There are many organic foods now available, including fruit, vegetables, meat, flour, and many processed foods which contain only organic ingredients and no additives.

Organic products are usually more expensive as they are more costly to produce, but the extra expense is worthwhile for the peace of mind they afford. It could be argued that we are actually paying a lot more for conventionally produced foods in terms of health risks, pesticide pollution, damage to soil and government subsidies.

The benefits of organic foods

Better for the environment The soil maintains a natural balance of nutrients and dangerous chemicals are not leeched into rivers.

More nutritious Organic foods contain more nutrients than conventionally produced foods because of the superior soil fertility.

Better animal welfare Organically farmed animals have more space and are not injected with hormones and antibodies as a matter of course. They are fed on natural foods.

Foods in season Organic foods are harvested in season, so the produce ripens on the plant leading to more nutrients and flavour.

No toxic chemicals We don't know what effect agricultural chemicals have on us in the long term, but the evidence is not encouraging.

Where to buy organic

Supermarkets Many now offer a good selection of organic fruits and vegetables, meats, and processed foods. Check the labels.

Box schemes Some companies deliver a seasonally varied selection of organic vegetables or meat, once a week or month.

Health food shops Health food shops are often good sources of organic products and staff should be knowledgeable.

Mail order Many small specialist producers offer a mail order service for their products. This is a convenient way to shop.

The internet This can be a useful way to find organic producers.

GM foods

Genetically modified (GM) foods are made by taking genes from one species and inserting them into another. For example, genes from an arctic fish which has 'antifreeze' properties may be inserted into a tomato to protect it from frost damage. There has been much controversy about this technique as many believe it is impossible to control, and unpredictable effects can occur. So far there is little evidence to suggest this technique is dangerous, but equally little to suggest it is safe.

Top organic products

If you cannot buy organic food all the time, concentrate on choosing these products as a priority:

Milk – Cows are treated with hormones and other growth promoters. Organic milk is readily available and not too expensive.

Beef – Beef has been found to contain more growth promoters than other meats, so buy organic if you can.

Carrots – Carrots absorb a lot of chemicals in the soil, including those from potentially harmful pesticides and fungicides. Consumers have been advised to scrub or peel carrots, but buying organic is a much safer option.

Salmon – Conventionally farmed salmon are treated with pesticides to prevent mite infestations and there are fears that the chemicals become concentrated in the fish. Consumers have been warned against consuming too much non-organic salmon.

Apples, apple juice and pears – Apples and pears are sprayed with organophosphate insecticides and these pose a particular risk to young children who are often fed with apple products.

Organic versus free-range

Free-range produce is about animal welfare. With chickens, for example, it means that birds have a guaranteed amount of space to move around in, rather than being cramped in crowded conditions with the associated increased risk of disease and the need for antibiotics. The term 'organic' goes one step further and also refers to the food the animals are given, which must be produced without chemicals. Also, organically farmed animals are not given antibiotics on a regular basis so they develop a natural resistance to disease.

SEE ALSO:

→ Making juices, page 40

Making juices

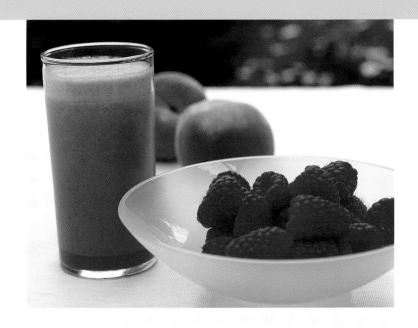

Fresh fruit and vegetables are inexpensive and packed with nutrients, and everyone knows we should eat plenty of them for the good of our health. So next time you want a quick snack why not consider a glass of juice (see recipes on pages 42–43) as a quick healthy option instead of crisps or biscuits? Go one step further and make freshly made juice a part of your regular routine – a daily dose of various fruit and vegetable combinations will ensure that your body receives its full quota of vitamins and minerals. The nutrients in juices are utilized by the body far more quickly than solid food and are therefore beneficial much earlier. The detoxifying effects of freshly made fruit and vegetable juices mean that they often form the basis of a detox diet (see page 98).

Although there are plenty of juices on the supermarket shelves, they bear little resemblance in taste or in nutritional value to those you make with a juicer. There are a few freshly squeezed juices available to buy and you can make do with these if you don't want to spend money on a juicer. However, once you've tasted real juice, you won't want shop-bought juices again.

Preparing the ingredients

When you make juice, try to use organic fruit and vegetables if you can as these will not have been treated with chemical fertilizers, pesticides or herbicides, which means that you can use the produce, skins and all. Choose fruit that is ripe, as it will be easier both to juice and to digest. Don't buy any produce that is bruised or obviously past its best, as the quality of the nutrients will have diminished.

If you are using organic produce, clean the fruit and vegetables thoroughly and use them whole – many nutrients are just below the surface of the skin. Some fruits such as pineapple, papaya, mango, bananas and citrus fruits need to be peeled, but many don't. Leaves,

Initial side-effects

When you first start drinking fresh juices regularly, you may find you are passing water more often than usual and that you have a slight headache. Once your body becomes accustomed to the detoxifying effects of the juices, however, these symptoms will pass.

tops and outer skins and peel on vegetables such as carrots, celery, beetroot and root vegetables all go in. Juice all the leaves – even the less appetizing outer ones on leafy green vegetables. If the produce is not organic, however, remove the skins, stems and roots. Large stones, such as those of cherries, plums, mangoes, apricots or peaches, should be removed but the smaller pips of melons, apples and grapes can be juiced, too.

Home-made juices do not look the same as those out of a carton. They may be a rather murky-looking colour and they may also have a much thicker consistency, sometimes with a froth on top, and a much more powerful taste. You don't need to strain the juice, even if it does have a froth – instead, just give it a stir and drink it as soon as you've made it as the juice starts to lose its nutritional value when it stands, even when stored in a refrigerator.

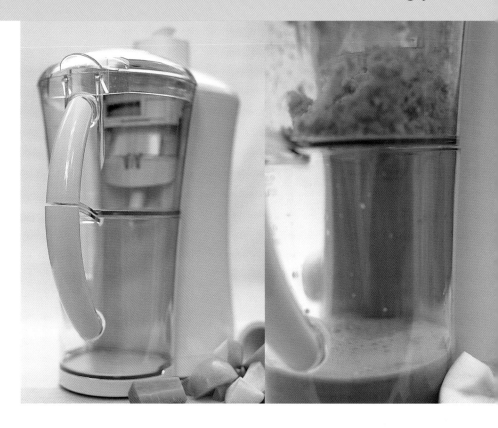

Buying a juicer

You can make juice with a blender or food processor only if there is a separate juicing attachment, otherwise the machine will make a purée of the whole fruit or vegetable. A dedicated juicer separates the fibrous pulp from the juice. Juicers are now very affordable but when it comes to choosing a juicer the other thing to bear in mind besides the price is the question of how trouble-free the juicer is to use. This is mainly down to how easy it is to clean – the pulps and fibres can become lodged in awkward corners so it's very important to get a machine that you can take apart to clean and put together again without fuss.

There are a number of different types of juicers that carry out the job in different ways.

Citrus juicer This is the simplest type of juicer and suitable for extracting the juice from lemons, limes, oranges and grapefruit.

Centrifugal juicer Vegetables and fruits are grated into tiny pieces and spun around at high speed with the liquid being extracted by centrifugal force. The juice pours into a jug, while the fibrous pulp is left behind. Centrifugal juicers tend to be the lowest in price. You need to add the fruit and vegetables gradually so they don't block up. If you're juicing something very fibrous, an apple or carrot will help keep the machine clear.

Masticating juicer This tears up the vegetables and fruit and forces the pulp against a mesh. This juicer is slower than a centrifugal juicer, but extracts more juice and therefore offers a higher nutritional content. It is also more expensive than a centrifugal juicer and tends to take up more room in the kitchen.

Hydraulic juice press Presses use immense force to squeeze the juice out of fruits and vegetables. The juice comes out through a filter into a jug and has more nutrients than that from any other type of juicer. These machines are, however, the most expensive.

Juice supplements

There are three supplements worth adding to juices for their concentrated vitamins and minerals and immunity-boosting and energizing properties:

- Aloe vera
- Spirulina
- Wheatgrass

SEE ALSO:

→ Vitamins, page 24

→ Minerals, page 26

→ Antioxidant foods, page 28

→ Organic foods, page 38

→ 7-stage detox diet, page 98

Juice recipes

Follow the recipes here (all the recipes make a glassful), or better still, buy whatever fruit and vegetables look freshest and best, and experiment. Be cautious about mixing fruit and vegetables, with the exception of carrot and apple, which will both mix with just about anything.

Citrus juice has a high acid content and therefore a very powerful scouring effect so is best diluted with water or combined with other fruit. Vegetable juices are not as deliciously sweet as the fruit juices but they have a much more powerful cleansing and healing effect. The right combinations can be very palatable, too, but you need to consider the taste of the ingredients. Don't mix lots of very strong-tasting vegetables together – you may find the result difficult to drink. If you are using vegetables that are very peppery or bitter, add carrots or cucumber to the recipe to dilute and sweeten them.

Strawberry and kiwi juice

Nutritious food, fast... These fruits, in particular the banana, create a feeling of fullness and they help to rebalance your sugar levels and thus your energy levels. Your sugar levels will also be helped by the protein in the linseeds. The high levels of vitamin B in this juice will increase your energy as well.

250 g (8 oz) strawberries
125 g (4 oz) kiwi fruit
100 g (3½ oz) banana
1 tablespoon spirulina
1 tablespoon linseeds
1–2 ice cubes
redcurrants, to decorate (optional)

1 Juice the strawberries and kiwi fruit and whiz in a blender with the banana, spirulina, linseeds and a couple of ice cubes. Decorate with redcurrants, if liked.

5-fruit juice

A sharp clean-tasting drink full of vitamin A, vitamin C, selenium and zinc.

150 g (5 oz) grapefruit
50 g (2 oz) kiwi fruit
175 g (6 oz) pineapple
50 g (2 oz) frozen raspberries
50 g (2 oz) frozen cranberries
raspberries, to decorate (optional)

1 Juice the grapefruit, kiwi fruit and pineapple. Whiz in a blender with the frozen berries. Decorate with raspberries, if liked, and drink with a straw.

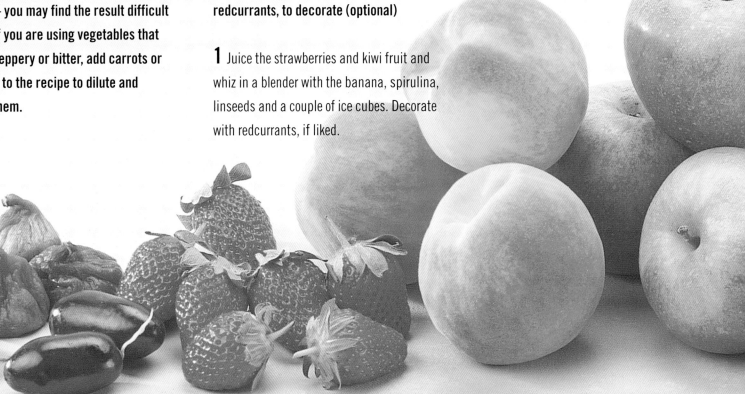

Watermelon and strawberry juice

High in zinc and potassium, two great eliminators useful for detoxification.

200 g (7 oz) watermelon
200 g (7 oz) strawberries
1–2 ice cubes
mint leaves and strawberries, to decorate
  (optional)

1 Juice the fruit and whiz in a blender with a couple of ice cubes. Serve decorated with mint leaves and whole or sliced strawberries, if liked.

Apple and blueberry juice

Blueberries contain anthocyanidins, which are lethal to the bacteria that can cause upset stomachs.

250 g (8 oz) apple
125 g (4 oz) blueberries, fresh or frozen

1 Juice the apple, then whiz in a blender with the blueberries. Serve in a tumbler.

Beta-carotene buzz

A drink bursting with beta-carotene

100 g (3½ oz) red pepper
125 g (4 oz) strawberries
50 g (2 oz) tomato
125 g (4 oz) mango
125 g (4 oz) watermelon
3 ice cubes
mango slices, to decorate (optional)

1 Juice all the ingredients, whiz in a blender with the ice cubes and serve in a tall glass. Decorate with mango slices, if liked.

Fruit, lettuce and celery juice

Pineapple and grapes give a boost of blood sugar, which can help to induce sleep. Lettuce and celery relax the nerves and muscles.

125 g (4 oz) pineapple (without skin)
125 g (4 oz) grapes
50 g (2 oz) lettuce
50 g (2 oz) celery
lettuce leaves, to decorate (optional)

1 Juice all the ingredients and serve in a tall glass over ice. Decorate with lettuce leaves, if liked.

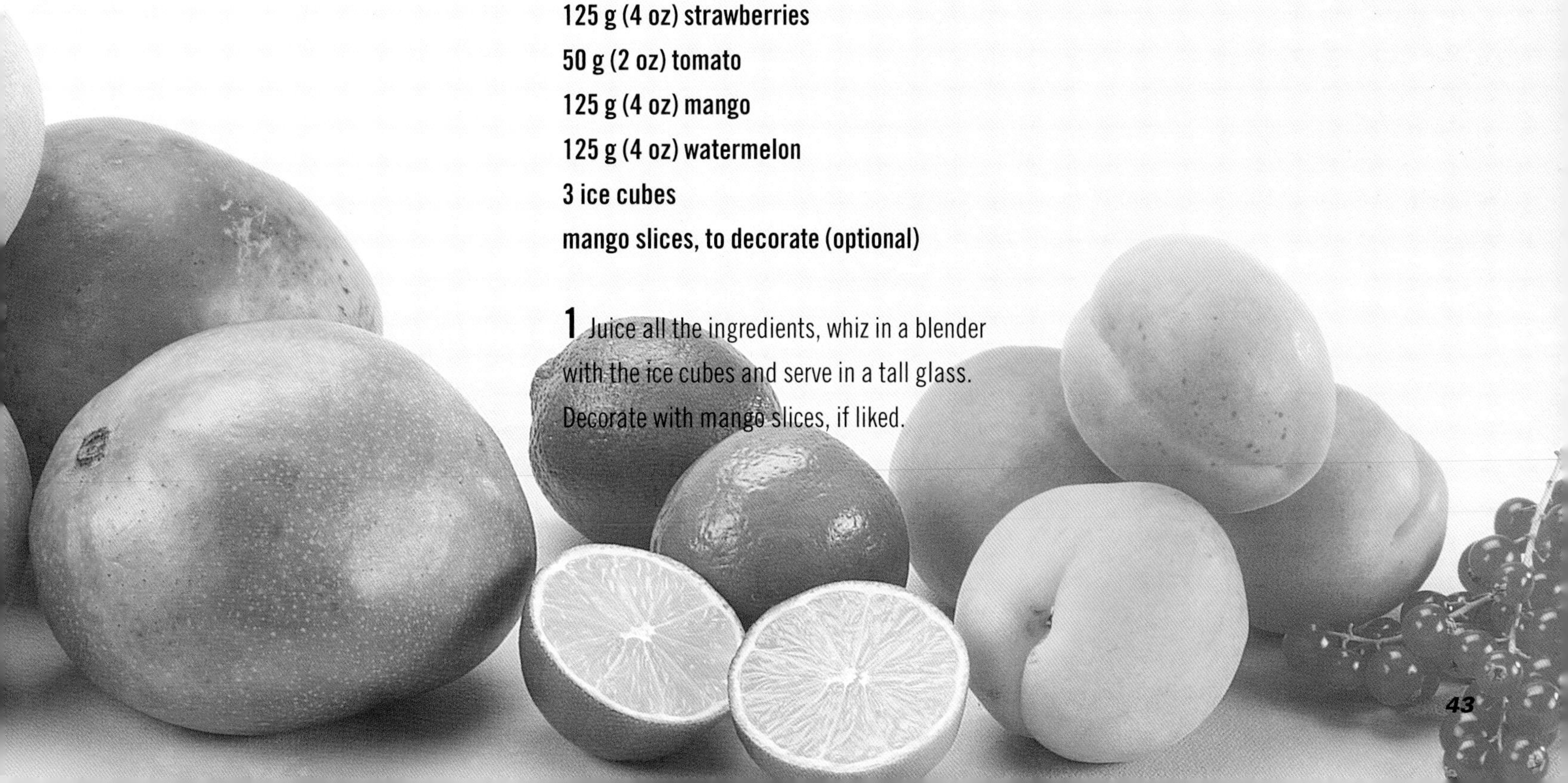

Herbal teas

Many herbs make deliciously flavoured teas, which are soothing, relaxing, refreshing or invigorating. These healthy wholesome drinks can be taken warm in winter and cooled in summer. They make a valuable addition to the daily diet if taken on a regular basis, and are a healthier alternative to ordinary caffeinated tea. While many herbs are taken for their therapeutic properties, most are very pleasant to drink and can continue to be taken after the treatment is finished.

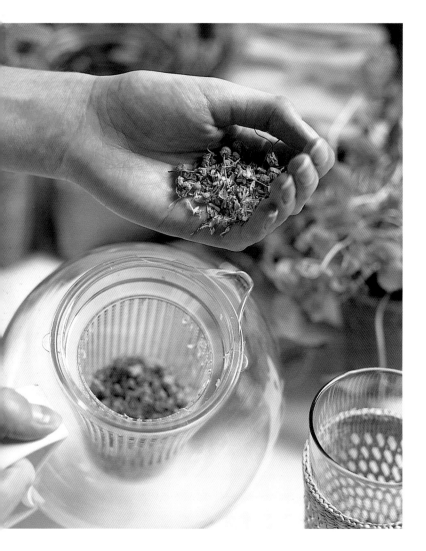

You can buy ready-made herb teabags or make your own herbal tea using fresh or dried herbs. If you use dried herbs, make sure you store them in dry containers that are airtight and made of dark glass or pottery since dried herbs deteriorate in bright sunlight. Just as ordinary tea suffers from being too long in the pot, so can a herb tea: overlong steeping can ruin a delicate flavour. If stronger tea is desired, add more herb at the outset. For average strength tea use one teaspoon of dried herb per teacup. If using fresh herbs, allow three teaspoons and crush the leaves before adding boiling water. Cover the cup and leave to stand for five minutes before straining and drinking. For iced tea, follow the same method, and leave to cool in a refrigerator for about one hour. Add ice cubes and a slice of lemon or some borage or mint leaves to make a refreshing drink.

Some spice teas are made by adding bruised seeds to a pan of boiling water and simmering for five minutes. All teas can be sweetened with a spoonful of honey if necessary.

As well as the huge variety of herb teas now on offer, there are also many fruit tea bags. These come in many flavours, including lemon, blackcurrant, raspberry and apple. There are also many combinations of different fruits, herbs and spices, which make palatable and tempting alternatives to normal tea and coffee.

Green tea

Green tea comes from the same plant as ordinary tea, but its leaves are treated differently – instead of being fermented they are pan-fried or steamed. Green tea contains much less caffeine and has some minerals and vitamins including antioxidants (see page 28). Green tea is believed to reduce the risk of certain cancers and to aid weight loss.

5 top teas

There is an endless variety of herbal teas. The following are just a few worth trying.

Peppermint This is very soothing for the digestive system and also a good early-morning pick-me-up. Make the tea using whole, slightly crushed leaves for a subtle taste. Peppermint milk makes a good nightcap and is made by pouring 300 ml (½ pint) boiling milk over 1 tablespoon of crushed leaves.

Camomile This very delicately flavoured tea is made from the flowers only, dried or fresh. Do not allow to steep for more than 3–5 minutes. It is very calming and, when drunk last thing at night, should guarantee you a good night's sleep.

Ginger Chop up some pieces of root ginger and steep for about 10 minutes in hot water. This calms the digestive system, expels gas and is very warming.

Rosehip This attractive-looking, sweet-tasting tea contains vitamin C. It is made from very finely crushed dried rosehips. Allow the tea to steep for 5–7 minutes.

Ayurvedic These teas, made according to Indian Ayurvedic medicine, are spicy and delicious. Different types for sleep, energy and even detox are available from health food shops.

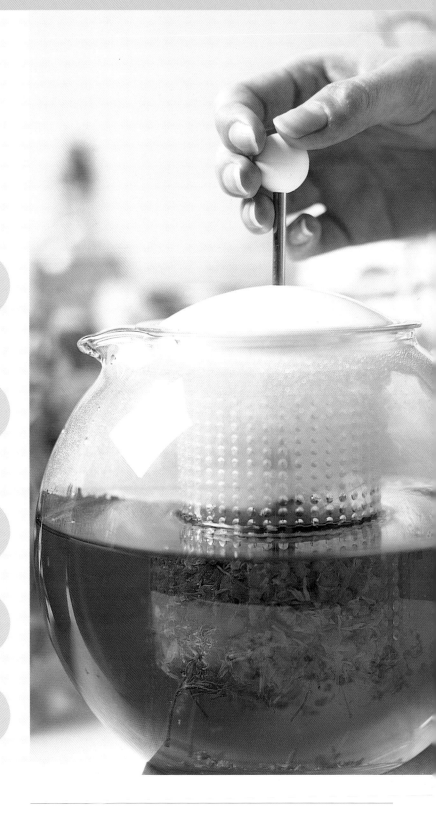

SEE ALSO:

→ Antioxidant foods, page 28

→ Everyday toxins, page 94

→ 7-stage detox diet, page 98

7-day menu planner

Previous pages in this chapter have emphasized how important it is to eat a balanced and varied diet every day to obtain the nutrients your body needs. With this in mind, the daily menus below have been compiled to provide examples of the balance of foods required on a daily basis. Together they comprise menus for a week of healthy and enjoyable eating suitable for you and your family, and should hopefully inspire you to continue eating healthily for life.

DAY	BREAKFAST/BRUNCH	LUNCH/SNACK	DINNER
1	Orange juice Coffee with semi-skimmed milk **Wheatgerm, honey and raisin muffins** (see page 49)	**Greek pitta wraps** (see page 56) Tomatoes with a light French dressing Banana	**Hot spiced stew with potatoes and cauliflower** (see page 74) **Vegetable carpaccio with parmesan shavings** (see page 68) **Fruit and nut crumble** (see page 81)
2	**Hot fruit salad** (see page 53) and natural yogurt **Smoked salmon and poached egg salad on blinis** (see page 57) Tea with semi-skimmed milk	**Strawberry and kiwi juice** (see page 42)	**Beetroot borscht with soured cream and chives** (see page 64) **Chicken with ginger** (see page 76) **Stir-fried Chinese cabbage** (see page 63) Boiled white rice **Wholemeal pear tart** (see page 82)
3	3 tablespoons **Granola** (see page 50) Banana and natural yogurt Wholemeal bread with polyunsaturated margarine and marmalade **5-fruit juice** (see page 42)	**Rocket, tuna and haricot bean salad** (see page 58) Crusty white bread	**Caldo verde** (see page 65) **Lentil moussaka** (see page 73) Crusty white bread **Lychee and apricot compôte** (see page 85)

DAY	BREAKFAST/BRUNCH	LUNCH/SNACK	DINNER
4	**Mixed rice kedgeree with kippers** (see page 55) Orange juice	**Pumpkin soup with crusty cheese topping** (see page 67) Apple **Tropical fruit salad** (see page 83)	**Zucchini al forno** (see page 69) **Mushroom crêpes** (see page 72) Green salad
5	3 tablespoons **Banana muesli** (see page 51) Yogurt Tea with semi-skimmed milk	**Prawn, mango and mozzarella salad** (see page 59) Crusty white bread **Watermelon and strawberry juice** (see page 43)	**Red pepper and ginger soup** (see page 66) **Noodles with smoked tofu and vegetables** (see page 75) **Baked braeburns with lemon** (see page 86)
6	**Honeyed ricotta with summer fruits** (see page 52) Wholemeal bread and butter Tea with semi-skimmed milk	**Marinated courgette and bean salad** (see page 61) with toasted bread **Beta-carotene buzz** (see page 43)	**Baked field mushrooms** (see page 70) **Green beef curry** (see page 77) Boiled rice **Yogurt with figs and passion fruit** (see page 84)
7	**Potato cakes** (see page 54) Yogurt and fruit Tea with semi-skimmed milk	**Rocket risotto** (see page 62)	**Carrot and coriander pâté** (see page 71) **Poached salmon steaks with hot basil sauce** (see page 78) **Courgette and mixed leaf salad** (see page 60) **3-fruit compôte** (see page 80) **Fruit, lettuce and celery juice** (see page 43)

Recipes

The recipes on the following pages have been nutritionally analyzed, with the amounts of carbohydrate, protein and fat (per portion) displayed below each recipe. Do note, however, that anything listed as 'optional' in the ingredients column has not been included in the nutritional analysis.

Follow the 7-day menu planner (see page 46) or simply experiment with healthier cooking, such as steaming and grilling, and try some of these recipes. You will soon discover that a sensible diet will boost energy and vitality and doesn't necessarily mean hours of preparation and cooking.

Fresh stock recipes

You will find it useful to refer to the following instructions for making chicken and vegetable stock as they are required for some recipes. Once made, the stocks can be frozen when cooled. Freeze in small batches in plastic tubs or ice cube trays. When frozen, the cubes can be transferred to plastic bags for ease of storage. Label the bags clearly with contents and date.

Chicken stock

Chop a cooked chicken carcass into three or four pieces and place it in a large saucepan with the raw giblets and trimmings, 1 roughly chopped onion, 2 large roughly chopped carrots and 1 roughly chopped celery stalk, 1 bay leaf, a few lightly crushed parsley stalks and 1 sprig of thyme. Cover with 1.8 litres (3 pints) of cold water.

Bring to the boil, removing any scum from the surface. Lower the heat and simmer for 2–2½ hours. Strain the stock through a muslin-lined sieve and leave to cool completely before refrigerating.

Makes **1 litre (1¾ pints)**
Preparation time: **5–10 minutes**
Cooking time: **about 2½ hours**

Vegetable stock

Place 500 g (1 lb) chopped mixed vegetables, such as carrots, leeks, celery, onions and mushrooms in a saucepan, using about an equal quantity of each one, and add 1 garlic clove, 6 peppercorns, 1 bouquet garni (2 parsley sprigs, 2 thyme sprigs and 1 bay leaf). Cover with 1.2 litres (2 pints) of water. Bring to the boil and simmer gently for 30 minutes, skimming when necessary. Strain the stock and ensure it is completely cool before refrigerating.

Makes **1 litre (1¾ pints)**
Preparation time: **5–10 minutes**
Cooking time: **about 45 minutes**

Breakfasts

Wheatgerm, honey and raisin muffins

125 g (4 oz) wheatgerm

2 teaspoons baking powder

pinch of salt

75 g (3 oz) raisins

4 tablespoons clear honey

50 g (2 oz) butter or margarine, melted

2 small eggs

about 6 tablespoons milk

1 Put the wheatgerm, baking powder, salt and raisins in a bowl, then add the honey, butter or margarine and eggs. Mix until blended, then stir in enough milk to make a fairly soft mixture which drops heavily from the spoon when you shake it.

2 Put heaped tablespoons of the mixture into a greased 12-bun tin, dividing the mixture between the 12 sections. Bake in a preheated oven at 180°C (350°F), Gas Mark 4, for 15–20 minutes, until the muffins have puffed up and feel firm to a light touch. Serve warm.

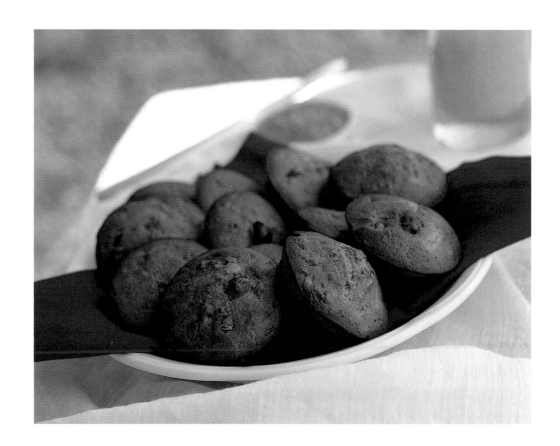

MAKES 12

Preparation time: **15 minutes**

Cooking time: **15–20 minutes**

Oven temperature: **180°C (350°F), Gas Mark 4**

NUTRITION FACT – Wheatgerm comes from the embryo of the wheat grain, where the essential nutrients for germination of the seed are stored. Wheatgerm is high in vitamin E and the B vitamins, all of which are needed for normal cell growth and metabolism.

carbohydrate 16 g / **protein** 4 g / **fat** 5 g / **kJ** 524 / **kcal** 125

Granola

100 ml (3½ fl oz) safflower oil

40 ml (1½ fl oz) malt extract

75 ml (3 fl oz) clear honey

325 g (11 oz) rolled oats

250 g (8 oz) jumbo oats (large oat flakes)

50 g (2 oz) hazelnuts

25 g (1 oz) desiccated coconut

50 g (2 oz) sunflower seeds

25 g (1 oz) sesame seeds

1 Place the oil, malt and honey in a large saucepan and heat gently until the malt is runny. Mix in the remaining ingredients and stir thoroughly.

2 Turn into a large roasting tin and bake in a preheated oven at 190°C (375°F), Gas Mark 5, for about 20 minutes, stirring occasionally, until golden brown. Leave to cool, then separate into pieces with your fingers.

3 Store in an airtight container. Serve with natural yogurt at breakfast time, or use as a topping for fresh fruit salad or stewed fruits.

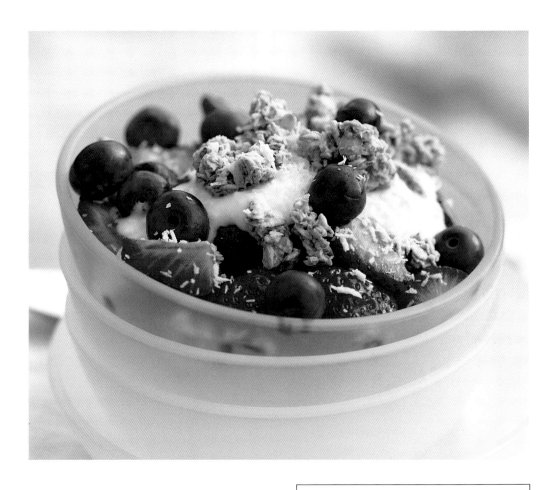

SERVES 18

(3 heaped tablespoons per portion)

Preparation time: **10 minutes, plus cooling**

Cooking time: **20 minutes**

Oven temperature: **190°C (375°F),**

  Gas Mark 5

NUTRITION FACT – Malt extract is prepared from malted barley; it is a carbohydrate in which the main sugar is maltose. In some types of malt there is an enzyme present which was believed to aid the digestion of starchy foods, but today malt is used mainly to add flavour to breakfast cereals and other foods.

carbohydrate 26 g / **protein** 5 g / **fat** 12 g /**kJ** 944 / **kcal** 225

Banana muesli

125 g (4 oz) rolled oats

50 g (2 oz) sunflower seeds

300 ml (½ pint) water

2 tablespoons clear honey

2 large bananas, peeled and sliced

250 g (8 oz) black grapes, halved and
deseeded

grated rind of 1 large orange

grated rind of 1 large lemon

50 g (2 oz) flaked almonds, toasted

GARNISH

pared strips of orange rind (optional)

pared strips of lemon rind (optional)

1 Put the rolled oats and sunflower seeds in a bowl with the water and leave to soak, overnight if possible.

2 Mix well until creamy, then add the honey, bananas, grapes and orange and lemon rind. Spoon into a large serving dish or 4 small ones and sprinkle with toasted almonds. Serve garnished with orange and lemon rind, if liked.

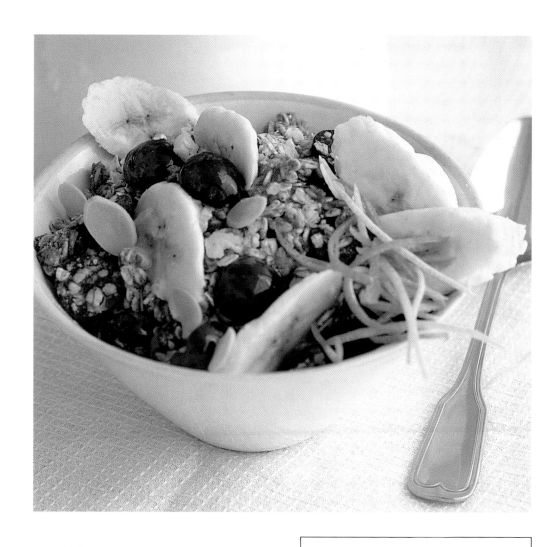

SERVES 4

Preparation time: **10 minutes, plus soaking**

NUTRITION FACT – Many nuts are good sources of vitamin E, and **almonds** have a particularly high content. Vitamin E is an antioxidant and there is some evidence that it may have a protective effect against coronary heart disease and some cancers.

carbohydrate 58 g / **protein** 10 g / **fat** 16 g / **kJ** 1680 / **kcal** 399

Honeyed ricotta with summer fruits

125 g (4 oz) raspberries

2 teaspoons rosewater

2 tablespoons pumpkin seeds

250 g (8 oz) ricotta cheese

250 g (8 oz) mixed summer berries

2 tablespoons clear honey with honeycomb

pinch of ground cinnamon

1 Rub the raspberries through a fine strainer to purée, then mix with the rosewater. Alternatively, process them together in a food processor or blender and then sieve to remove the pips. Toast the pumpkin seeds.

2 Slice the ricotta into wedges and arrange on plates with the berries. Drizzle over the honey and raspberry purée, adding a little honeycomb, and serve scattered with the pumpkin seeds and a pinch of cinnamon.

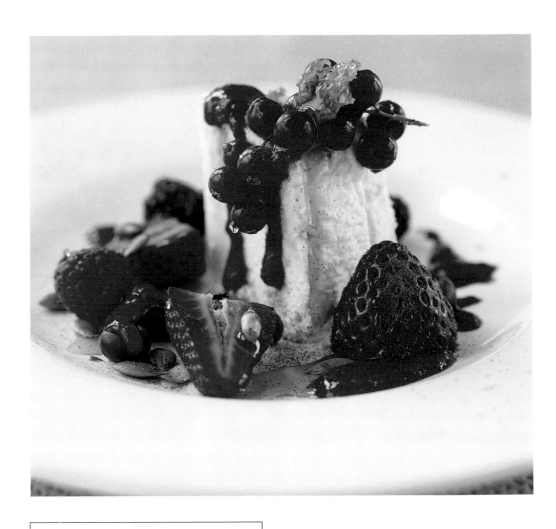

SERVES 4

Preparation time: **10 minutes**

NUTRITION FACT – **Berries** are rich in antioxidant vitamins C, E and beta-carotene, which is converted into vitamin A in the body.

carbohydrate 17 g / **protein** 8 g / **fat** 9 g / **kJ** 750 / **kcal** 179

Hot fruit salad

175 g (6 oz) dried apricots

150 g (5 oz) dried prunes

150 g (5 oz) dried figs

600 ml (1 pint) apple juice

2 tablespoons Calvados or brandy
 (optional)

25 g (1 oz) walnuts, coarsely chopped

low-fat natural yogurt, to serve (optional)

1 Place the dried fruits in a bowl with the apple juice and leave to soak overnight.

2 Transfer to a saucepan and simmer for 10–15 minutes. Turn into a bowl and pour over the Calvados or brandy, if using. Sprinkle with the walnuts and serve immediately with low-fat natural yogurt, if liked.

SERVES 6

Preparation time: **10 minutes, plus soaking**

Cooking time: **10–15 minutes**

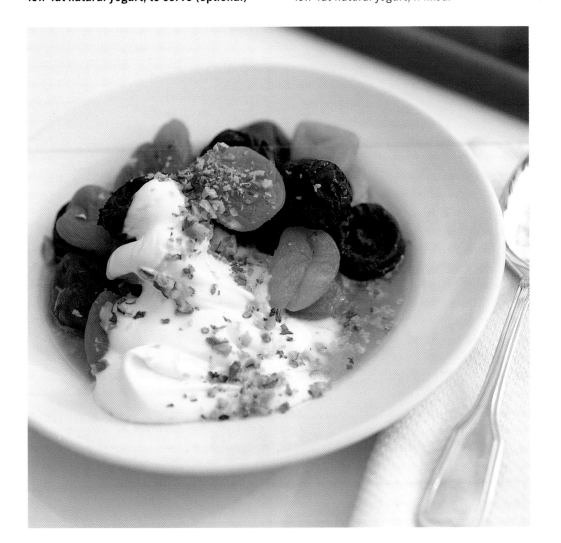

NUTRITION FACT – Dried fruits are rich in potassium, which is an essential element in the diet. Potassium is involved in the function of body cells, and is needed for growth and repair of lean body tissue.

All animal proteins are good sources of potassium. For vegetarians, good sources are potatoes, Brussels sprouts, cauliflower, peas and mushrooms.

carbohydrate 44 g / **protein** 4 g / **fat** 4 g / **kJ** 944 / **kcal** 222

Potato cakes

500 g (1 lb) potatoes, grated
1 onion, chopped
2 tablespoons chopped parsley
2 eggs, beaten
salt and pepper
2 tablespoons olive oil

1 Put the grated potatoes in a colander and rinse under cold running water to remove excess starch. Pat dry with a clean tea towel.

2 Place the potatoes in a bowl with the onion, parsley, eggs and salt and pepper to taste. Mix thoroughly.

3 Heat the oil in a 20–23 cm (8–9 inch) heavy-based frying pan. Add the potato mixture and pat lightly into a cake. Fry gently for about 8–10 minutes until the underside is crisp and brown.

4 Slide the potato cake on to a plate then invert it back into the pan and fry the other side for 10 minutes until crisp and brown. Using a cutter, stamp the potato cake into rounds. Alternatively, cut the potato cake into wedges. Season with salt and pepper and serve immediately.

SERVES 4
Preparation time: **10 minutes**
Cooking time: about **20 minutes**

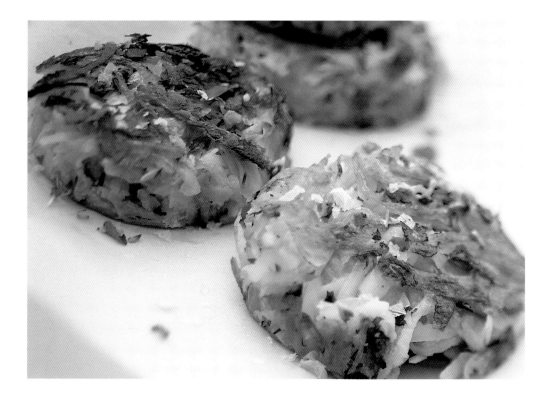

NUTRITION FACT – **Potatoes** are a good source of vitamin C in the diet, if eaten frequently and in medium to large portions. New potatoes have the highest amount. Vitamin C content falls gradually the longer potatoes are stored before eating: after three months storage the vitamin C content is less than half the freshly harvested content.

carbohydrate 25 g / **protein** 6 g / **fat** 9 g / **kJ** 813 / **kcal** 194

Mixed rice kedgeree with kippers

75 g (3 oz) wild rice

175 g (6 oz) basmati rice

325 g (11 oz) kipper fillets

25 g (1 oz) butter

1 small onion, chopped

1 small garlic clove, chopped

grated rind and juice of 1 lemon

1 tablespoon hot curry paste

1 teaspoon ground turmeric

4 ripe tomatoes, skinned, deseeded and
 diced

50 g (2 oz) cashew nuts

2 tablespoons chopped fresh coriander

2 tablespoons chopped parsley

salt and pepper

GARNISH

1 hard-boiled egg, shelled and quartered

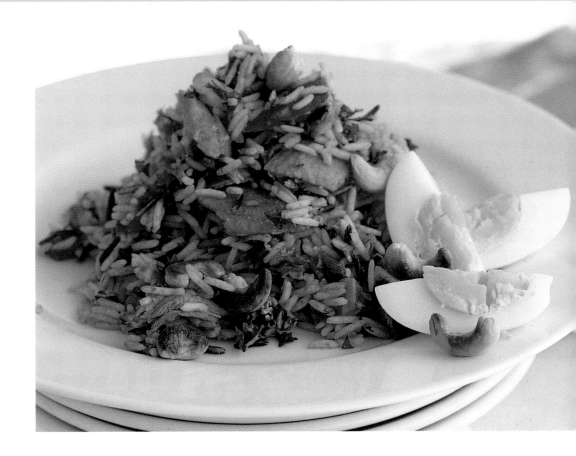

1 Cook the wild rice according to packet instructions, and drain. Cook the basmati rice in plenty of lightly salted boiling water for 15 minutes; drain, refresh under cold water and drain again. Spread both rices on a baking sheet and leave to dry for 30 minutes.

2 Steep the kippers in a bowl filled with boiling water for 8–10 minutes until they are cooked. Drain well and pat dry, skin the fillets and discard any large bones, then carefully flake the flesh.

3 Melt the butter in a saucepan and fry the onion, garlic, lemon rind and juice, curry paste and turmeric for 5 minutes, add the tomatoes and cashew nuts and fry for a further 10 minutes. Add the coriander and parsley, season with salt and pepper to taste and continue to stir over a low heat for 4–5 minutes until warmed through.

4 Stir the rice and kippers through the mixture and transfer to warmed serving plates. Garnish with the egg quarters and serve immediately.

SERVES 4

Preparation time: **15 minutes, plus drying**

Cooking time: **30–50 minutes**

NUTRITION FACT – Kippers are oily fish and a rich source of a particular type of polyunsaturated fat found only in the oils of such fish. These fish oils may protect against coronary heart disease. Kippers also contain vitamins A and D.

carbohydrate 56 g / **protein** 30 g /
fat 24 g / **kJ** 2335 / **kcal** 560

Light meals and side dishes

Greek pitta wraps

4 large pitta breads
125 g (4 oz) cooked lamb, finely shredded
1 small bunch spring onions, trimmed and
   chopped
2 lettuce leaves, chopped
2 tomatoes, peeled, deseeded and chopped
4 black olives, halved and pitted
75 g (3 oz) feta cheese, crumbled
4 lettuce leaves
salt and pepper

DRESSING
2 tablespoons natural yogurt
2 tablespoons olive oil
¼ teaspoon Dijon mustard
¼ teaspoon honey
salt and pepper

1 Carefully cut a slit across the top of each pitta bread. Gently open out each bread to form a pocket. Mix the dressing ingredients together in a small bowl, and season with salt and pepper to taste.

2 Mix the lamb with the spring onions, chopped lettuce, tomatoes, olives, feta cheese, dressing and salt and pepper to taste, blending well.

3 Divide the lamb, salad and feta mixture equally between the pitta pockets.

4 Cook under a preheated moderate grill for about 2–3 minutes until the filling is bubbling, turning once. Add the fresh lettuce leaves and quickly roll up the pittas in greaseproof paper to serve.

MAKES 4
Preparation time: **10 minutes**
Cooking time: **2–3 minutes**

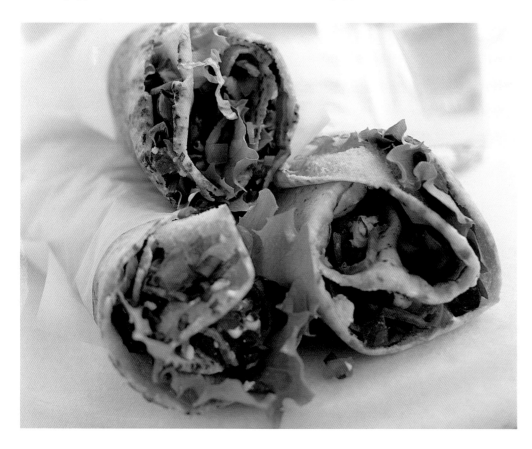

NUTRITION FACT – Feta cheese is made from sheep and goats' milk and has a higher water content than many hard cheeses. The fat and calorie content of feta is therefore quite a bit lower (by weight of portion) than that of, for example, Cheddar-type cheeses.

carbohydrate 60 g / **protein** 19 g /
fat 29 g / **kJ** 2346 / **kcal** 560

Smoked salmon and poached egg salad on blinis

1 tablespoon distilled white vinegar

4 eggs

4 blinis, about 10 cm (4 inches) in diameter

25 g (1 oz) Anchovy Butter (see box right)

125 g (4 oz) frisée lettuce

200 g (7 oz) smoked salmon

1 tablespoon poppy seeds

fresh chives, to garnish

DRESSING

2 teaspoons Champagne or white wine
  vinegar

1 teaspoon Dijon mustard

1 tablespoon snipped chives

6 tablespoons extra virgin olive oil

2 ripe tomatoes, skinned, deseeded and
  diced

salt and pepper

1 Bring a small frying pan of water to a gentle simmer, add the vinegar and then carefully break in the eggs to fit closely together. Remove the pan from the heat and leave the eggs in the water to poach until just set.

2 Meanwhile, toast the blinis for 1 minute. Spread anchovy butter on one side.

3 Blend together all the dressing ingredients except the tomatoes, season with salt and pepper to taste, and toss half of the dressing with the frisée lettuce. Stir the diced tomato into the remaining dressing.

4 Arrange the blinis on serving plates, top each one with some smoked salmon and dressed frisée. Carefully remove the poached eggs from the water with a slotted spoon, drain on kitchen paper and sprinkle over the poppy seeds. Place 1 egg on top of each blini. Pour the tomato dressing around each one and serve immediately, garnished with the chives.

SERVES 4

Preparation time: **20 minutes**

Cooking time: **15 minutes**

COOK'S TIP – To make **Anchovy Butter**, purée 1–2 anchovy fillets using a mortar and pestle. Place in a bowl; add pepper, 2 teaspoons lemon juice and 25 g (1 oz) unsalted butter. Mix with a fork.

carbohydrate 18 g / **protein** 23 g / **fat** 30 g / **kJ** 2030 / **kcal** 490

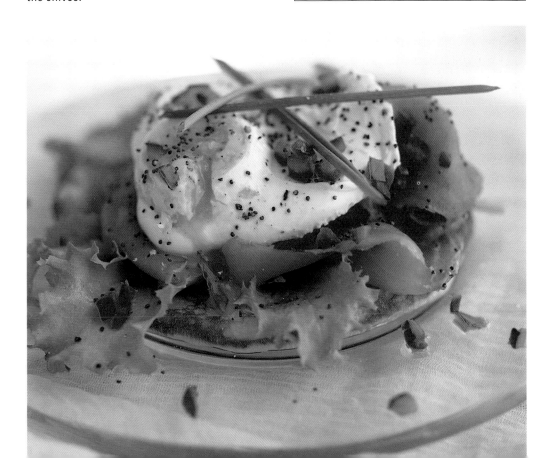

Rocket, tuna and haricot bean salad

4 tomatoes, skinned, deseeded and roughly chopped

125 g (4 oz) rocket

400 g (13 oz) can haricot beans, drained

200 g (7 oz) can tuna in spring water, drained

1 red onion, chopped

125 g (4 oz) artichoke hearts in olive oil, drained except for 1 tablespoon of oil

2 young celery sticks with leaves, chopped

1 tablespoon pitted black olives

4 tablespoons lemon juice

1 tablespoon red wine vinegar

¼ teaspoon crushed dried chillies

handful of flat leaf parsley, roughly chopped

salt and pepper

TO SERVE

French bread (optional)

salad leaves

lemon wedges

1 Put the tomatoes in a large salad bowl with the rocket. Stir in the beans and tuna, roughly breaking the tuna into large chunks. Stir in the chopped red onion.

2 Add the artichoke hearts, with 1 tablespoon of oil from the jar, the celery, olives, lemon juice, vinegar, chilli and parsley. Season with salt and pepper to taste.

3 Mix all the ingredients together well and allow to stand for 30 minutes for the flavours to mingle. Serve the salad at room temperature with crusty bread, if liked.

SERVES 4

Preparation time: **15 minutes, plus standing**

NUTRITION FACT – **Tuna** may be bought canned in oil, brine or spring water. The advantage of the spring water variety is that it does not have added fat or salt. High salt intakes may be linked to high blood pressure and it is sensible to limit the amount of salt added to food.

carbohydrate 10 g / **protein** 17 g / **fat** 5 g / **kJ** 623 / **kcal** 147

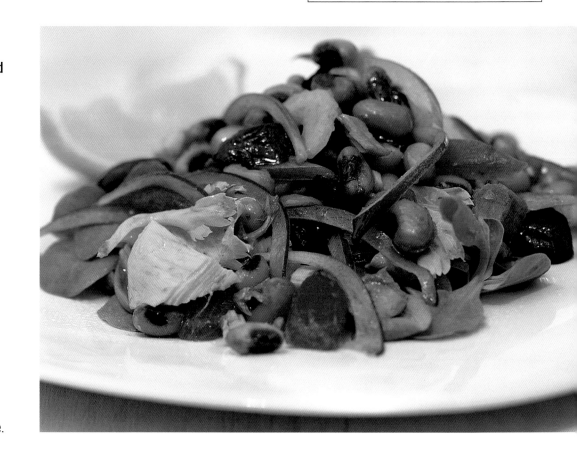

Prawn, mango and mozzarella salad

125 g (4 oz) salad leaves

25 g (1 oz) radicchio, shredded

1 large ripe mango, peeled, stoned and
  thinly sliced

150 g (5 oz) mozzarella cheese, sliced

12 large cooked peeled prawns

1 tablespoon extra virgin olive oil

GRILLED PEPPER SALSA

1 large red pepper

½ tablespoon balsamic vinegar

pinch of sugar

1 tablespoon extra virgin olive oil, plus
  extra for brushing

salt and pepper

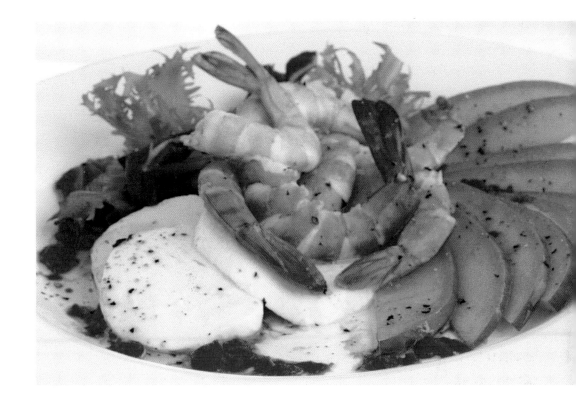

1 Start by making the grilled pepper salsa.
Brush the pepper with a little oil and cook
under a preheated hot grill for 10–12
minutes, turning frequently until charred all
over. To simplify removing the skin, place the
pepper in a plastic bag, seal and set aside
until cool enough to handle.

2 Skin and deseed the pepper over a bowl to
catch the juices, then roughly chop the flesh.
Place it in a blender or food processor with
the juices, vinegar and sugar and blend
until smooth. Transfer to a bowl and whisk
in the oil. Season with salt and pepper to
taste and set aside.

3 Arrange the salad leaves and radicchio on
a plate with the mango slices fanned out and
the mozzarella slices and the prawns in the
middle. Drizzle over the grilled pepper salsa
and a little olive oil. Serve garnished with
black pepper.

SERVES 4
Preparation time: **15 minutes**
Cooking time: **10–12 minutes**

NUTRITION FACT – **Mango** is a rich
source of iron and vitamin A. It also
contains some of the B vitamins and
vitamin C.

carbohydrate 9 g / **protein** 16 g /
fat 14 g / **kJ** 934 / **kcal** 224

Courgette and mixed leaf salad

4 tablespoons light French dressing

1 garlic clove, crushed

275 g (9 oz) courgettes, thinly sliced

500 g (1 lb) salad leaves

50 g (2 oz) green or black olives, halved
   and pitted

1 tablespoon pine nuts

salt and pepper

1 Put the French dressing and garlic in a salad bowl. Add the sliced courgettes and toss well. Leave to stand for 30 minutes to allow the courgettes to absorb the flavour of the dressing.

2 Tear the salad leaves into manageable pieces and add to the courgettes and dressing with the olives and pine nuts. Season with salt and pepper to taste. Toss the salad thoroughly before serving.

SERVES 6

Preparation time: **15 minutes, plus standing**

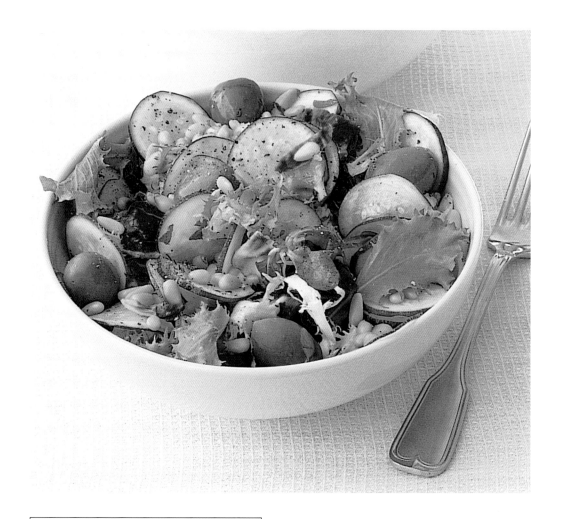

NUTRITION FACT – **Pine nuts** are high in protein and essential fatty acids. They contain magnesium, potassium, zinc and some B vitamins.

carbohydrate 5 g / **protein** 2 g / **fat** 4 g / **kJ** 235 / **kcal** 56

Marinated courgette and bean salad

250 g (8 oz) green beans

375 g (12 oz) courgettes, diced

475 g (15 oz) can blackeye beans, drained

2 tablespoons olive oil

2 tablespoons lemon juice

1 garlic clove, crushed

2 tablespoons chopped parsley

salt and pepper

crusty bread, sliced and toasted, to serve
  (optional)

1 Cut the green beans into 2.5 cm (1 inch) lengths and cook in lightly salted boiling water for 5 minutes. Add the courgettes and cook for a further 5 minutes. Drain thoroughly and place in a bowl with the blackeye beans.

2 Add the remaining ingredients, with salt and pepper to taste, while still warm and mix well to combine. Leave to cool and serve with toasted slices of crusty bread, if liked.

SERVES 4

Preparation time: **10 minutes, plus cooling**

Cooking time: **10 minutes**

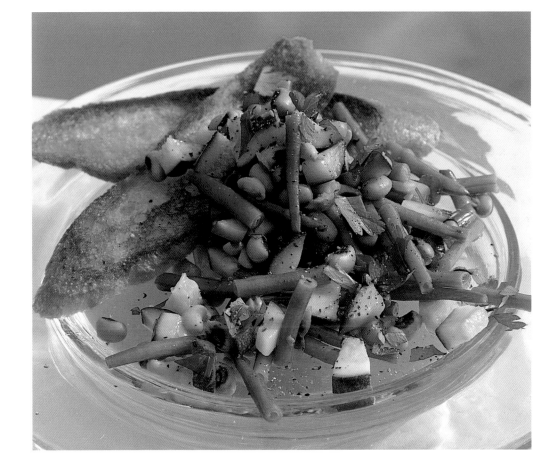

NUTRITION FACT — Blackeye beans have a high nutritional value and contain soluble dietary fibre, which helps to control the level of cholesterol in the blood.

carbohydrate 29 g / **protein** 13 g / **fat** 7 g / **kJ** 927 / **kcal** 220

Rocket risotto

1 teaspoon olive oil

1 onion, finely chopped

300 g (10 oz) arborio rice

1.2 litres (2 pints) Vegetable Stock (see page 48)

50 g (2 oz) rocket leaves

salt and pepper

1 Heat the oil in a nonstick frying pan, add the onion and fry for a few minutes until softened. Pour in the rice and stir well to coat the grains.

2 With the pan set over a medium heat, gradually add a little vegetable stock. Stir continuously while the stock is absorbed into the rice. Keep on adding the stock a little at a time – this will take about 20 minutes.

3 Stir in the rocket, reserving 4 leaves for garnish, and cook just until the leaves start to wilt. Season to taste and serve each portion garnished with a rocket leaf.

SERVES 4

Preparation time: **5 minutes**

Cooking time: **20–25 minutes**

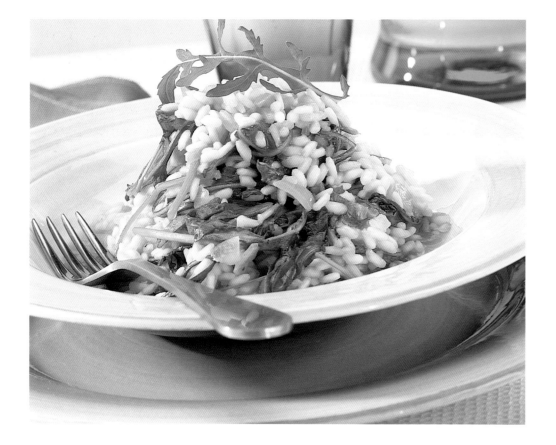

COOK'S TIP – For a main meal, add some diced, cooked chicken, a handful of prawns, or some grated Parmesan cheese and a few chopped nuts, when you add the rocket. Make sure all the ingredients are heated through thoroughly before serving.

carbohydrate 63 g / **protein** 6 g / **fat** 1 g / **kJ** 1223 / **kcal** 290

Stir-fried chinese cabbage

8–10 large Chinese cabbage leaves

2 tablespoons oil

125 g (4 oz) canned bamboo shoots,
  drained and sliced

1 onion, sliced

1 celery stick, sliced

lemon juice

salt and pepper

lemon slices, to garnish

1 Cut the Chinese cabbage leaves diagonally into thin strips.

2 Heat the oil in a nonstick frying pan or wok. Add all the vegetables and fry gently for about 8 minutes, stirring frequently. Add a little lemon juice and season with salt and pepper to taste. Garnish with lemon slices and serve.

SERVES 4

Preparation time: **10 minutes**

Cooking time: **8 minutes**

FOOD FACT — There are many types of **Chinese leaf vegetables**. Chinese cabbage forms a large, dense head of pale green leaves, much like a Cos lettuce. Pak choi and bok choi form smaller, open heads of dark green leaves with long, white edible stems. Any of them can be used for this dish.

carbohydrate 5 g / **protein** 2 g / **fat** 6 g / **kJ** 323 / **kcal** 78

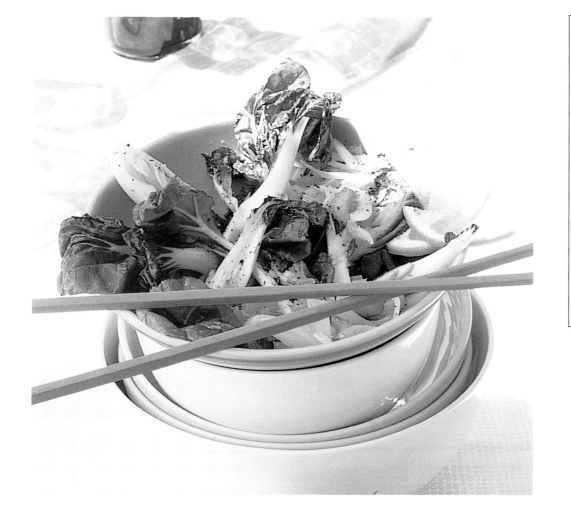

Soups and starters

Beetroot borscht with soured cream and chives

750 g (1½ lb) fresh raw beetroot, washed

1 carrot, grated

1 onion, grated

2 garlic cloves, crushed

1.5 litres (2½ pints) Vegetable Stock
  (see page 48)

4 tablespoons lemon juice

2 tablespoons sugar

1 large cooked beetroot

salt and pepper

GARNISH

150 ml (¼ pint) soured cream

1 teaspoon snipped chives

whole chives

1 Scrape young beetroot, or peel older ones with a potato peeler, then coarsely grate the flesh into a large saucepan. Add the carrot, onion, garlic, stock, lemon juice and sugar and season with salt and pepper to taste. Bring to the boil. Cover the pan, reduce the heat and simmer for 45 minutes.

2 Meanwhile, cut the whole cooked beetroot into matchsticks about 4 cm (1½ in) long. Cover and refrigerate until required.

3 When the soup vegetables are tender, strain the contents of the saucepan through a sieve lined with muslin. Discard the vegetables. (At this stage, the beetroot juice can be cooled and stored in the refrigerator until required. It will keep for several days. It can also be frozen.)

4 Put the beetroot juice into a saucepan with the beetroot matchsticks. Gently bring to the boil, then simmer for a few minutes to warm the beetroot through. Season with salt and pepper to taste, ladle into warmed soup bowls and serve with a spoonful of soured cream on top and with snipped chives and some whole chives tied in a small bundle.

SERVES 6

Preparation time: **25 minutes**

Cooking time: **1 hour**

> **NUTRITION FACT** – The benefits of **Beetroot** are both powerful and wide-ranging. It has a very high antioxidant content and stimulates the circulation. It also has a high folate content, but this diminishes with cooking and pickling.
>
> **carbohydrate** 20 g / **protein** 4 g / **fat** 5 g / **kJ** 566 / **kcal** 135

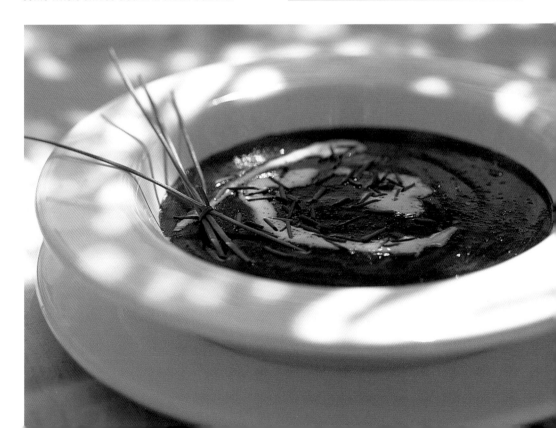

Caldo verde

2 tablespoons olive oil

1 large onion, chopped

2 garlic cloves, chopped

500 g (1 lb) potatoes, cut into 2.5 cm
  (1 inch) cubes

1.2 litres (2 pints) water or Vegetable Stock
  (see page 48)

250 g (8 oz) spring greens, finely shredded

2 tablespoons chopped parsley

salt and pepper

long croûtons, to serve

1 Heat the oil in a large frying pan and fry
the onion for 5 minutes until softened but not
brown. Add the garlic and potatoes and cook
for a few minutes, stirring occasionally.

2 Add the water or stock, season with salt
and pepper to taste and cook for 15 minutes
until the potatoes are tender. Mash the
potatoes roughly in their liquid, then add the
greens and boil, uncovered, for 10 minutes.
Add the parsley and simmer for 2–3 minutes
until heated through. Serve with long croûtons.

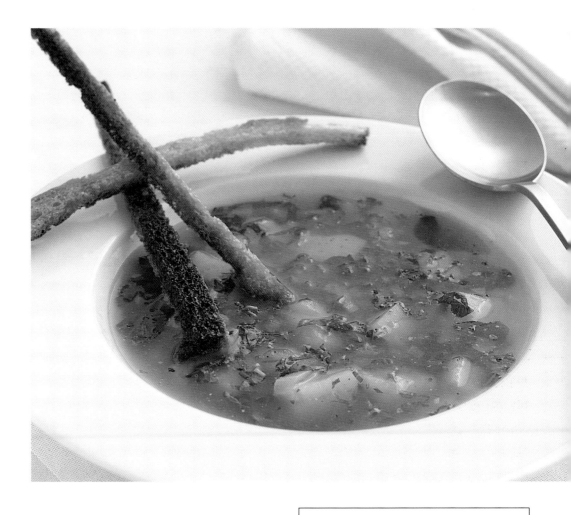

SERVES 6

Preparation time: **10 minutes**

Cooking time: **40 minutes**

NUTRITION FACT — Like many green
vegetables, **spring greens** contain
folate (folic acid). Folate is necessary
for normal cell growth and for the
prevention of a particular form of
anaemia. Folate diminishes with
storage, so choose leafy vegetables
that are as fresh as possible.

carbohydrate 19 g / **protein** 4 g /
fat 4 g / **kJ** 523 / kcal 123

Red pepper and ginger soup

3 red peppers, halved, cored and deseeded

1 red onion, quartered

2 garlic cloves, unpeeled

1 teaspoon olive oil

5 cm (2 inch) piece of fresh root ginger, grated

1 teaspoon ground cumin

1 teaspoon ground coriander

1 large potato, chopped

900 ml (1½ pints) Vegetable Stock (see page 48)

4 tablespoons low-fat fromage frais

salt and pepper

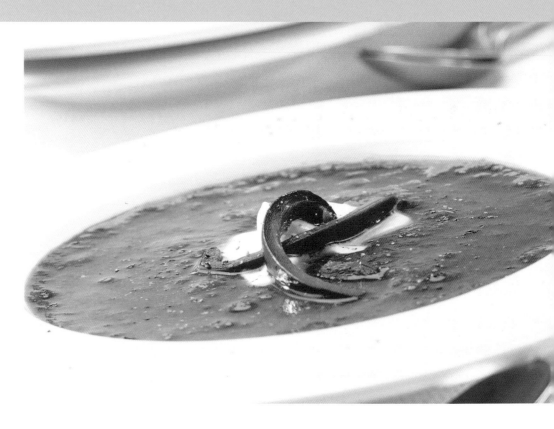

1 Place the peppers, onion and garlic cloves in a nonstick roasting tin. Roast in a preheated oven, 200°C (400°F), Gas Mark 6, for 40 minutes, or until the peppers have blistered and the onion quarters and garlic are very soft. If the onion quarters start to brown too much, cover them with the pepper halves.

2 Meanwhile, heat the oil in a saucepan and fry the ginger, cumin and coriander over a low heat for 5 minutes, until softened. Add the potato and stir well, season and pour in the vegetable stock. Simmer, covered, for 30 minutes.

3 Remove the cooked vegetables from the oven. Place the peppers in a plastic bag. Tie the top and leave to cool. (The steam produced in the bag makes it easier to remove the skin when cool.) Add the onions to the potato mixture and carefully squeeze out the garlic pulp into the saucepan, too. Peel the peppers and add all but one half to the soup. Simmer for 5 minutes.

4 Pour the soup into a blender or food processor and blend, in batches if necessary, for a few seconds until quite smooth. Return to the saucepan and thin with a little water, if necessary, to achieve the desired consistency.

5 Spoon into warmed bowls. Slice the remaining pepper and lay on top of the soup with a spoonful of fromage frais.

SERVES 4

Preparation time: **20 minutes, plus cooling**

Cooking time: **45 minutes**

Oven temperature: **200°C (400°F), Gas Mark 6**

NUTRITION FACT – Peppers are a good source of vitamin C and beta-carotene, which is converted into vitamin A in the body. They are believed to give you a boost by increasing energy supplies, and can help protect against heart disease, high blood pressure and cancers.

carbohydrate 17 g / **protein** 4 g / **fat** 2 g / **kJ** 385 / **kcal** 92

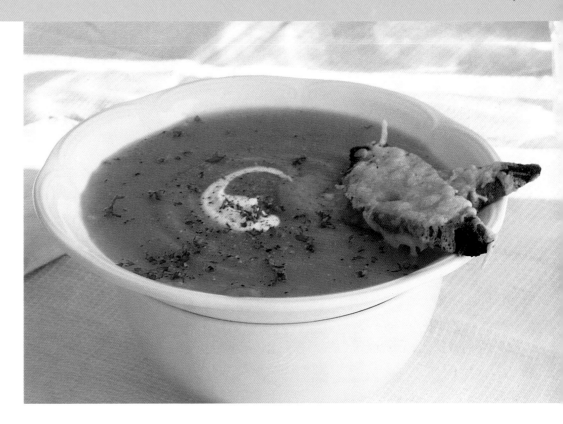

Pumpkin soup with crusty cheese topping

1 tablespoon sunflower or olive oil

1 large onion, finely chopped

3 garlic cloves, crushed

2 celery sticks, chopped

750 g (1½ lb) pumpkin flesh, roughly
   chopped

750 ml (1¼ pints) Vegetable or Chicken
   Stock (see page 48)

pinch of grated nutmeg

1 bay leaf

a few parsley stalks

65 ml (2½ fl oz) single cream

1–2 tablespoons finely chopped parsley,
   plus extra to garnish

salt and pepper

single cream or crème fraîche, to serve
   (optional)

GARNISH

1 small French stick

50 g (2 oz) Gruyère or fontina cheese,
   grated

1 Heat the oil in a saucepan and fry the
onion and garlic until soft but not brown. Add
the celery and pumpkin flesh and fry for
10–15 minutes to draw out the flavours. Stir
in the stock and nutmeg. Tie the bay leaf and
parsley stalks together, add and bring to the
boil. Reduce the heat and simmer for about
30 minutes until the vegetables are soft.

2 Remove the bouquet of herbs and purée the
soup in a blender or food processor, or pass it
through a fine sieve. Return the purée to the
saucepan, bring to the boil and season with
salt and pepper. Stir in the cream and finely
chopped parsley, return to the boil, then
reduce the heat and keep the soup warm
while preparing the garnish.

3 Slice the bread into 8, place on a baking
sheet and toast both sides under a preheated
moderate grill until golden. Leave the grill on.

4 Pour the hot soup into 4 deep ovenproof
bowls. Arrange 2 pieces of French bread in
each one, overlapping them slightly. Sprinkle
the bread with grated cheese. Set the bowls
on the baking sheet and cook quickly under
the grill until the cheese is golden brown and

bubbling. Garnish with parsley and a small
swirl of single cream or crème fraîche, if
liked. Serve immediately.

SERVES 4
Preparation time: **25 minutes**
Cooking time: **1¼ hours**

NUTRITION FACT – Like many yellow
and red vegetables **pumpkin** is a good
source of carotene, from which our
bodies can make vitamin A, which is
important for the health of soft tissue
and helps prevent night blindness.

carbohydrate 38 g / **protein** 11 g /
fat 12 g / **kJ** 1229 / **kcal** 293

Vegetable carpaccio with parmesan shavings

12 small radishes, trimmed and sliced

1 green pepper, cored, deseeded and cut into thin strips

1 red pepper, cored, deseeded and cut into thin strips

2 small carrots, thinly sliced

3 celery sticks, thinly sliced

1 small fennel bulb, thinly sliced

1 tablespoon extra virgin olive oil

25 g (1 oz) Parmesan cheese, shaved

pepper

1 Divide the vegetables between 4 large plates and arrange in attractive mounds in the centre.

2 Drizzle the vegetables with enough olive oil to lightly moisten them. Scatter the Parmesan shavings around them and garnish with a few grindings of black pepper.

SERVES 4

Preparation time: **15 minutes**

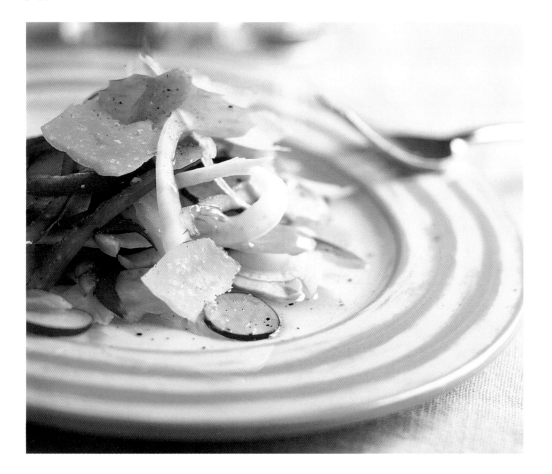

NUTRITION FACT – The main nutritional difference between old **carrots** and young carrots is their carotene content. Carotene is stored in the growing root, so that old carrots have a very high carotene content.

carbohydrate 6 g / **protein** 4 g / **fat** 5 g / **kJ** 354 / **kcal** 85

Zucchini al forno

4 large or 8 small courgettes

1 teaspoon oil

1 garlic clove, finely chopped

500 g (1 lb) canned tomatoes

50 g (2 oz) canned anchovies, drained

salt and pepper

TO SERVE

lemon slices

mixed salad

GARNISH

1 teaspoon chopped thyme

1 teaspoon chopped rosemary

1 Halve the courgettes lengthways, and scoop out the seeds and pulp with a spoon. Sprinkle the inside of each one with salt and leave to drain upside down on kitchen paper.

2 Heat the oil in a saucepan and lightly fry the garlic. Rub the tomatoes through a sieve to remove the seeds and add the pulp to the saucepan. Bring to the boil and cook vigorously until reduced by half. Remove from the heat and stir in one chopped anchovy fillet. Season with salt and pepper to taste.

3 Wipe the insides of the courgettes with absorbent kitchen paper to remove the salt and set them in a large baking dish. Fill each one with some tomato sauce and arrange an anchovy fillet on top. Grind over plenty of black pepper and bake in a preheated oven at 200°C (400°F), Gas Mark 6, for about 40 minutes. Allow to cool then serve with lemon slices and salad leaves and garnished with the thyme and rosemary.

SERVES 4

Preparation time: **15 minutes, plus cooling**

Cooking time: **55 minutes**

Oven temperature: **200°C (400°F),**
  Gas Mark 6

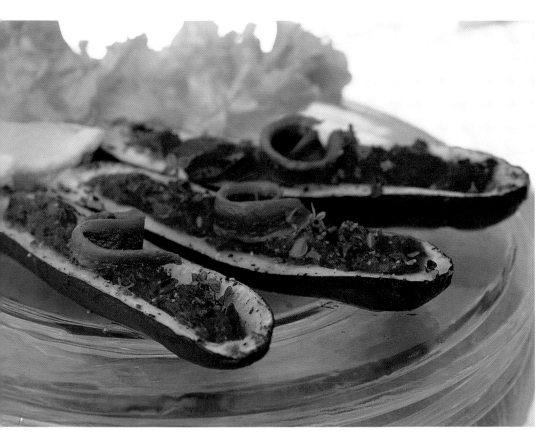

NUTRITION FACT – Courgettes retain essential vitamins in the skin, such as K and B12, which are lost when they are peeled.

carbohydrate 11 g / **protein** 7 g / **fat** 4 g / **kJ** 420 / **kcal** 100

Baked field mushrooms

5 large mushrooms
DRESSING
4 tablespoons balsamic vinegar
1 tablespoon wholegrain mustard
TO SERVE
75 g (3 oz) watercress
salt and pepper
Parmesan shavings, to garnish (optional)

1 Remove the stalks from 4 of the mushrooms and reserve them. Place the 4 mushrooms in a small roasting tin, their gills facing uppermost. Cook in a preheated oven, 200°C (400°F), Gas Mark 6, for 15 minutes.

2 Meanwhile, make the dressing. Finely chop the remaining mushroom and reserved stalks and mix in a small bowl with the balsamic vinegar and mustard. Season with salt and pepper.

3 Remove the mushrooms from the oven and spoon the dressing over each mushroom. Return to the oven and continue to cook for 25 minutes, covering the tin with foil after 10 minutes.

4 When cooked, lift the mushrooms on to a plate and keep warm. Tip the watercress into the hot juices and toss well. Spoon piles of watercress on to 4 warmed plates. Place a mushroom on top and garnish with Parmesan shavings, if liked.

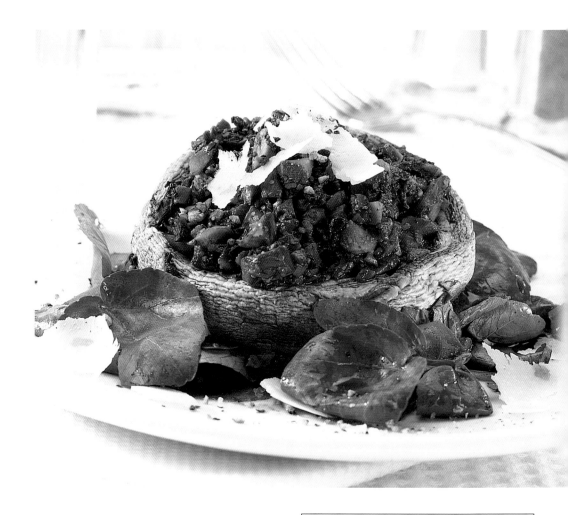

SERVES 4
Preparation time: **5 minutes**
Cooking time: **40 minutes**
Oven temperature: **200°C (400°F), Gas Mark 6**

COOK'S TIP – Use large field or open-cap mushrooms for this dish. Portobello mushrooms are also widely available and have a good flavour.

carbohydrate 1 g / **protein** 2 g / **fat** 1 g / **kJ** 63 / **kcal** 15

Carrot and coriander pâté

500 g (1 lb) carrots, grated
1 tablespoon ground coriander
175 ml (6 fl oz) freshly squeezed orange
  juice
300 ml (½ pint) water
50 g (2 oz) medium-fat soft cheese
30 g (1¼ oz) fresh coriander leaves
salt and pepper
country bread, to serve (optional)

1 Place the grated carrots in a saucepan with the ground coriander, orange juice and water. Cover with a lid and simmer for 40 minutes until the carrots are cooked. Cool and transfer to a blender or food processor with a little of the cooking liquid.

2 Add the soft cheese and coriander leaves; blend until smooth. Season to taste and blend again. Spoon into small dishes and chill before serving with country bread, if liked.

SERVES 4
Preparation time: **5 minutes, plus chilling**
Cooking time: **40 minutes**

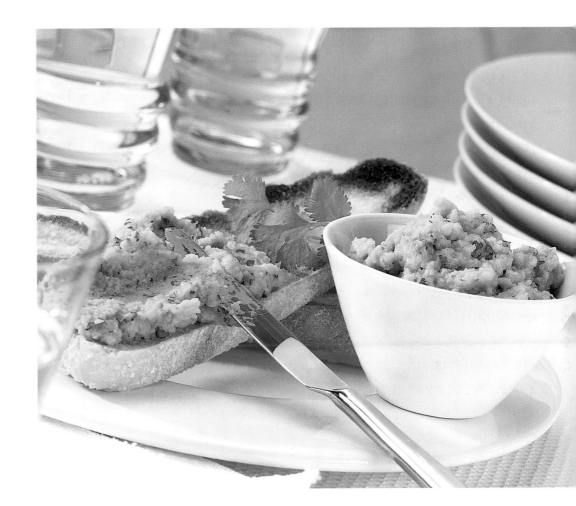

COOK'S TIP — This pâté has a smooth texture because it has been blended thoroughly. If you prefer a coarser texture, blend briefly.

carbohydrate 14 g / **protein** 2 g / **fat** 2 g / **kJ** 352 / **kcal** 84

Main meals

Mushroom crêpes

50 g (2 oz) plain flour
150 ml (¼ pint) skimmed milk
1 small egg, beaten
1 teaspoon olive oil
salt and pepper
flat leaf parsley sprigs, to garnish
FILLING
300 g (10 oz) chestnut mushrooms, chopped
1 bunch of spring onions, finely chopped
1 garlic clove, chopped
400 g (13 oz) can chopped tomatoes,
   drained
2 tablespoons chopped oregano

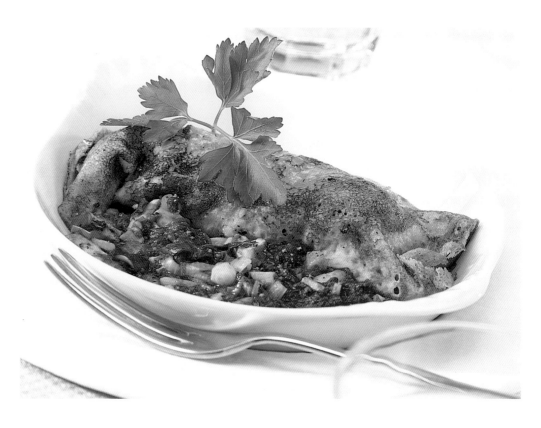

1 To make the crêpe batter, place the flour, milk, egg and seasoning in a blender or food processor and blend until smooth, or whisk the batter by hand.

2 Pour a few drops of oil in a frying pan. Heat the pan, pour in a scant covering of batter and cook for 1 minute. Carefully flip the pancake and cook the second side. Slide out of the pan on to greaseproof paper. Make 3 more pancakes in the same way, adding a few more drops of oil to the pan between each pancake, and stack them in between sheets of greaseproof paper.

3 Now make the filling: put all the ingredients into a small saucepan and cook, stirring occasionally, for 5 minutes. Season to taste and divide the filling between the pancakes, reserving a little of the mixture to serve, and roll them up. Transfer the pancakes to an ovenproof dish and cook in a preheated oven, 180°C (350°F), Gas Mark 4, for 20 minutes. Serve with the remaining mixture on top and garnish with the parsley.

SERVES 4
Preparation time: **20–25 minutes**
Cooking time: **35 minutes**
Oven temperature: **180°C (350°F),
   Gas Mark 4**

COOK'S TIP – Serve the pancakes with some lightly steamed vegetables.

carbohydrate 16 g / **protein** 7 g / **fat** 3 g / **kJ** 470 / **kcal** 111

Lentil moussaka

3 tablespoons vegetable oil

1 onion, chopped

4 celery sticks, chopped

1 garlic clove, crushed

400 g (13 oz) can chopped tomatoes

250 g (8 oz) green lentils

2 tablespoons Japanese soy sauce

900 ml (1½ pints) water

500 g (1 lb) aubergines, sliced

salt and pepper

1 tablespoon oregano, to garnish

TOPPING

2 eggs, beaten

150 ml (¼ pint) low-fat fromage frais

1 tablespoon grated Parmesan cheese

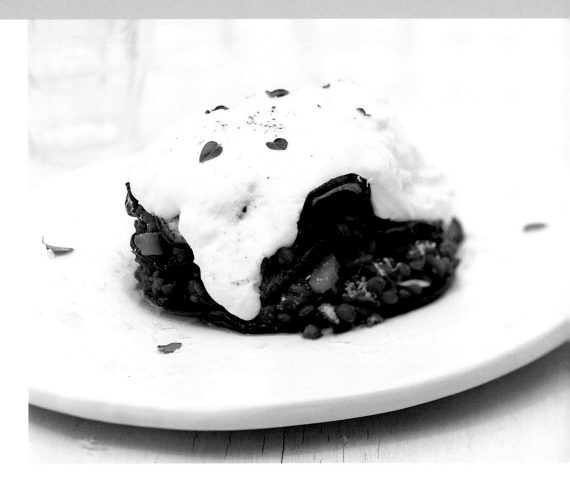

1 Heat 1 tablespoon of the oil in a saucepan, add the onion and cook until softened. Add the celery, garlic, tomatoes with their juice, lentils, soy sauce, ¼ teaspoon pepper and water. Cover and simmer for 50 minutes, until cooked.

2 Heat the remaining oil in a griddle pan, add the aubergine slices in batches and cook on both sides until golden. Alternatively, cook under a preheated moderate grill.

3 Cover the base of a shallow ovenproof dish with the lentil mixture and arrange a layer of aubergine slices on top. Repeat the layers, finishing with a layer of aubergine slices.

4 Mix the eggs and fromage frais for the topping, season with salt and pepper to taste, and pour over the aubergines. Top with the cheese and bake in a preheated moderate oven at 180°C (350°F), Gas Mark 4, for 30–40 minutes, until golden. Serve garnished with oregano leaves.

SERVES 4

Preparation time: **20 minutes**

Cooking time: **1¼–1½ hours**

Oven temperature: **180°C (350°F), Gas Mark 4**

NUTRITION FACT – Lentils are a useful source of iron in the vegetarian diet. Iron from vegetable sources is not as easily absorbed as iron from animal sources. However, a source of vitamin C (salad, peppers, fruit juice) taken at the same time aids the absorption of vegetable iron.

carbohydrate 43 g / **protein** 26 g / **fat** 14 g / **kJ** 1625 / **kcal** 385

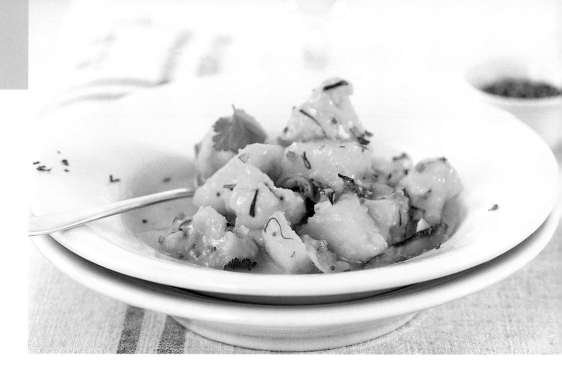

Hot spiced stew with potatoes and cauliflower

375 g (12 oz) whole lentils or split yellow
   peas, rinsed and soaked in water for
   15 minutes

1.8 litres (3 pints) Vegetable Stock (see
   page 48)

3 tablespoons vegetable oil

2 large onions, cut into wedges

1–1.25 kg (2–2½ lb) potatoes, cut into
   chunks

1 cauliflower, cut into florets and stalks
   removed

3–4 garlic cloves, crushed

2 teaspoons turmeric

2 tablespoons black mustard seeds

1–2 tablespoons fennel seeds

1–2 small green chillies, deseeded and
   chopped

1 teaspoon saffron threads, soaked in
   2 tablespoons warm water

125 g (4 oz) coconut cream

2 tablespoons chopped coriander

salt and pepper

1 Rinse the lentils or split peas under cold
running water, drain and put into a large
saucepan with half of the stock. Bring to the
boil, then reduce the heat and simmer for
30 minutes until the lentils or split peas are
soft and all the liquid has been absorbed.

2 Meanwhile, prepare and cook the
vegetables. Heat the oil in a large saucepan,
add the onions and fry over a low heat for
about 8 minutes, stirring frequently. Add the
potatoes and cauliflower to the pan with the
garlic and cook for 1 minute. Stir in the
turmeric, mustard and fennel seeds and the
chopped chillies, mixing them in the pan. Add
the remaining stock and the soaked saffron
threads with their water and bring to the boil.
Reduce the heat and cook gently for
10–15 minutes or until the vegetables are
almost cooked.

3 When the lentils or split peas are cooked,
mash them with a potato masher to form a
thick purée, leaving a few whole. Add the
coconut cream and stir well to mix. Add this
thick purée to the vegetables and stir well to
combine. This will make the stew rich and
thick. Season with salt and pepper and cook
gently until the vegetables are completely
tender and the flavours combined. Stir in the
coriander and serve immediately.

SERVES 6
Preparation time: **15 minutes, plus soaking**
Cooking time: **45 minutes**

NUTRITION FACT – The fat content of
the different commercial brands of
coconut cream available in the
supermarket varies enormously –
from about 22 to 68 per cent. For
healthier eating, choose the lower-fat
varieties. Although a vegetable,
coconut is unusual in that its fat
content is almost entirely saturated.

carbohydrate 70 g / **protein** 23 g /
fat 15 g / **kJ** 2077 / **kcal** 494

Noodles with smoked tofu and vegetables

175 g (6 oz) dried thread egg noodles

sunflower oil, for deep-frying

250 g (8 oz) firm smoked tofu, cubed

1 onion, finely chopped

1 teaspoon grated fresh root ginger

2 garlic cloves, crushed

1 small red chilli, deseeded and finely sliced

250 g (8 oz) broccoli florets

175 g (6 oz) baby sweetcorn, cut in half
 lengthways

175 g (6 oz) fresh bean sprouts

2 red chillies, deseeded and cut in half, to
 garnish

SAUCE

250 ml (8 fl oz) teriyaki sauce

2 tablespoons sake (Japanese rice wine)

2 tablespoons lemon juice

2–3 teaspoons sweet chilli sauce

2 teaspoons brown sugar

1 Cook the noodles in a large saucepan of boiling water according to packet instructions until just tender. Drain and refresh under cold running water until very cold. Leave to drain.

2 Heat about 5 cm (2 in) sunflower oil in a heavy-based frying pan or wok and fry the tofu cubes for 3–4 minutes until crisp and lightly golden. Drain on kitchen paper and keep warm. Remove all but a few tablespoons of the oil from the wok and fry the onion, ginger, garlic and chilli until soft but not brown. Remove from the heat.

3 Blanch the broccoli in a large saucepan of boiling water for about 1 minute, drain and refresh under cold water. Drain again and pat dry with kitchen paper. Combine all the sauce ingredients in a bowl and mix well.

4 Return the frying pan or wok with the onion mixture to the heat. When reheated, add the broccoli and stir-fry for 2–3 minutes. Add the sweetcorn and bean sprouts and stir-fry for about 3 minutes. Add the sauce, toss to combine, then add the noodles and the fried tofu. Cook for another 1 minute until heated through. Serve garnished with chilli halves.

SERVES 4

Preparation time: **20 minutes**

Cooking time: **20 minutes**

NUTRITION FACT – **Tofu** is a curd made from soya beans and is a good protein source for vegetarians. It has a similar protein content to beans and lentils and can be a rich source of calcium, depending on the method that is used to make it.

carbohydrate 48 g / **protein** 26 g / **fat** 17 g / **kJ** 1827 / **kcal** 436

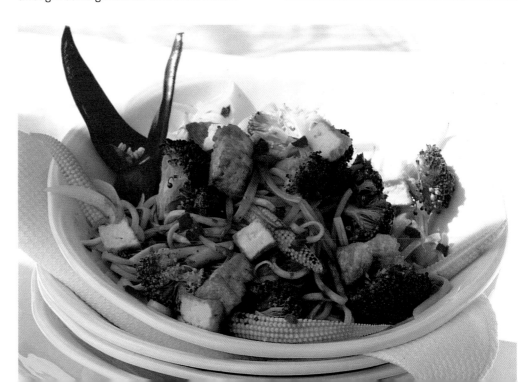

Chicken with ginger

375 g (12 oz) boneless, skinless chicken
breasts

1 tablespoon dry sherry

4 spring onions, chopped

2 large carrots, thinly sliced

2.5 cm (1 inch) piece of fresh root ginger,
peeled and finely chopped

1 tablespoon oil

1–2 garlic cloves, thinly sliced

2 celery sticks, diagonally sliced

1 small green pepper, cored, deseeded and
sliced

1 small yellow pepper, cored, deseeded and
sliced

2 tablespoons light soy sauce

2 tablespoons lemon juice

grated rind of 2 lemons

½ teaspoon chilli powder

1 Cut the chicken into 7 cm (3 inch) strips.
Combine the sherry, spring onions, carrots
and ginger, add the chicken and toss well to
coat, then set aside for 15 minutes.

2 Heat the oil in a large nonstick frying pan
or wok. Add the sliced garlic, celery and green
and yellow peppers and stir-fry for 1 minute.
Add the chicken pieces and their marinade
and cook for 3 minutes more. Stir in the soy
sauce, the lemon juice and rind and the chilli

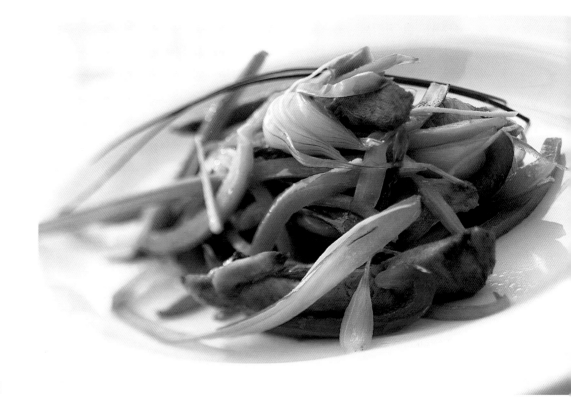

powder and cook the mixture for a further
1 minute. Divide between 4 warmed serving
plates, and serve immediately.

SERVES 4

Preparation time: **20 minutes, plus
marinating**

Cooking time: **5 minutes**

NUTRITION FACT – **Ginger** can be
bought fresh or dried. The fresh variety
does not keep for very long, and should
be wrapped in foil and stored in the
refrigerator. Dried ginger has a much
longer shelf life, but should be kept in
an airtight container to retain its
flavour. Ginger contains calcium,
magnesium, phosphorus and
potassium. It improves circulation and
prevents nausea.

carbohydrate 5 g / **protein** 22 g /
fat 6 g / **kJ** 698 / **kcal** 166

Green beef curry

300 g (10 oz) beef fillet, finely sliced

1 red onion, cut into thin wedges

1–2 tablespoons Thai green curry paste

125 g (4 oz) mangetout, thinly sliced
  lengthways

150 ml (¼ pint) water

small bunch of basil leaves

boiled rice, to serve (optional)

1 Preheat a nonstick wok or large frying pan. Dry-fry the beef for 2 minutes, then remove with a slotted spoon, leaving the juices in the pan.

2 Reheat the pan and stir-fry the onion for 1 minute until softened. Add the curry paste and stir-fry for another minute or so. Now add the mangetout and water. Return the meat to the pan and stir-fry for a further 5 minutes. When the beef has cooked, throw in the basil and stir-fry for 30 seconds. Serve immediately with boiled rice, if liked.

SERVES 4

Preparation time: **5 minutes**

Cooking time: **10 minutes**

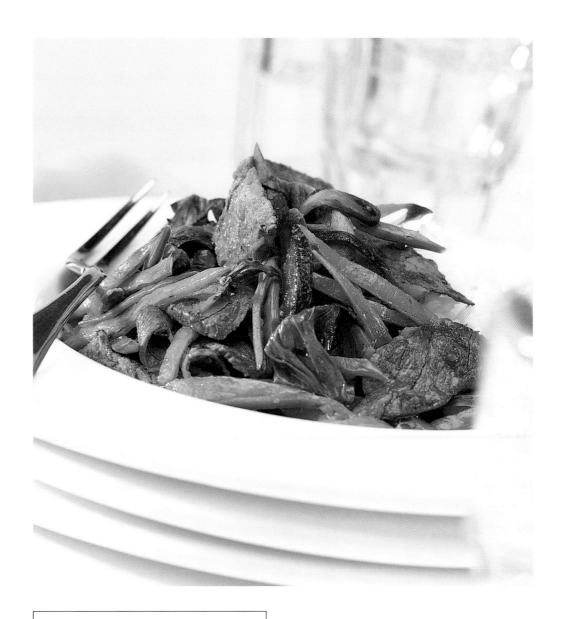

COOK'S TIP — Choose a lean cut of beef as it will contain less saturated fat. Trim the meat of all visible fat when you slice it.

carbohydrate 7 g / **protein** 17 g / **fat** 5 g / **kJ** 580 / **kcal** 139

Poached salmon steaks with hot basil sauce

1 large bunch of basil

4 celery sticks, chopped

1 carrot, chopped

1 small courgette, chopped

1 small onion, chopped

6 salmon steaks, about 125 g (4 oz) each

75 ml (3 fl oz) dry white wine

125 ml (4 fl oz) water

1 teaspoon lemon juice

15 g (½ oz) unsalted butter

salt and pepper

lemon slices, to serve

basil leaves, to garnish

1 Strip the leaves from half the basil and set aside. Spread all the chopped vegetables over the bottom of a large flameproof casserole dish with a lid, press the salmon steaks into the vegetables and cover them with the remaining basil. Pour over the wine and water and season with salt and pepper. Bring to the boil, cover and simmer for about 10 minutes. Transfer the salmon steaks to a warmed serving dish.

2 Bring the poaching liquid and vegetables back to the boil and simmer for 5 minutes.

Strain into a blender or food processor and add the uncooked basil. Blend to a purée and return to a saucepan. Bring the purée to the boil and reduce by half, until thickened. Remove the saucepan from the heat, add the lemon juice and stir in the butter. Pour the sauce over the salmon steaks and serve with lemon slices and garnished with basil leaves.

SERVES 6

Preparation time: **15 minutes**

Cooking time: **25 minutes**

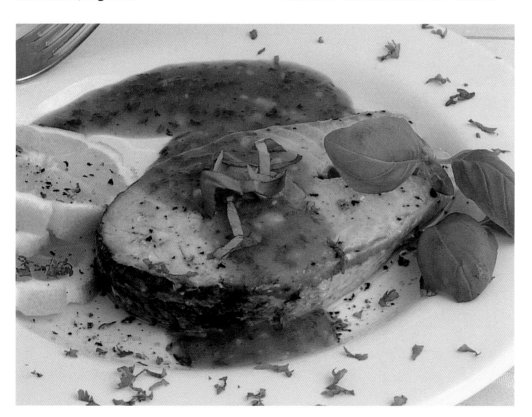

NUTRITION FACT — **Salmon** is a good source of vitamin D, which we need for the absorption of calcium. The major vitamin D source is the action of sunlight on the skin, and for most people vitamin D from the diet is unimportant. However, some people such as housebound elderly people, could suffer a deficiency if they do not get sufficient vitamin D from dietary sources.

carbohydrate 3 g / **protein** 24 g / **fat** 17 g / **kJ** 1130 / **kcal** 272

Grilled cod steaks with mint pesto

4 cod steaks, about 175 g (6 oz) each

olive oil, to baste

lemon juice

salt and pepper

lime wedges, to garnish

MINT PESTO

6 tablespoons chopped mint

1 tablespoon chopped parsley

1 garlic clove, chopped

1 tablespoon grated Parmesan cheese

1 tablespoon single cream

1 teaspoon balsamic vinegar

3 tablespoons extra virgin olive oil

1 Brush the cod steaks with oil and squeeze over a little lemon juice. Season with salt and pepper and cook under a preheated moderate grill for 3–4 minutes on each side until golden and cooked through.

2 Meanwhile, place all the ingredients for the pesto in a blender or food processor and blend until fairly smooth. Season with salt and pepper to taste and transfer to a bowl. Alternatively, pound the ingredients together with a mortar and pestle.

3 Serve the cod steaks topped with a spoonful of the pesto and garnish with the lime wedges.

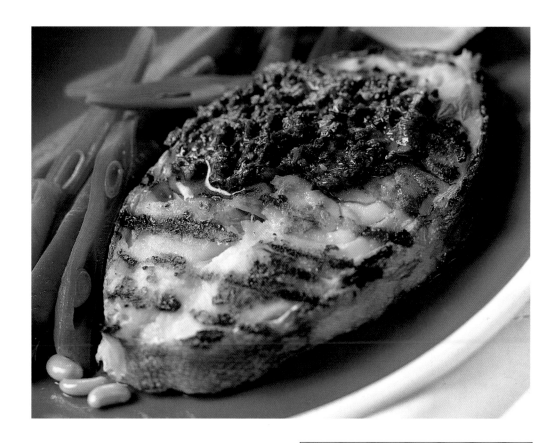

SERVES 4

Preparation time: **10 minutes**

Cooking time: **about 8 minutes**

NUTRITION FACT – Cod is rich in magnesium. This fragrant pesto is a particularly good partner for cod. Serve with a selection of steamed green vegetables drizzled with extra virgin olive oil and lime juice and garnished with sprigs of mint, if wished.

carbohydrate 1 g / **protein** 32 g / **fat** 12 g / **kJ** 1008 / **kcal** 240

Desserts

3-fruit compôte

2 ripe pears, peeled, cored and quartered
250 ml (8 fl oz) freshly squeezed orange
   juice
50 ml (2 fl oz) dark rum
½ cinnamon stick
175 g (6 oz) seedless black grapes, halved
½ firm honeydew melon, peeled, deseeded
   and cut into large chunks
ground cinnamon, to dust
dessert biscuits, to serve

1 Put the pears, orange juice, rum and
cinnamon stick into a large saucepan. Cover
and simmer for 5 minutes. Add the remaining
fruit and simmer for a further 5 minutes.

2 Remove from the heat and transfer to a
bowl. Chill overnight and remove the
cinnamon before serving. Decorate with a
dusting of ground cinnamon, if liked. Serve
with dessert biscuits.

SERVES 4
Preparation time: **5 minutes, plus chilling**
Cooking time: **10 minutes**

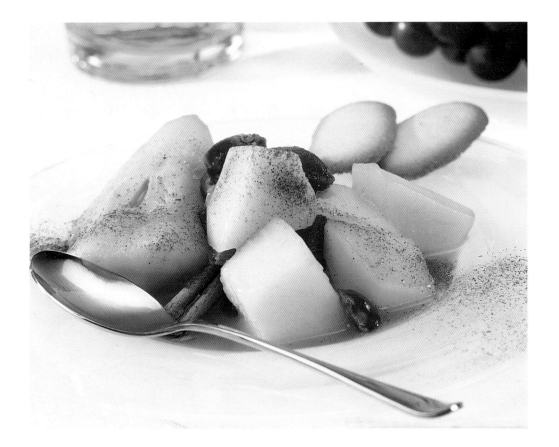

COOK'S TIP — If you like, use different
fruits in this recipe, such as apples,
blackberries, plums, raspberries,
blueberries or peaches.

carbohydrate 28 g / **protein** 1 g /
fat 0 g / **kJ** 593 / **kcal** 140

Fruit and nut crumble

175 g (6 oz) dried apricots
125 g (4 oz) dried pitted prunes
125 g (4 oz) dried figs
50 g (2 oz) dried apples
600 ml (1 pint) apple juice
100 g (3½ oz) wholemeal flour
50 g (2 oz) margarine
50 g (2 oz) muscovado or soft brown
   sugar, sifted
50 g (2 oz) hazelnuts, chopped
low-fat yogurt, to serve (optional)
rosemary sprigs, to garnish

SERVES 6

Preparation time: **15 minutes, plus soaking**
Cooking time: **35–50 minutes**
Oven temperature: **200°C (400°F),**
   Gas Mark 6

NUTRITION FACT – Dried fruit such as
apricots and **prunes** add to the iron
content of the diet. Absorption of iron
is aided by vitamin C, but inhibited by
a number of other factors, including
tea-drinking.

carbohydrate 67 g / **protein** 6 g /
fat 13 g / **kJ** 1663 / **kcal** 394

1 Place the dried fruits in a bowl with the
apple juice and leave overnight to soak.
Transfer to a saucepan and simmer for
10–15 minutes, until softened. Turn into
an ovenproof dish.

2 Sift the flour into a bowl and rub in the
margarine until the mixture resembles
breadcrumbs. Stir in the sugar, reserving a
little to serve, and the hazelnuts, then
sprinkle the crumble mixture over the fruit.

3 Bake in a preheated oven at 200°C
(400°F), Gas Mark 6, for 25–30 minutes.
Serve with low-fat yogurt, if liked, sprinkled
with the reserved sugar and garnished
with rosemary.

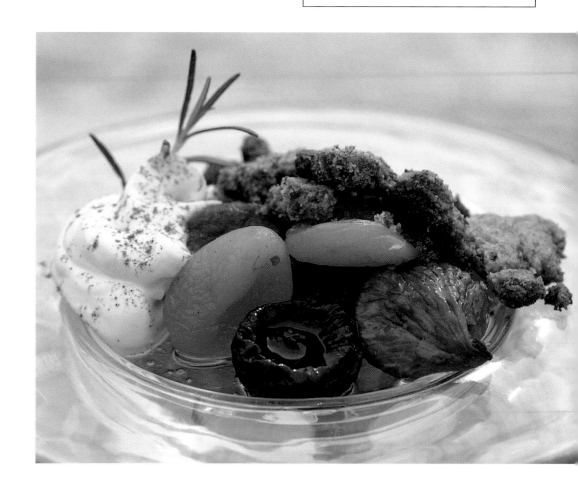

Wholemeal pear tart

PASTRY

100 g (3½ oz) plain flour, sifted

100 g (3½ oz) wholemeal plain flour

100 g (3½ oz) sunflower margarine

2–2½ tablespoons cold water

FILLING

2 tablespoons raspberry jam (optional)

2 teaspoons custard powder

½–1 tablespoon caster sugar

150 ml (¼ pint) skimmed milk

425 g (14 oz) canned pear halves in natural juice, drained

1 tablespoon clear honey, warmed, to glaze

redcurrants, to decorate

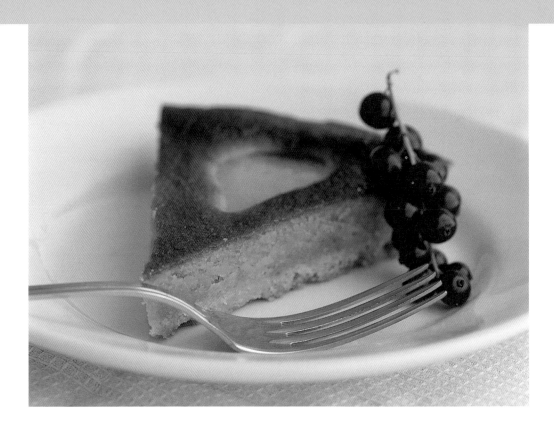

1 To make the pastry, place the flours in a mixing bowl. Rub in the margarine until the mixture resembles fine breadcrumbs. Add water, mix to make a firm dough and knead until smooth. Roll out two-thirds of the pastry to a circle large enough to line an 18 cm (7 in) greased flan ring, reserving the rest.

2 Trim the edges from the ring. Place in the refrigerator for 10–15 minutes to chill. Prick the base of the pastry case with a fork and bake blind in a preheated oven at 200°C (400°F), Gas Mark 6, for 10 minutes. Leave to cool, then spread the jam, if using, over the pastry base.

3 To make the custard filling, blend the custard powder and sugar with 1 tablespoon of the milk in a small bowl. Bring the rest of the milk to the boil in a small saucepan and pour it over the custard, stirring until thickened and smooth. Pour the custard into the flan and allow to set slightly. Arrange the pear halves around the edge of the pastry, rounded sides up.

4 Roll out the remaining pastry to fit the flan ring. Dampen the edge of the pastry base. Place the pastry top on the flan and press gently to seal the edges. Trim and flute the edges. Bake in the oven for 30–40 minutes.

5 Remove from the oven, take off the flan ring and brush the tart with warmed honey. Serve decorated with redcurrants.

SERVES 6

Preparation time: **30 minutes, plus chilling**

Cooking time: **40–50 minutes**

Oven temperature: **200°C (400°F), Gas Mark 6**

NUTRITION FACT – **Pears** are a source of vitamins B and C and they also contain potassium.

carbohydrate 44 g / **protein** 5 g / **fat** 14 g / **kJ** 1304 / **kcal** 311

Tropical fruit salad

2 kiwi fruit, peeled and sliced

1 starfruit, sliced

2 mangoes, peeled and cubed

1 small papaya, peeled and cubed

6 lychees, peeled

1 banana, sliced

shredded rind of 1 lime, to garnish

DRESSING

25 g (1 oz) sugar

100 ml (3½ fl oz) water

2 tablespoons lime juice

pulp and seeds of 2 passion fruit

SERVES 4–6

Preparation time: **15 minutes, plus chilling**

Cooking time: **7 minutes**

NUTRITION FACT – Kiwi fruit are quite high in vitamin C, about the same as oranges, weight for weight. Fruits have varying contents of vitamin C, with blackcurrants and guavas among the highest and plums and grapes among the lowest.

carbohydrate 38 g / **protein** 2 g / **fat** 1 g / **kJ** 675 / **kcal** 158

1 First make the dressing. Put the sugar and water in a saucepan and heat until the sugar has dissolved. Add the lime juice and simmer for 5 minutes. Remove from the heat and set aside to cool. When the dressing is cool, stir in the passion fruit pulp and seeds.

2 Gently mix all the prepared fruit in a large bowl. Pour the dressing over the fruit and chill for 15 minutes. Serve garnished with shreds of lime rind.

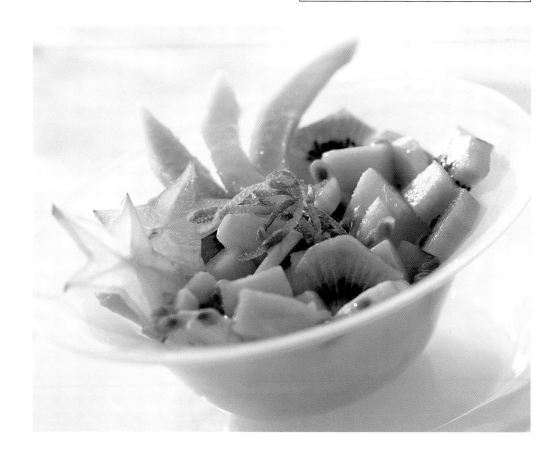

Yogurt with figs and passion fruit

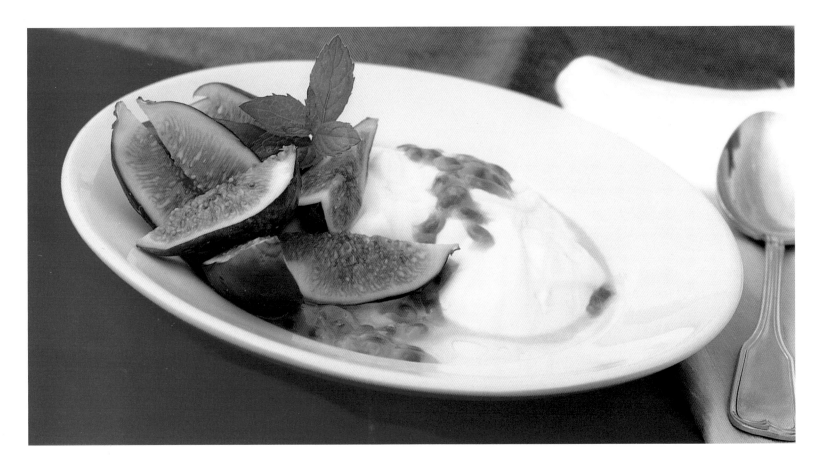

2 passion fruit
1 tablespoon clear honey
4 fresh figs
250 ml (8 fl oz) Greek yogurt
mint sprigs, to decorate

1 Cut the passion fruit in half, scoop out the seeds and mix with honey.

2 Cut each fig into 4 segments, peeling the fruit first if preferred. Serve the figs with the yogurt and the passion fruit mixture, and decorate with mint sprigs.

SERVES 4
Preparation time: **10 minutes**

NUTRITION FACT – **Figs** contain vitamins A, B and C. They also have digestive properties.

carbohydrate 9 g / **protein** 5 g / **fat** 6 g / **kJ** 442 / **kcal** 105

Lychee and apricot compôte

425 g (14 oz) canned lychees
175 g (6 oz) dried or Hunza apricots
2 large oranges
2 tablespoons pine nuts, toasted

1 Drain the lychees and make the liquid up to 300 ml (½ pint) with water. Put the apricots into a saucepan, pour over the liquid, cover and bring to the boil. Turn off the heat and leave to soak for 1 hour. Bring to the boil again, covered, simmer gently for 10 minutes and leave to cool. Turn into a glass bowl with the lychees.

2 Pare off thin strips of orange rind with a potato peeler and cut them into needle-fine shreds. Blanch in boiling water for 1 minute, then drain and dry on kitchen paper.

3 Peel the oranges with a serrated knife and cut into segments, removing all the pithy membranes. Add to the bowl and mix together gently.

4 Sprinkle the fruit with pine nuts and orange rind and serve chilled.

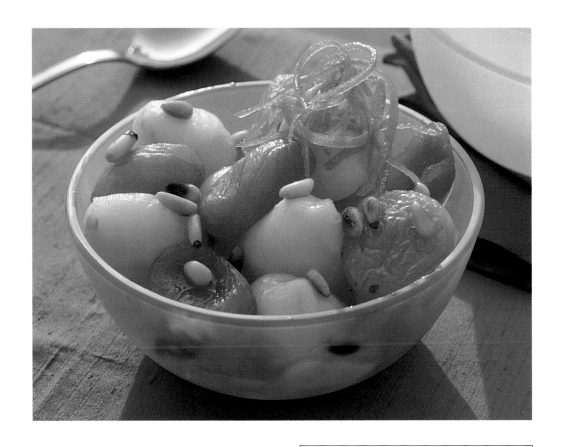

SERVES 6
Preparation time: **20 minutes, plus soaking and chilling**
Cooking time: **20 minutes**

FOOD FACT – Hunza are delicious baby apricots from the Hunza valley in northern India. They are much sweeter than ordinary dried apricots, so you may need to add a little lemon juice. Apricots contain powerful antioxidants.

carbohydrate 31 g / **protein** 3 g / **fat** 3 g / **kJ** 645 / **kcal** 152

Baked braeburns with lemon

4 large Braeburn apples

1 lemon cut into 4 segments

50 g (2 oz) light muscovado sugar

1 teaspoon cinnamon

low-fat fromage frais, to serve (optional)

1 Carefully remove the core from the middle of each apple. Using a small knife make the hole in the centre of each apple slightly larger. Put the lemon segments in a bowl and scatter the sugar and cinnamon over.

2 Once coated, push a lemon wedge into the centre of each apple. Arrange the apples in a small roasting tin lined with foil, then bake in a preheated oven, 180°C (350°F), Gas Mark 4, for 45 minutes. Serve with low-fat fromage frais, if liked.

SERVES 4

Preparation time: **10 minutes**

Cooking time: **45 minutes**

Oven temperature: **180°C (350°F), Gas Mark 4**

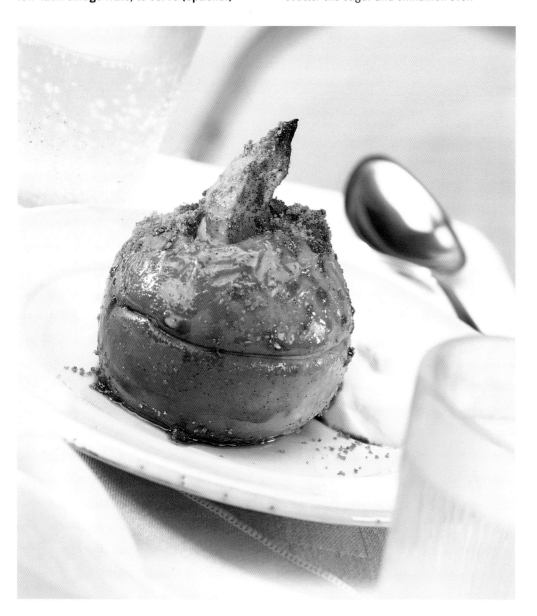

COOK'S TIP — If you cannot find Braeburn apples, use another variety instead, such as Cox's or Granny Smith's which will be just as good.

carbohydrate 31 g / **protein** 1 g / **fat** 0 g / **kJ** 515 / **kcal** 120

Hazelnut meringues with raspberries

2 egg whites
125 g (4 oz) icing sugar, sifted
50 g (2 oz) hazelnuts, finely chopped
TO SERVE
500 g (1 lb) raspberries
125 ml (4 fl oz) whipping cream, whipped
strawberry or mint leaves, to decorate
icing sugar, to dust (optional)

1 Whisk the egg whites until stiff and dry. Add the icing sugar a tablespoon at a time and continue to whisk until very thick.

2 Carefully fold in the hazelnuts. Pipe the meringue mixture on to a nonstick baking sheet in swirls.

3 Bake in a preheated oven at 180°C (350°F), Gas Mark 4, for 15–20 minutes. Leave to cool slightly, then transfer to a wire rack to cool.

4 Serve the meringues with the raspberries and whipping cream, decorate with the strawberry or mint leaves and dust with icing sugar, if liked.

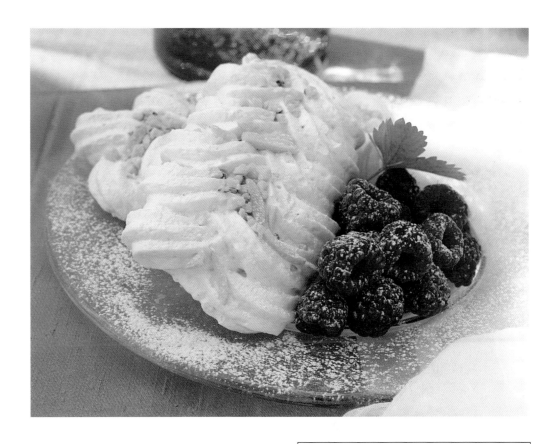

SERVES 6
Preparation time: **15 minutes**
Cooking time: **15–20 minutes**
Oven temperature: **180°C (350°F),**
  Gas Mark 4

NUTRITION FACT — There is very little nutritional difference between white and brown sugars. **Brown sugar** contains small traces of some minerals, but its main function in the diet, as with all sugars, is to add a pleasant sweetness to food.

carbohydrate 27 g / **protein** 4 g / **fat** 14 g / **kJ** 1000 / **kcal** 239

Detoxifying your body

Thanks to modern living, our bodies are under constant assault from pollution, stress, bad posture, sedentary jobs and bad eating habits. Over time, the effects build up and may manifest in many forms, from headaches and digestive problems to more serious conditions, such as ulcers, cancer and heart disease. Following a detox programme enables our bodies to repair, cleanse and restore balance to the entire system.

Why detox?

These days, we all live at a pace that would have seemed unbelievable, and indeed impossible, to our grandparents. We have demanding jobs – and often have to travel long distances to get to them – we keep later and longer hours, we run homes, bring up children and usually try to fit in hectic social lives, too. It's no surprise then that we become tired and run down, never feeling on top of things. And because time is the one thing most of us don't have enough of, we cut corners. We eat convenience or junk food, we don't get enough sleep, we can't fit in exercise and we often drink too much or smoke as a quick-fix way to relax. Although many of us probably recognize that this is no way to live, we may not be aware of the very real dangers this lifestyle presents.

Body renewal

Our bodies are extremely complex organisms in a state of constant growth and renewal on a cellular level. They get rid of old, damaged and dead cells and replace them with new ones on a daily basis. There is also a system of priorities for the metabolism – for instance, if we fall ill, our body concentrates its energies on repelling invading infections and the healing process. Similarly, when we pour toxins into our bodies, it treats these as a matter of urgency and works on processing them to render them harmless. What this means, however, is that there is less energy for the everyday processes of cleansing, healing and renewal. Over time, the body can't keep up the pace, the strain shows on the overworked liver and kidneys and the body's performance slows down.

If consuming toxins is inherently a bad thing, then a detoxification diet (see page 98) must by implication be a good thing. It allows two things happen. First, we stop overloading the body with harmful substances and, secondly, we give it plenty of

the right nutrients to actually speed up the elimination of old toxins and promote cell renewal. And, as the cells are rejuvenated, you become healthier and you look and feel younger! A tall order from just a change of diet? Far from it. It is universally accepted that high-fat, processed, salty foods are linked to heart disease and that many other serious conditions have also been linked to diet; the World Health Organization has found that around 85 per cent of adult cancers are avoidable and of these around half are related to dietary deficiencies. It isn't that we don't eat enough – most people in the developed world eat too much. But the food we tend to eat has lost much of its nutritional value through processing and is packed full of fat, sugar and nutritionally worthless preservatives, colourings and flavourings instead.

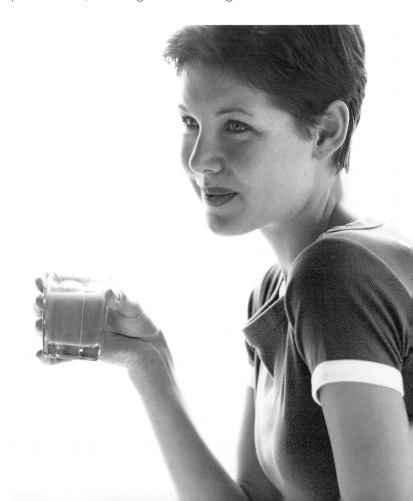

Are you intoxicated?

The person who is not carrying environmental toxins in their blood in the 21st century is living some self-sufficient rural idyll that most of us could only dream of and the rest of us would find numbingly boring. Modern urban life is toxic by definition. But is your body carrying many more toxins than it is built to handle? There are intrusive and expensive tests to find out, but running through the following questions on your diet and environment will give you a fair idea. You can then decide whether a detox diet is worth it. Simply put a tick or cross beside each.

If you have more than **15 ticks**, you need to reduce your exposure to and consumption of toxins with a detox diet. **Fewer than 10** and you are doing the best you can in the polluted world none of us can escape.

DIET

Do you regularly consume:
- ☑ Sugary snacks?
- ☑ Tea and coffee?
- ☐ Alcohol?
- ☑ Canned food?
- ☐ Fried food?
- ☐ Smoked or cured meat or fish?
- ☑ Fast food?
- ☑ Tap water?
- ☐ Fluoridated water?
- ☐ Water supplied through lead pipes?
- ☑ Commercially produced (non-organic) fruit, vegetables and meat?

ENVIRONMENT

Do you:
- ☐ Regularly smoke or work with smokers?
- ☐ Regularly take prescription drugs or painkillers?
- ☐ Have amalgam fillings?
- ☑ Use aerosol sprays?
- ☑ Use household cleaners?
- ☐ Exercise near busy roads?
- ☑ Drive in heavy traffic?
- ☐ Work with a VDU screen?
- ☐ Spend a lot of time in the sun?
- ☐ Take the Pill or hormone replacement therapy?
- ☐ Live near electricity pylons or a power station?

Super scavengers

Vitamins A, C and E are vital for health. These vitamins, together with the mineral selenium, are known as antioxidants (see page 28). They can protect us not only against minor infections but also against serious degenerative diseases such as cancer and heart disease, as well as conditions that come with premature ageing. They work by scavenging for free radicals. Free radicals are electrochemically unbalanced molecules, generated within our bodies by, among other things, pollution, cigarettes, pesticides, drugs, certain foods, overeating and stress. Free radical molecules are responsible, on a cellular level, for many of the things that go wrong with the body. They react with other, healthy molecules to make them unstable, too, and a chain reaction can start up, which leads to a process of cellular destruction and disease.

We clearly need as many antioxidants as we can get, and one of the best sources is in fresh fruit and vegetables. As many nutrients are destroyed by cooking, raw fresh produce is so much more effective – and is consequently at the core of any detox plan.

The detox process

Your body knows how to cleanse and restore itself – during detoxification, you are simply giving it a helping hand. For the deepest and swiftest detoxification, you should not only stop adding new toxins but help it in the cleansing process. The liver and kidneys, the main organs of detoxification, will do most of the work: the liver renders harmless the toxins that enter our body or eliminates them altogether, while the kidneys filter out toxins in the blood and eliminate them in the urine.

During a detox programme (see pages 98–101), there are no new toxins to be processed, giving these important organs the opportunity to work on the store of old ones. There is time to cleanse and repair long-standing damage and the body starts straight away. It rids itself of tissues that are diseased, damaged or dead, and the building up of new healthy cells speeds up.

Detoxification involves not only diet. Various body and skin treatments help the general detox process, including hydrotherapy (see page 170), facial exfoliation (see page 118), skin brushing (see page 168) and manual lymphatic drainage (MLD) massage (see page 106). Deep breathing exercises (see page 240) will help you to expel toxins more readily, too, by improving your circulation, enhancing lymph flow and massaging the liver in a way that stimulates its detox mechanisms. In addition, a detox programme aims to detox not just the body but to detox the mind as well. This may seem a rather strange idea – after all, it is the body that tries to digest the wrong food, breathes in polluted air or suffers the side-effects of antibiotics. However, stress can be regarded as the mind's toxin; it not only has the effect of making us anxious, depressed or insomniac, it also releases toxins into the body (see page 230). There are various effective therapies and techniques for combating stress and finding relaxation (see Chapter 6).

When to detox

The first few days of a detox diet can be an endurance test. You usually feel tired and get withdrawal symptoms from forsaken foods. These include muscle pains, mood swings, humdinger headaches and skin problems (see Side-effects, below). But remind yourself that these are positive signs of trapped toxins being released, and persevere: within a relatively short time you will feel re-energized and your skin will be glowing.

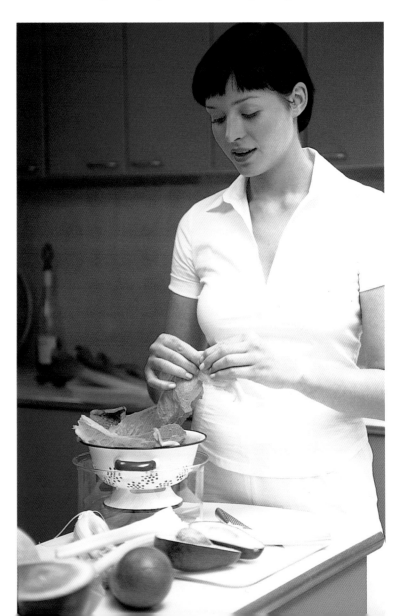

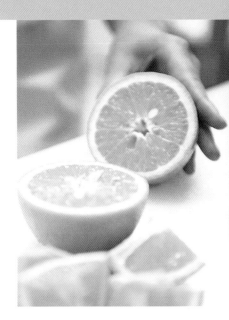

A detox programme is actually much easier than you think, but help yourself by choosing the right time to detox. Spring and summer are the ideal seasons to go on a detox diet: fresh, locally grown fruit and vegetables are in better supply and one feels less need to eat for comfort or warmth. Find a time when you are not going to be very busy or stressed or having a particularly social time – with all the temptations of food and drink that go with it! If you follow a juice fast (see page 40), try to fit the juice fast itself into a long weekend when you can find some quiet time on your own or with a friend who wants to do it with you. If you work, start the diet on a Friday so you are not wilting over the office desk during the enervating early days. (See Weekend home health spa, page 102.)

Detox 'nos'

You will have to cut out certain things in order for the detoxification process to work – in particular smoking, alcohol, over-the-counter drugs (but check with your doctor about prescribed drugs) and caffeine. After the first few days, when you may have withdrawal symptoms, you will feel better, look better and have much more energy. It really is worth it!

Side-effects

As soon as you start, some side-effects are inevitable as your body begins to clear itself of toxins. These are nothing to worry about – in fact, they are a sign that the detox is working. The following common side-effects are only temporary and they will be replaced by a feeling of general wellbeing by the end of the week.

Furry tongue This happens to everyone. Clean your teeth frequently and scrape your tongue with the toothbrush a few times.

Headache This is common if there was a lot of caffeine, chocolate, alcohol or sugar in your diet. Don't take any medication. Drink extra fluids, rest and dab some lavender essential oil (see Aromatherapy, page 278) on to your temples.

Irritability Try to limit outside stress where possible. Practise relaxation or meditation (see pages 242 and 244). Exercise can help, as does rest if tiredness is the cause.

Excessive elimination Great! It's not really excessive even having to urinate every half hour at times. This is just the toxins coming out and is particularly likely if you've had water retention. Loose bowels are also possible as with any change of diet and so, paradoxically, is constipation. These problems usually normalize within a few days.

Flu and cold symptoms Runny nose and eyes, aches and pains are all quite common and only temporary.

Skin eruptions Many toxins are eliminated through the skin, so you may get spots on the face or body. Baths or showers once or twice daily are important to wash the toxins away. The skin will clear by the end of the week, by which time it is usually glowing with health.

Tiredness You may feel tired, particularly if you've been under stress. Rest if you need to – higher energy levels will soon replace fatigue.

SEE ALSO:

→ Top foods for health, page 28

→ Exfoliation, page 118

→ Skin brushing, page 168

→ Hydrotherapy, page 170

→ Living with stress, page 230

→ Improve your breathing, page 240

→ Relaxation, page 242

→ Manual lymphatic drainage, page 106

→ Meditation, page 244

→ Aromatherapy, page 278

Everyday toxins

Modern life is necessarily toxic to some extent. Everyday we face a multitude of pollutants and chemicals in the air that we breathe and in the food and water we consume. While there are some everyday toxins you can do little about, there are certain choices you can make to limit your exposure to others. For example, avoid exercising near busy roads and wear a mask if cycling in heavy traffic to avoid inhaling exhaust fumes; choose organic foods; and replace chemical aerosols and household cleaning agents with natural products wherever possible.

Smoking

Carbon monoxide, arsenic, ammonia, formaldehyde, DDT and nitric acid are some of the more than 4000 chemicals found in cigarette smoke; there are just as many in cigar smoke. Inhaled carbon monoxide replaces the oxygen in the blood that is required by all the body's organs to function properly. Thus smoking increases the risk of serious chronic health problems, including heart disease, lung and respiratory diseases and certain cancers. The reduced amount of oxygen reaching the skin accelerates ageing, resulting in dull, sallow-looking skin and wrinkles. Smoking also robs the body of vital nutrients, in particular the B vitamins and vitamin C. Cigarette smoke can be just as dangerous for non-smokers so even if you are a non-smoker try and avoid smoky atmospheres.

If you want to give up smoking, seek advice from your doctor or a pharmacist on any of the treatments that might help. Enlist the help of friends and family and avoid situations in which you might be tempted to smoke. It's never too late to stop – even after many years of smoking, much of the damage done to the body can be reversed.

Acupuncture can been used to treat some people with addictions such as smoking and alcohol. Hypnotherapy is another possibility.

Caffeine

Caffeine is a stimulant found in coffee, tea, cola drinks and chocolate. It may provide a temporary lift, but should be taken with care. It is addictive, it stimulates the heart and central nervous system and often causes headaches, sleeping problems, anxiety and nervousness. Caffeine raises blood pressure and blood sugar levels, and irritates the gut. It also directly suppresses the immune system and is known to interfere with the body's absorption of many nutrients, including vitamin B1, biotin, potassium, zinc, calcium and iron.

Decaffeinated brands of both tea and coffee are now widely available, as are herb and fruit teas, chicory and dandelion coffee. Green tea (see page 44) is a good substitute for ordinary tea, while mineral water (see page 96) helps clear toxins from the body.

Alcohol

Alcohol is a sedative hypnotic drug that depresses the central nervous system. Taken in moderation, it is enjoyable and relatively harmless, but taken too often or to excess, it drastically reduces energy levels, suppresses the body's immune system and can overtax the liver's normal process of detoxification.

Alcohol inhibits the absorption of all nutrients in the body, especially vitamins B1 and B2. It interferes with a group of enzymes crucial to the body's detoxification process, acting as a 'master toxin', potentiating the effects of other toxins. Alcohol also contributes to fluctuations in blood sugar levels, which can result in depression, anxiety and nervousness. It is a diuretic, dehydrating skin as well as other tissues, and it increases the risk of developing food sensitivities.

Research suggests that a small amount – no more than two or three glasses per week – of red wine, which contains antioxidants, is beneficial for overall good health, particularly for the heart.

Top tips for a healthy liver and lymph

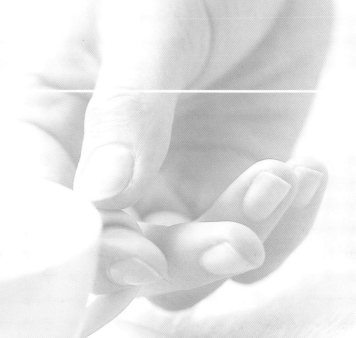

- Avoid any foods of which you suspect you may be intolerant. They will produce toxins in the gut that cause stress to the detoxification mechanisms.
- Chew your food well to help release the enzymes that aid digestion.
- Consume plenty of foods containing folate, flavonoids, magnesium, iron, sulphate and selenium and B vitamins 2, 3, 6 and 12 (see page 25), since toxicity in the body can be caused by deficiency of the nutrients that the liver needs for detoxification as much as by exposure to toxins.
- Cut down on stimulants such as tea and coffee, and depressants such as alcohol.
- Eat foods rich in antioxidants (see page 28), which aid the natural detox mechanisms.
- Take a daily dose of echinacea, milk thistle or dandelion root (as tablets, tincture or teas) – all herbs with a long-established reputation as blood cleansers and skin tonics.

- Don't use antibiotics or antacids unless absolutely necessary. Antibiotics can destroy the useful bacteria in the gut that eliminate toxins; antacids decrease the natural acidity that is necessary for complete digestion.
- Take a dose of activated charcoal twice a week. This is a medicinal form of charcoal with the capacity to absorb whatever molecules it encounters, including toxins. Don't take it with food or medicines though, or it will absorb them.

Processed foods

Some of the many colourings, flavourings and preservatives found in highly processed foods can produce food intolerances (see page 36), asthmatic attacks, skin rashes and swelling, especially in children.

Familiarize yourself with the ingredients typically found on food labels if you are concerned about the chemicals you are consuming. But remember that many additives are added in only minute quantities and not all E-numbered additives are bad for you (on the contrary some of the more widely used preservatives and antioxidants are essential).

More home cooking with fresh ingredients will mean you are more likely to know what is in the food that you eat. Organic foods are increasingly popular because of their lack of chemicals – organic fresh produce does not have the pesticide residues found in conventionally grown fruits and vegetables, which should always be washed or peeled before eating.

SEE ALSO:

→ A balanced diet, page 14

→ Fats, page 22

→ Vitamins, page 24

→ Minerals, page 26

→ Food allergies and intolerances, page 36

→ Organic foods, page 38

→ Making juices, page 40

→ Herbal teas, page 44

→ Improve your complexion, page 122

→ Sun safety, page 154

→ Aromatherapy, page 278

Water

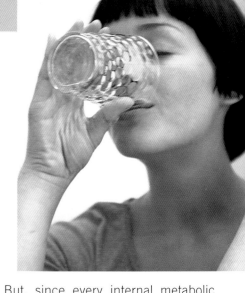

In the course of a normal day, without breaking sweat, the average body loses at least 1.5 litres (2½ pints) of water through the skin, lungs, gut and kidneys. It has to do this to eliminate toxins – among them those that cause dark bags under the eyes and those that congregate under the skin to erupt as spots. At the same time as it is expelling water, the body also needs to produce about 350 ml (12 fl oz) of water to burn glucose for energy.

The amount of water we use and lose obviously varies from one person to another, according to their size and level of activity. But, since every internal metabolic reaction relies on water, the average person needs to take in at least 1.8 litres (3 pints) of water a day to function optimally.

Few people drink anything like that quantity. It may seem as if you do, but social custom dictates that a lot of liquid is drunk as coffee, tea, beer, coke and saccharine-sweetened sodas. All are diuretics, so much of the liquid you take in enters the sewerage system within an hour or two of putting down your cup. It does not have time to hydrate brain cells, let alone be absorbed by the dermis (just below the top layer of skin), which comes low down the list in the body's order of priorities. Consequently, most people, without knowing it, are chronically dehydrated. The effects, while hardly life-threatening, can greatly impinge on everyday activity. Fatigue, headaches, indigestion and joint pain are the most common symptoms of dehydration, though we usually attribute them to other causes.

How thirsty is your body?

Whether you are detoxing or not, you should drink about 1.8 litres (3 pints) of filtered or bottled water every day, taken in small amounts regularly throughout the day. Don't include drinks made with water such as tea and coffee as part of the ideal daily water intake. These, and other drinks, require filtration by the kidneys, whereas pure water does not.

This average of about 1.8 litres (3 pints) is required by your body on a day of normal activity in cool weather. When the sun is out and you are digging the garden or jogging, you can add half as much again.

Don't forget that you can eat water, too. Most fruit and vegetables consist of about 90 per cent water, and four pieces of fruit and four servings of vegetables – just over 1 kg (2 lb) in weight – can provide 1 litre (1¾ pints) of water.

Although it is important to drink enough water, don't drink too much with meals. This has the effect of forcing food down rapidly, causing indigestion, and dilutes the digestive juices, making them less effective.

Bottled or tap water?

Fears about the quality of the water that repeatedly negotiates the sewerage network before spurting out of our domestic taps have fuelled a boom in sales of the bottled variety.

In principle, there is good reason to swap tap water for bottled. Hundreds of chemical contaminants have been identified in tap water, the most common being nitrates, lead, aluminium and pesticides. But bottled water is not always the pure and simple substance it sounds.

Rehydrating your body

Water is the quickest and purest way of flushing toxins out of your system, and keeping your body in top condition. Drinking more water results in:

- Improved skin and hair condition
- Healthier body systems, for example the circulatory, urinary, and digestive systems
- Increased energy levels and vitality
- Increased concentration and stamina
- Less susceptibility to stress, anxiety and exhaustion
- Slowing down of the signs of ageing, thanks to stimulation of the production of growth hormone from the brain's pituitary gland
- Reduced water retention and puffiness
- More effective fat-burning
- More powerful and flexible muscles

Bottled water can be classified as table water, spring water or natural mineral water. Only the last is guaranteed to be from an unpolluted underground source; it is untreated and contains naturally occurring minerals, which have passed into the water as it flows through various layers of earth and rock to wells or springs, and which should be listed on the label. 'Spring water' is usually subterranean, too, but it does not have to be bottled on the spot and might well be treated to remove bacteria. 'Table water' is the least well defined and could be a mixture of water from many sources, including tap water. However, it has usually been purified and often has minerals added. Sparkling waters are carbonated with naturally occurring carbon dioxide.

But don't think of mineral water as a liquid nutritional supplement. Spring or tap water is often artificially carbonated, a process that can cause carbon molecules to bind to minerals in the body and rob it of nutrients. Even the mineral content of true mineral water is small and not always a healthy balance. If the water is high in sodium, for example, it will also have a mild dehydrating effect. On the analysis label, look for a high calcium-to-sodium ratio. If you buy bottled water, opt for glass, as chemicals from plastic bottles left in the sunlight can often leak into the water.

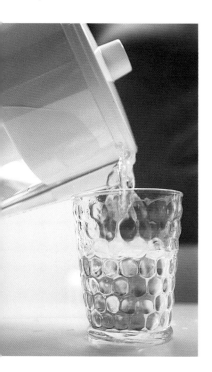

Filtering water

Filtering tap water is another increasingly popular option and results in clearer-looking and fresher-tasting water. Most jug filters, which contain activated carbon and ion-exchange resins, remove metals, chlorine and water hardness. But filtration also removes some of the naturally occurring minerals, such as calcium, along with the impurities. Filters also remove the chlorine put in tap water to destroy bacteria, so you should not keep the water standing in the jug for more than a day, or be sure to refrigerate it. Change the filter regularly or the harmful residues caught inside the filter can start to leach back into the jug.

A permanent filter can be plumbed under the kitchen tap to remove heavy metals, chemicals and bacteria. A more expensive option – but one that guarantees the purest water – is reverse osmosis, whereby water is passed under pressure through a porous membrane to separate the water from the other elements it contains.

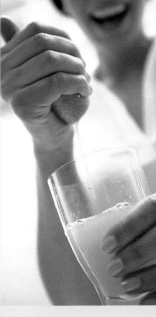

7-stage detox diet

Unlike most detox diets, which set down exact time limits within a strict plan, this one can be adapted to last anything from one to four weeks. The questionnaire on page 91 will help you assess your level of need; the more profound your problem, the longer your diet should be. The plan is split into seven stages. If you are initially trying out just a week-long detox, each stage will last one day, while in a two-week regime each stage will last two days and so on. Obviously, the longer the plan the greater the effect. It is important to follow the plan in the order given. After the liquids-only stage (Stage 1) you must come back to food slowly or you will overload the digestive system, undo all you have achieved and even feel quite unwell.

The 7 stages are:

1. **Stage 1** Liquids only
2. **Stage 2** Liquid and fruit only
3. **Stage 3** Add raw vegetables
4. **Stage 4** Add cooked vegetables and brown rice
5. **Stage 5** Add beans, lentils, nuts and seeds
6. **Stage 6** Add grains and live yogurt
7. **Stage 7** Add fish

CAUTION: This diet is designed for a normal, healthy adult and should not be undertaken without prior consultation with a doctor by anyone who is pregnant, on long-term prescription drugs or has dietary restrictions.

Stage 1 Liquids only

Traditionally, this would be just water, which is the quickest and purest means of flushing out the system (see page 96). But adding a squeeze of fresh lemon to warm water helps to neutralize acidity and stimulate the bowels.

If you find this too restricting, there are other liquids that have supplementary benefits. For example:

- **Freshly made fruit and vegetable juices** (see pages 40–3) are packed with the nutrients, often destroyed in processing and cooking, that help cleanse and regenerate the entire system. Choose the fruits that have special detox powers (see **Stage 2**, below). Using a juicer will not only broaden your choices and maximize the nutritional value of the juices, but leave behind a pulp that you can use as an instant face pack (see page 120).
- **Herbal or spice teas** (see page 44) are another option. Not only do they ease the tedium of the liquid-only stage but they can also act as useful detoxifiers or circulatory stimulants. For herbal teas, choose from ginger, dandelion, fennel or yarrow (but unsweetened – not even with honey).
- **The final option is broth**, ideally made from vegetables (see box, opposite). If you decide to follow the detox diet for four weeks, then you can base it on fresh meat or fish stock.

Many people worry about fasting, thinking that if you miss a meal, you'll faint or fade away. On the contrary – you will feel more energetic, not less. Some people, however, should not fast. They include pregnant or breastfeeding women, children, the frail and elderly, anyone with diabetes, TB, advanced heart disease, kidney dysfunction, or any degenerative disease, and anyone who is underweight. Everyone should, in any case, have a check-up with their doctor first before undertaking a detox programme that lasts for longer than a week.

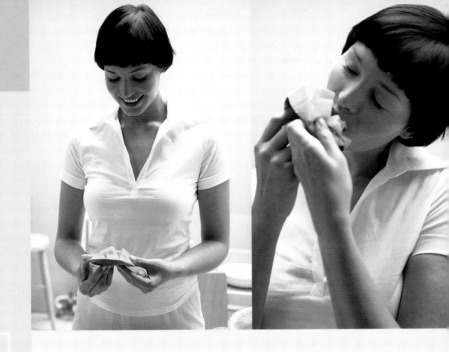

Vegetable broth

Freshly made each day, vegetable broth makes a cleansing and alkalizing hot drink, supplying vitamins, minerals and trace elements. As always, organic produce is best, but if this is not available make sure you clean the vegetables particularly well.

2 large potatoes

2 carrots

4 celery sticks, including leaves

2 beetroots (uncooked), including leaves

at least two other vegetables, one of them green, such as cabbage, turnips, spinach, spring greens, parsnips, sweet potatoes, leeks, onion

flavourings – no salt but fresh herbs and spices, such as parsley, rosemary, sage, root ginger, chillies (the last two make it quite hot)

1.8 litres (3 pints) filtered water

Wash all the ingredients thoroughly, but don't peel and keep any leaves. Put the water into a large pan. Chop the vegetables roughly and add immediately so that there is no time for them to be oxidized by exposure to the air. Bring to the boil, cover and simmer for 45 minutes. Remove from the heat and stand for 15 minutes more. Strain the liquid and discard the vegetables.

Stage 2 Liquid and fruit only

Although they often taste acidic, fruits are generally very alkaline foods so they help neutralize the acidic waste that is produced when you begin to detoxify. With their high fibre content, fruits are also good laxatives and will help shift some of the estimated 3–4 kg (6½–9 lb) of decayed material in the intestines. As with vegetables (Stage 3), buy organic if you can or you will only be replacing some of the toxins you are eliminating with pesticide residues.

The following fruits all have helpful detox properties:

- **Apples** contain a lot of pectin, which helps to remove toxins, and tartaric acid, which aids digestion.
- **Pineapple** contains the enzyme bromelin, which helps to produce acids that destroy bad bacteria in the gut, encourage the growth of 'good' bacteria that are important for digestion, and support tissue repair.
- **Mango** also contains bromelin, and an enzyme called papain, which helps to break down protein wastes.
- **Grapes** help to counter the production of mucus, which can clog up tissues; and cleanse the liver and kidneys. Their high fructose content also provides instant energy.
- **Watermelon** is a diuretic, and therefore speeds the passage of fluids carrying toxins through the system.

Stage 3 Add raw vegetables

Include bean sprouts (best grown yourself), as sprouting increases the nutritional content of seeds five-fold. Use raw garlic, which is an excellent blood cleanser – but at your discretion!

Vegetables share many of the properties of fruit, and some of the ones that can be eaten in salads have particular detox powers:

- **Fennel** helps to improve digestion in general and also prevents flatulence.
- **Watercress** contains betacarotene and sulphur, both of which are liver tonics.
- **Dandelion leaves** are a liver and kidney tonic and also act as a diuretic.
- **Parsley** is a mild diuretic and contains zinc and trace minerals that aid liver function.

Top detox foods

- **Apples**
- **Beetroot**
- **Brown short-grain rice**
- **Cayenne pepper**
- **Dandelion leaves**
- **Fennel**
- **Garlic**
- **Ginger**
- **Globe artichoke**
- **Grapes**
- **Jerusalem artichoke**
- **Leafy green vegetables**
- **Leeks**

- **Mango**
- **Onions**
- **Parsley**
- **Pineapple**
- **Watercress**
- **Watermelon**

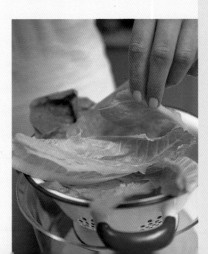

Stage 4 Add cooked vegetables and brown rice

Cook the vegetables with as little water and for as short a time as possible to retain their maximum nutritious value. Steaming is the best method, followed by stir-frying.

Cruciferous vegetables (leafy green vegetables) are particularly good for an overtaxed liver. The rice should always be brown short-grain as this kind is by far the most absorbent; it soaks up toxins from the gut and is the most easily digested and contains the most fibre.

Among the spices you can cook with include cayenne pepper and ginger, both of which stimulate digestion and encourage the elimination of toxins through the skin.

Vegetables normally eaten cooked that have detox properties include the following:

- **Leeks**, onions and garlic contain sulphur compounds that bind to and speed the elimination of toxic metals.
- **Globe artichoke** stimulates the liver's production of bile, which speeds up digestion.
- **Jerusalem artichoke** contains inulin, which aids the growth of beneficial bacteria in the gut. But beware of their deserved reputation for flatulence!
- **Beetroot** is an acidic (as opposed to acid-forming) food, which stimulates the production of enzymes that aid digestion in the stomach.

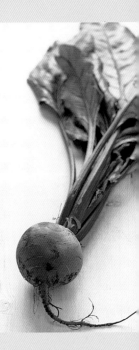

Stage 5 Add beans, lentils, nuts and seeds

Beans and lentils are a good source of protein but should not be eaten with rice at this stage since mixing starch and protein can slow digestion. Try to leave four hours between the consumption of the two food types.

Nuts should be eaten raw and unsalted. Like seeds, they provide useful calories in the form of essential fatty acids (EFAs), which are needed by all the cells in the body but which it cannot manufacture. EFAs also stimulate the flow of bile, which speeds up digestion. Sesame, sunflower and linseeds are all rich sources.

Stage 6 Add grains and live yogurt

The yogurt should be goat's or sheep's, which are easier to digest than live cow's yogurt but have the same beneficial action on the gut.

The grains should always be wholegrains, which provide fibre to help move wastes through the intestines and trace minerals useful for liver function. Choose from rye, buckwheat, barley or oats – anything but wheat. All help to deliver a slow and steady supply of glucose into the blood, enabling the liver to build up a supply of glycogen, which it needs to carry out its detox functions effectively as well as to deliver sugar into the blood for emergency energy.

Stage 7 Add fish

Any fresh fish will do but your skin will benefit from the essential fatty acids (EFAs) in oily, cold-water fish. By this stage, you should begin to feel more relaxed and not in a hurry to eat everything you have been missing.

Ideally, introduce excluded food types with at least a day between each. By this stage you should be more in tune with your body, which will help you to decide what and when. Add dairy products (cheese, cream, milk) and meat gradually, as they are high in saturated fats, which slow down digestion. Add wheat last. If you reintroduce these complex foods too quickly, you increase the chances of digestive problems.

Food intolerances

A growing range of ailments including skin problems, digestive disorders, depression and excess weight are now linked to food intolerances (see page 36). During a detox diet, you may identify a food intolerance. Because a particular food has been removed, long-term problems, such as headache or eczema, may disappear. Watch carefully for any reappearance as you return more foods to your diet. If the symptoms recur, you should be able to pinpoint the intolerance and adapt your diet.

SEE ALSO:

→ Antioxidant foods, page 28

→ Top foods for health, page 28

→ Food intolerances, page 36

→ Making juices, page 40

→ Herbal teas, page 44

→ Water, page 96

→ Detoxing weekend home health spa, page 102

Weekend home health spa

Does the idea of having a relaxing, pampered weekend at home – a couple of days where *you* come first – appeal to you? The Weekend Home Health Spa programme occupies an entire weekend. It is deeply cleansing and restorative for body and mind. This is the programme for you if you feel you have a poor diet of rich or junk foods or too much alcohol, or if you are continually battling against a polluted smoky atmosphere. It is also very helpful if you have decided to stop smoking; you will feel so purified by the end of the weekend, you may be very reluctant to spoil it all with a cigarette.

The first thing you need to do is make the necessary time for yourself. Choose a weekend that will be just for you, and don't make any other arrangements. Because this weekend's cleansing diet depends on fresh, preferably organic, fruit and vegetables, buy these on Thursday or Friday so that they are at their best. Keep them in the refrigerator until you need them. A skin brush and Moor mud should be available from your local chemist or health shop. Don't forget to book your lymph massage session if you are going to a professional therapist, and the sauna and steam rooms for Sunday, if you need to do this in advance.

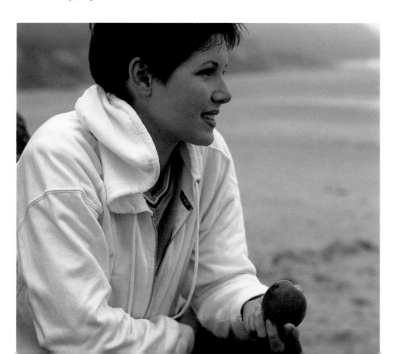

Weekend Schedule

Friday
7.00 pm
Evening meal
8.00 pm
Visualization
9.00 pm
Moor mud treatment
10.00 pm
Bed

Saturday
8.00 am
Juice: juice of a lemon squeezed into hot water
9.00 am
Skin brushing; herbal tea or water
9.30 am
Hydrotherapy
10.30 am
Juice: apple and carrot juice
11.00 am
Pilates
12.00 pm
Juice: tomato juice
2.00 pm
Herbal tea or water
3.00 pm
Manual lymphatic drainage

4.00 pm
Juice: raspberry and peach juice
5.00 pm
Herbal tea or water
6.00 pm
Visualization
6.30 pm
Juice: apple and carrot juice
8.00 pm
Herbal tea or water
10.00 pm
Bed

Sunday
8.00 am
Pilates
9.00 am
Breakfast
11.00 am
Swim, sauna and steam
1.00 pm
Lunch
3.00 pm
Hair and skin cleanse
6.00 pm
Evening meal
8.00 pm
Epsom bath
10.00 pm
Bed

Friday

7.00 pm
Evening meal
8.00 pm
Visualization
9.00 pm
Moor mud
treatment
10.00 pm
Bed

You begin your detox tonight. From now on, throughout the rest of the weekend, you will be eating and drinking only fresh and, if possible, organic fruit and vegetables. Because this is such a deeply cleansing diet, you will be throwing off toxins at quite a rate, so you may experience some unexpected side-effects (see page 93). These can include headaches, skin eruptions and strange-smelling urine. You may also feel tired. None of these is anything to worry about. Take it easy as much as possible and, if you do get a headache, put some lavender essential oil in a burner (see page 278) and rest to ease it, rather than taking over-the-counter drugs. After your supper, visualization session and therapeutic bath, go to bed early, allowing the body to get started on the detox without any distractions.

7.00 pm Evening meal

You begin the main detox tomorrow with a day of fasting and drinking only juice, herbal tea and water. However, tonight you can eat. Make yourself a big plate of salad using fruit and vegetables only (see recipes pages 58–61). Eat slowly, savouring the fresh flavours. Allow plenty of time for your food to digest by relaxing in a peaceful atmosphere. Part of the aim of this weekend is that your mind should free itself of all negative, stressful thoughts. To achieve this, you need to reverse the all-too-common feeling that we need to be going at full throttle all the time.

You should also start to increase your liquid intake tonight. Drink plenty of bottled or filtered water, or herbal tea (see page 44) throughout the evening. This will help to flush out the system and get the detoxing process off to a good start.

8.00 pm Visualization

Visualization is a form of meditation. Like all meditation, it helps to calm and focus the mind and has many additional benefits: it can improve memory and concentration, relieve stress and any addictive tendencies. If you find yourself craving particular foods or nicotine this weekend, you may well find that visualization will help.

As its name suggests, visualization is all about seeing an image in your mind's eye.

There are three ways in which you can achieve this aim: by focusing, by mental visualization and by colour visualization (see page 250). You may want to try all three methods during the course of the weekend, but limit yourself to one particular approach each session.

Ideally, your visualization session should last for 20 minutes. If, however, you find this too difficult at first, begin with 10 minutes and try to extend the session a little each time. There will be two sessions a day for the rest of the weekend and the cumulative effect of these is most beneficial. By the fifth session on Sunday evening you should find your mind is becoming much clearer and calmer. When each session is finished, don't jump up immediately. Remain seated for a few minutes, breathing slowly, and try to retain the tranquillity the session brings for the rest of the evening.

9.00 pm Moor mud treatment

Therapeutic mud is one of the oldest forms of treatment for various ailments and beauty applications and is therefore particularly useful for detoxification. Take a Moor mud drink and soak in a Moor mud bath (see page 172) for 20–30 minutes immediately before you go to bed.

8.00 am
Juice: juice of a lemon squeezed into hot water
9.00 am
Skin brushing; herbal tea or water
9.30 am
Hydrotherapy
10.30 am
Juice: apple and carrot juice
11.00 am
Pilates
12.00 pm
Juice: tomato juice
2.00 pm
Herbal tea or water
3.00 pm
Manual lymphatic drainage
4.00 pm
Juice: raspberry and peach juice
5.00 pm
Herbal tea or water
6.00 pm
Visualization (as Friday)
6.30 pm
Juice: apple and carrot juice
8.00 pm
Herbal tea or water
10.00 pm
Bed

Saturday

Today is the main day of your detoxing, with a juice fast at its centre (see box opposite for recipes). Don't be too daunted by a liquid-only day; many people find that they rather enjoy it. Fresh juices have a remarkably cleansing and regenerating effect on the entire system as they retain all of the nutrients that are often destroyed in processing and cooking. Low in calories and high in fibre, they are packed with antioxidants to accelerate healing and are particularly effective at cleansing the gut. Juices are very easily assimilated by the body and contain all the nutrients present in raw fruit and vegetables. And, because it's easier to drink juice than it is to eat huge quantities of raw vegetables or fruit, you include a larger quantity of fresh, natural nutrients in your diet than usual.

You cannot make juice with a food processor or liquidizer unless there is a separate juicing attachment. These machines will make a fruit or vegetable purée, while a juicer separates the fibrous pulp from the juice. If you do not have a juicer, you can purchase fresh juice in supermarkets or health food shops (adapt the 'juice menu' provided according to availability), but before you buy check the ingredients list to make sure these juices do not have any additives.

The important thing to remember when it comes to making juices is that they must be fresh – fresh ingredients and freshly made. Always drink the juice the moment you've made it. Don't be tempted to make double the quantity and store some for later; even sealed or in the fridge, it will start to lose vital nutrients. The ultimate detox juice is probably carrot and apple – the best all-rounder for cleansing and boosting the immune system as well as simply being delicious.

Topping up the liquids

Even though you are having nothing but liquid during the course of the day, juice alone will not be enough. You need to drink about 1.8 litres (3 pints) of filtered or bottled water as well (see page 96), to help flush the toxins out of your system. If you want something warm, herbal teas are an excellent way of increasing your fluid intake. They do not contain tannin or caffeine as they are made from pure herbs or, in some cases, spices. You can either make your own with herbs from the garden or supermarket (see page 44) or buy them ready-made. Whether you use fresh or dried herbs or tea bags, you should let them infuse for at least five minutes in boiling water before you drink them.

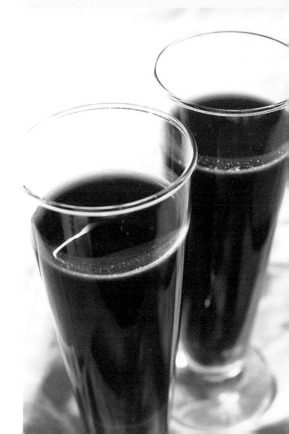

JUICE RECIPES

Wash the fruit and vegetables to be juiced, and chop smaller if necessary so as to fit in the juicer. (Remove the stones from the peaches.) Juice and drink immediately.

Apple and carrot juice

4 carrots

2 green apples

The ultimate detox juice, this is the best general tonic for cleansing and boosting the immune system. If you choose only one juice, this is the one.

Tomato juice

6 tomatoes

A delicious bright red juice, best drunk on its own. Tomatoes contain betacarotene, which helps to boost the body's immunity to disease.

Raspberry and peach

1 small punnet of raspberries

2 peaches

A thick, sweet, restorative juice, particularly good if you are overtired or anaemic. If you find it too thick, add an apple or two.

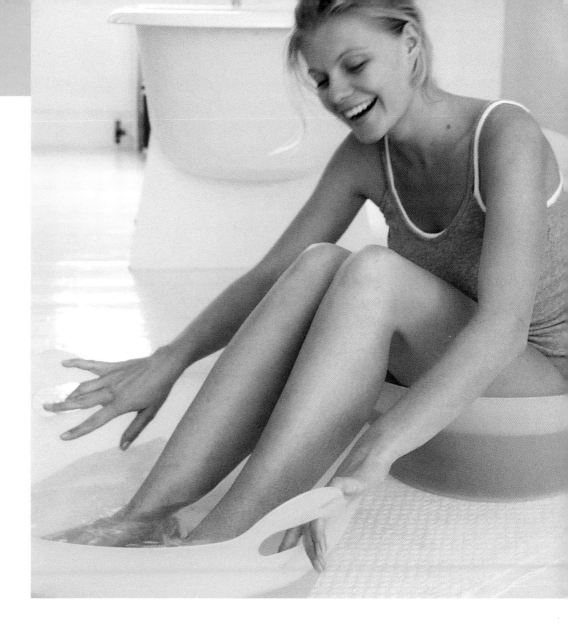

9.00 am Skin brushing

The skin is the largest organ of the body, and the largest area from which toxins are eliminated. There are a number of treatments to stimulate this elimination, of which skin brushing (see page 168) is one. It improves the circulation of blood and lymph (see below), which helps the body to slough off toxins more quickly and efficiently.

Carry out skin brushing in the bathroom, as you will have your hydrotherapy shower and treatments immediately after. Skin brushing always comes first, as it is always done on dry skin.

9.30 am Hydrotherapy

Hydrotherapy also stimulates the circulation of the blood and lymph and destroys circulating toxins. It incorporates a wide range of treatments involving water.

After the skin brushing take a hydrotherapy shower (see page 170). If you find it tiring, rest until your next session, the Pilates body toning. However, if you find the shower stimulating, you might want to try one or two other hydrotherapy treatments – try a sitz bath or water treading (see page 170). Both are beneficial during detoxification and will often give you a boost if you are feeling tired.

Saturday

11.00 am Pilates

When fasting, even for one day, over-energetic exercise is not appropriate, but some gentle exercise will help the detoxification process and also make you feel good, and if you were to lie in bed all day, your system would become sluggish, which is exactly the opposite of what you need while detoxing. Exercise also lifts the spirits, so it helps, too, to overcome feelings of tiredness or lethargy.

The Pilates exercises for today (see pages 184–197) are very focused. You concentrate on using specific muscle groups correctly to tone, strengthen and elongate and at the same time release tension and improve posture. Wear loose, comfortable, preferably cotton clothing, and use a warm but not stuffy room.

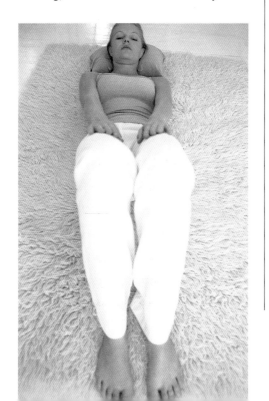

3.00 pm Manual lymphatic drainage

Any type of massage will help you to relax. However, this weekend, manual lymphatic drainage (MLD), in particular is the greatest help in the actual process of detoxification, as well as contributing to a feeling of wellbeing. It is a very gentle, rhythmical technique which, by stimulating the lymphatic system, accelerates the process of shedding toxins. MLD is now widely available; ask at your local sports centre, gym or pool for an MLD-trained therapist and book an appointment for a treat.

The lymphatic system resembles the circulation system, the major difference being that it does not have a central organ, like the heart in the circulatory system, to keep the lymph moving. Rather, the lymph moves as a result of the muscles contracting and relaxing, hence the beneficial effects of exercise on the lymphatic system. Keeping the lymph moving is vital because it plays such a central part in the health of the immune system. Essentially, it is the body's waste disposal system. It gets rid of toxins and dead cells, particles of pollution and antibiotics. So, by stimulating the lymphatic system, detoxification becomes more efficient, too.

By accelerating the workings of the lymphatic system, MLD reduces many of the symptoms caused when it is overstretched. These include bloating, premenstrual tension and cellulite. It is also an extremely relaxing therapy, and the very gentle strokes that are used make it ideal during fasting when you may be feeling particularly sensitive.

If you are unable to find an MLD therapist, there are other effective ways of stimulating the lymphatic system. One is rebounding – jumping on a mini-trampoline – for about 10–15 minutes. Alternatively, a brisk walk is an excellent way of stimulating the lymph – the more pleasant the surroundings, the better. Wear loose, comfortable clothes and low-heeled shoes. Walk at a brisk pace, but don't try jogging. Enjoy your surroundings, breathe deeply and spend at least an hour.

The remainder of the day...

After the massage, spend the rest of the day relaxing. Between resting and juices, you should fit in another visualization session for 20 minutes. Before bed, if you wish, have a relaxing bath to put you in the mood for a restful night's sleep. Try either a Moor mud bath (see page 172) or an Epsom bath (see page 152). Alternatively, for something a little more sensual, you could try an aromatherapy bath (see page 282). Whatever you decide, aim to be in bed by about 10.00 pm.

Sunday

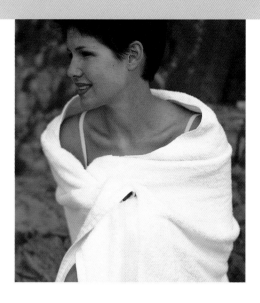

8.00 am
Pilates (as Saturday)
9.00 am
Breakfast
11.00 am
Swim, sauna and steam
1.00 pm
Lunch
3.00 pm
Hair and skin cleanse
6.00 pm
Evening meal
8.00 pm
Epsom bath
10.00 pm
Bed

Today you will be eating solid food, but the detoxification will continue as you are eating only raw food, and some very lightly cooked fruit and vegetables. Drink just as much water as yesterday and include herbal teas whenever you like. The greater the quantity of these fluids you drink, the quicker the toxins will be flushed through the system. Any fruit is good for breakfast, sliced and mixed with a little honey or unsweetened fruit juice, if liked. You can just mix up whatever appeals to you and looks good when you go shopping. Try to buy organic produce whenever possible and make sure it is ripe and therefore at its most delicious. You can have fruit juice to drink, too.

Sauna and steam Many sports centres now have saunas and steam baths. If yours has a pool with a sauna or a steam bath adjacent, this is ideal. Alternating saunas and steam baths with a cold shower or a swim in the pool works on the hydrotherapy principle of stimulating the circulation of blood and lymph by changing the temperature. Of course, you sweat off waste in the sauna or steam bath, too, helping the detoxification process further. However, remember that a very light diet combined with sudden changes of temperature may make you light-headed, so move from one to the other slowly. If you want to have a fairly lengthy swim, do this first.

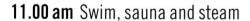

11.00 am Swim, sauna and steam

Sunday's hydrotherapy treatment takes you out to your local gym or swimming pool. Ideally, you should look for a leisure centre that has a swimming pool, sauna and steam room. You can, however, improvise. The other alternative, if you don't have a local pool, or you simply don't feel like going out, is to repeat yesterday's hydrotherapy at home.

Swimming Swimming is the ideal exercise for a detoxing weekend. You use most of the muscle groups in your body if you vary your strokes, but your muscles and joints are supported by the water, so you are not going to injure yourself, as you might do in an overly energetic aerobics class. It is not necessary to swim at a furious pace or for a long period of time and, if you alternate swimming with the other hydrotherapy methods, your mind and body will feel completely relaxed afterwards.

You can also do the exercises over the page in the water – they are particularly beneficial if your joints are stiff. They also help to improve muscle tone, as you are working against the resistance of the water. Warm up first with a couple of lengths and, if you start to feel cold, swim a few more.

If you do this in the afternoon, ensure at least two hours have passed since lunch.

Alternate five to ten minutes of heat with one or two lengths of the pool, and repeat a few times. If you don't have a pool, have a cool to cold shower and rest for a few minutes before returning to the heat treatment. Drink plenty of water throughout. Dry yourself gently, then rest, lying down, before getting dressed.

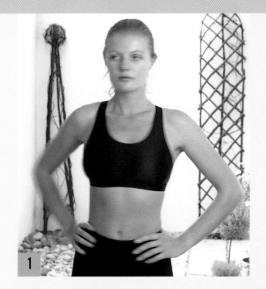

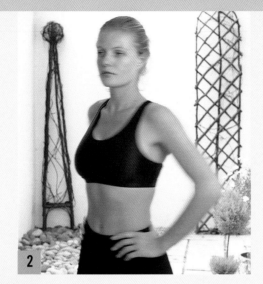

Exercises for the upper body

These exercises are best done in the water, but are shown on land here for clarity.

1 Standing a little way away from the edge of the pool, with your feet apart, place your hands on your hips.

2 Turn as far as you can to the right and then to the left. *Repeat 10 times*, alternating from side to side.

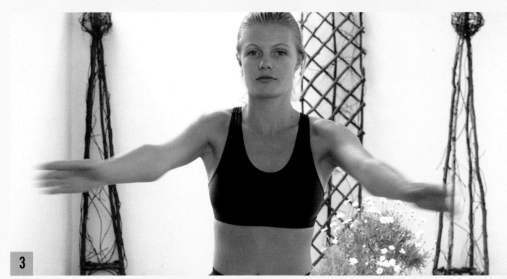

3 With your shoulders under the water (you can kneel for this if the water is very shallow) take your arms out to your sides so that they are just under the water.

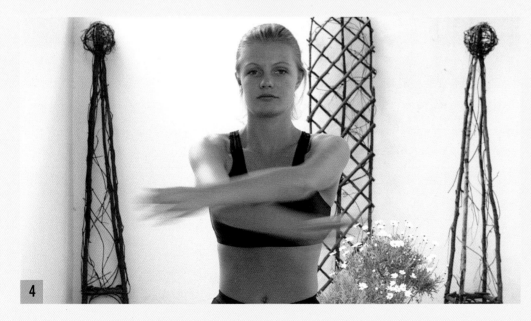

4 With a slight curve from shoulder to your wrist, slowly bring your hands together against the resistance of the water. When your forearms meet, there should be a large circle of water between your arms – enough to encompass a beach ball. *Slowly repeat the exercise 10 times*.

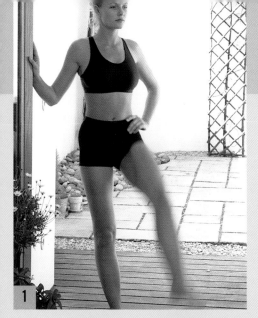

1

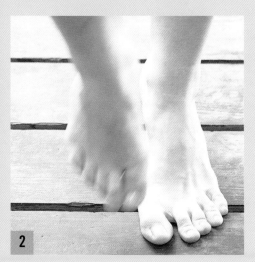

2

Exercises for legs and hips

1 Stand so that your side is next to the edge of the pool and hold on to the handrail. With a straight back, lift your outside leg and swing it back and forth as far as you can. *Repeat 10 times*, then turn round and change legs.

2 Walk on the spot, feeling your feet go down from your toes to your heels on the floor of the pool. Gradually make the steps bigger, with your knees coming higher each time. If you can, after two minutes, turn this into a run. Continue running for two minutes.

Sunday

1.00 pm Lunch and evening meal

Eat salad for Sunday's lunch and evening meal. If you can, eat at least one salad meal a day for the week following your detox and drink plenty of water; this will allow the cleansing process to continue.

3.00 pm Skin and hair cleanse

The afternoon treatment is a relaxing, deep cleanse for the skin and hair (see pages 117 and 146). It helps eliminate toxins, many of which are lost through the skin during detoxification. Keep drinking as much water as you can to speed up the process of flushing the toxins out of your body.

Once you have rinsed off the mask and applied a moisturizer, relax until supper time.

8.00 pm Epsom bath

An Epsom salts bath (see page 152) probably does not sound like a very glamorous end to your weekend. However, it is one of the most cleansing and relaxing late-night treatments.

Do not use Epsom salts if you have eczema, psoriasis or broken skin. Have a soothing aromatherapy bath instead (see page 282).

After your bath, get into bed for another early night of peaceful sleep, ready to awake in the morning fully refreshed and revitalized for the week ahead.

SEE ALSO:

→ Antioxidant foods, page 28

→ Making juices, page 40

→ Herbal teas, page 44

→ Water, page 96

→ Skin cleanse, page 117

→ Aromatherapy hair treatment, page 146

→ Skin brushing, page 168

→ Epsom bath, page 152

→ Moor mud treatment, page 172

→ Hydrotherapy, page 170

→ Pilates, page 184

→ Visualization, page 250

→ Aromatherapy bath, page 282

→ Aromatherapy, page 278

Face and hair

Our faces tend to be the most graphic representation of the person we are, in body and soul. As the most exposed part of the body, it is our faces that age the fastest. There are off-the-shelf potions and lotions galore to help you care for your skin, but equally there are plenty of measures you can take yourself to look after your complexion – both externally and from within. Get both your hair and your skin in tiptop condition and you have the perfect combination for a feeling and appearance of good health and wellbeing.

3

Face facts

Your face doesn't take up much space. Of the 2 square metres (21½ square feet) of skin that contours the body, that covering the face accounts for just 4.5 per cent. Yet it attracts more attention, generates more concern and fuels more commercial enterprise than any other part of the body.

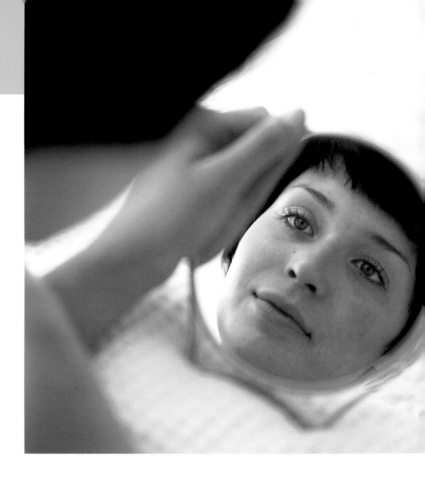

The imbalance somehow makes sense, however, because every face tells a story. The unique features that a face develops through accidents of inheritance and experience, be they laughter lines or wilting eyes, offer myriad insights into the interior life of their wearer. Most significantly, perhaps, it reveals age. The skin is the body's only visible organ and the face its most exposed part.

The face is also the most expressive part of the body, capable of a wider range of movements than any other, and it rarely rests, resulting in wrinkles and furrows. As the population ages more rapidly than ever, creases and jowls are becoming the norm and people are flocking as never before to clinics, pharmacies and beauticians in search of ready-to-wear cures. Consumers are constantly persuaded to believe that newly synthesized chemicals, cutting-edge technology or state-of-the-art surgery will help rejuvenate their skin.

Self-help for your skin

However, there are easy steps you can take yourself to look after your facial skin that involve no consultations of plastic surgeons, pharmacists or cosmetic technicians. If facial massage and exercise (see pages 126–139) are all you do, you will keep your looks longer than most. But add to them the occasional internal spring clean (see Chapter 2) and a diet that feeds your skin (see Chapter 1), and your complexion will bloom. Water it regularly outside (see page 152) and in (see Water, page 96) to keep it that way.

Instead of buying a foundation cream to conceal your skin, build a natural foundation with well-toned muscle. Instead of putting energy into looking for the ultimate crow's feet cream, put it into eye exercises. Instead of buying a new blusher brush, achieve a rosy glow by boosting your circulation. Instead of paying for a high-tech moisturizer, turn on the kitchen tap. And rather than covering up creases, smooth them away with some gentle massage.

There will always be other things you could usefully do in that time – mow the lawn, dust the furniture or make a meal – but none of their effects will endure. Spend the time on a few minutes of exercise, massage and cleansing and the results will still be looking back at you from the mirror next year. If you follow this programme, you won't have any glitzy packaging to brighten your bathroom shelf, but you might have an enviable complexion that belies your age.

SEE ALSO:

→ Water, page 96

→ 7-stage detox diet, page 98

→ Improve your complexion, page 122

→ Facial massage, page 126

→ Facial exercise, page 134

Your beauty secrets revealed

1 What is your haircare routine?

☐ **A**: I wash my hair every day.

☑ **B**: I wash and condition my hair every 2–3 days.

☐ **C**: I like trying out new colours and products so it varies.

2 How often do you massage your face?

☐ **A**: Every day.

☐ **B**: Every week.

☑ **C**: Hardly ever.

3 How do you remove your make-up at the end of the day?

☐ **A**: I use soap, then a moisturizer.

☐ **B**: I use a cleanser and toner, followed by a moisturizer.

☑ **C**: I usually use a cleanser but if it's late I leave it till morning.

4 What is your dental routine?

☐ **A**: I brush morning and night.

☐ **B**: I brush and floss morning and night.

☑ **C**: I brush in the morning and use minty chewing gum during the day.

5 What do you drink during the day?

☑ **A**: Juice, tea and coffee.

☐ **B**: Water and herbal tea.

☐ **C**: Fizzy drinks, occasionally some wine with my lunch.

6 How much time do you sit in the sun?

☑ **A**: Quite a lot when the weather's good, but I always use a sun cream.

☐ **B**: I cover up, especially in the hottest part of the day.

☑ **C**: I love sun bathing on holiday and my skin tans easily.

7 How many fresh fruits and vegetables do you eat each day?

☑ **A**: I love fruit but I'm not a big veg fan.

☐ **B**: I try to have a balanced five fruit and vegetables a day.

☐ **C**: I tend to eat on the move so it depends what is available.

8 How often do you do facial exercises?

☐ **A**: Every week.

☐ **B**: Every day.

☑ **C**: Hardly ever.

9 When do you wear sunglasses?

☑ **A**: I always wear them in the summer.

☐ **B**: I wear dark glasses that block out the harmful rays, even in the winter.

☐ **C**: I've got a whole range of fashion sunglasses for every occasion.

10 How often do you exfoliate?

☐ **A**: Every day.

☑ **B**: Every week.

☐ **C**: Hardly ever.

HOW YOU SCORED

MOSTLY As

You are certainly trying to keep your skin and hair in good condition but sometimes you try too hard. For instance, it is great to exfoliate your skin and have clean hair but every day is a bit too much – you'll actually damage them in the long run. In the sun, make sure your sun cream has a high sun protection factor (SPF) and wear sunglasses. Your teeth will benefit from flossing at least once a day. Try to eat more vegetables – a side salad or carrot juice will increase your intake. Substitute some water for tea and coffee during the day. For facial fitness, swap round the exercises and massage – massage weekly and exercise daily.

MOSTLY Bs

Your skin- and haircare programme is almost too good to be true! If it is too much of an effort, you can relax some aspects of it. For instance, a glass of wine or a little sun (with a high SPF, of course) actually do you good. However, you are aware of what your routine should be and you follow it. Keep your water intake up and you should be looking radiant.

MOSTLY Cs

Oh dear. You have a lot of fun but it will be at the expense of your skin and hair. Don't follow all of the advice in this chapter in one go but you need to make some changes. Always take off your make-up at night and use a night-time moisturizer. Always use a high SPF sun cream in the sun. Be sure to feed your hair with conditioner and have it cut regularly. Eat more fruit and vegetables and less processed food and drink a litre bottle of water every day.

Skincare basics

Your face needs cleansing thoroughly at least once, preferably twice, a day to remove grime and the dead skin cells that continuously accumulate. A cleansing, toning and moisturizing routine should become as natural as brushing your teeth. When you first start, the odd spot may appear initially as dirt is flushed out from below the surface of the skin. Any spots should soon go and your skin will look clearer and feel silkier and smoother after just a week or two of such cleansing.

Soap story

Cheap, compact and versatile, soap is the most fundamental of all toiletries. All soaps consist of a fat (tallow or vegetable oil) to lift oil and grease, and an alkaline compound to dissolve the soap-dirt mixture in water for removal. Other ingredients may include moisturizing cream (for mild soaps), glycerine and alcohol (for transparent soaps), antibacterial agents (for deodorant soaps), aloe vera, vitamin E or oatmeal.

Bar soap has an effective cleansing action and generally has a high perfume and colour content. It is often condemned for its drying effects. If you do experience problems with facial dryness, flaking or discomfort, swap your soap for a 'superfatted' one that contains substances such as cocoa butter or olive oil or for a gentle, hypo-allergenic facial cleanser, or specialist facial cleansing bar. Glycerine soap, which is also higher in fat than normal soap, is the best choice for oily skin.

A basic skincare routine

- **Cleansing** – twice daily
- **Toning** – twice daily
- **Moisturizing with UV protective cream** – every morning
- **Moisturizing with a specialist night cream** – every night
- **Exfoliating** (see page 118) – weekly
- **Special treatments** (such as facial masks or pore cleansing strips) – weekly or monthly

Cleansing, toning and moisturizing

There are a whole host of products for cleansing, moisturizing and toning to suit every type of skin – dry, normal, oily and sensitive – and you may have to experiment until you find the ones that suit you best. Some new all-in-one products remove make-up, cleanse, exfoliate and tone. Cleansers are used to remove all traces of make-up, dirt and atmospheric pollutants. Toners remove any remaining make-up (and the cleanser itself), and freshen and prepare the skin to receive the moisturizer. Moisturizers are absorbed into the skin to soften and nourish it.

• **Cleansing** For the simplest cleansing treatment, gently press a hot clean flannel against your face to open the pores. Then, with your eyes closed, massage a little vegetable oil (see What oil should I use?, page 127) very gently into your skin using your fingertips, in small circular motions over your whole face and your neck. This massaging action improves circulation (which aids the removal of toxins) and helps firms up the facial muscles. Rinse the flannel then wipe off the oil and accompanying grime thoroughly.

Of the commercial cleansers there are two basic kinds – foaming cleansers and milks or creams. For the former, create a foam between wet hands before applying it to your damp face using your

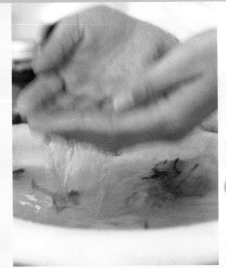
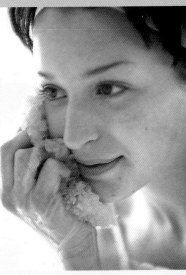

Tips and tricks

- Use warm not hot water for washing your face, since hot water can encourage the development of extra blood vessels, resulting in a ruddy complexion. If you have a tendency to thread veins, avoid steam baths, excessive alcohol, hot spices and caffeine.
- Do not substitute soap for a cleansing lotion as part of your basic skincare routine. Soap and water can strip facial skin of its acidic film and dry it out.
- Always remove make-up at the end of the day. Use eye make-up remover and cream cleanser as appropriate with plenty of cotton wool, taking care not to pull and drag the skin, especially around the eyes.
- Avoid using tissues for cleansing as they are made from wood pulp and contain microscopic splinters of wood that can become embedded in the skin. Use flannels or cotton wool pads instead.
- Keep your hair away from your face with a hairband when applying cleansers and creams.
- If you have dry skin, avoid washing your face too often and avoid dry environments. Use a wipe-off cream cleanser rather than a foaming facial wash. Use specialist rich cream moisturizer and night cream and don't use face masks (which dry out on the skin), facial scrubs or astringent toner.
- If you have oily skin or a tendency to large pores, wash your face three times a day. Cleanse with a foaming facial wash and use pore cleansing strips. Use an astringent, such as rosewater, to close the pores morning and night. Moisturize with a light, oil-free lotion (if you need one at all). Avoid using facial scrubs too often. Use dry powder make-up and oil-free cosmetics.
- If you have sensitive skin use a fragrance-free cream cleanser and moisturize with emollient cream or sensitive skin cream. Avoid using any fragranced products not indicated for sensitive skin.

fingertips in circular motions as above. Splash with tepid or cool water to remove. To use a milky or creamy cleanser, dot it over your forehead, cheeks, nose and chin, and proceed as above. Remove by splashing with water or with damp cotton wool.

- **Toning** Apply a few drops to damp cotton wool and wipe gently over your face and neck. If necessary pat dry with a clean dry towel.
- **Moisturizing** Lastly, use a good-quality moisturizer both to apply water to your skin and to prevent it from evaporating. Moisturizers contain varying proportions of oil and water and include a variety of ingredients. Many daytime moisturizers now contain a sun protection factor, as well as antioxidants (see page 28). A good night cream will help repair and nourish your skin overnight. Dot cream around your face, over your neck and down to below your collar bone, and gently rub it in using your fingertips.

SEE ALSO:

→ Aromatherapy facial, page 116

→ Exfoliation, page 118

→ Improve your complexion, page 122

→ Facial massage, page 126

→ Facial exercise, page 134

Aromatherapy facial

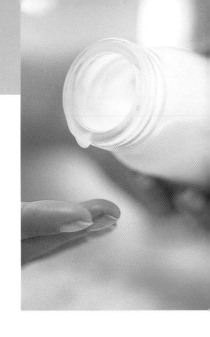

This facial deep-cleanses and rejuvenates the skin. You can buy over-the-counter products that have essential oils added, or make those described in the box below using aromatherapy oils and other natural ingredients.

Before you begin the facial, you might like to apply an aromatherapy treatment to your hair (see page 146). If so, make up the recipe and apply the mixture to your whole head, massaging it well into your scalp and making sure that all of your hair is covered. Wrap a towel around your hair and continue with the facial. Leave the hair oil on for at least as long as the facial, although you could leave the treatment on overnight and wash your hair when you shower the following morning.

Home-made skin treatments

CLEANSING MASKS

Choose one of the following recipes according to your skin type and blend the ingredients together well before use.

For dry skin
2 teaspoons clear, runny honey
2 drops lavender oil
2 drops rose oil

For normal to oily skin
2 teaspoons natural yogurt
2 drops lemon oil
2 drops cypress oil

FACIAL TONERS

Pour 50 ml (2 fl oz) of bottled water into a small, clean mist sprayer. Add the essential oils below according to your skin type and shake well to mix. Spray over your face and throat with your eyes closed.

For normal to dry skin
4 drops lavender oil
4 drops rose oil
2 drops geranium oil

For oily skin
4 drops lavender oil
4 drops vetivert oil
2 drops bergamot oil

ESSENTIAL OIL SKIN CONDITIONERS

The recipe is for a larger quantity than you will need for just one application. Blend the following essential oils in 50 ml (2 fl oz) of carrier oil. Use any cold-pressed vegetable oil or, if you have dry or problem skin, calendula or wheatgerm oil.

For dry skin
10 drops rose oil
10 drops lavender oil
5 drops sandalwood oil

For normal to oily skin
10 drops lemon oil
10 drops lavender oil
5 drops cypress oil

For mature skin
10 drops frankincense oil
10 drops neroli oil
5 drops rose oil

EYE COMPRESS SOLUTION

Put 1 drop camomile essential oil into 1 litre (1¾ pints) cold water. Mix well.

Skin cleanse

1 Begin by **cleansing** your skin thoroughly using a cleanser that can be removed with water. You can then exfoliate your skin with a mini-loofah, specifically designed for use on your face, while your skin is still wet. Use gentle, small circular movements, avoiding your eye area and concentrating on your forehead, nose, chin and cheeks. Rinse well with clean water.

2 Tone your skin by spraying it with floral water. If you are using a proprietary brand, look for a toner that is alcohol free, as alcohol is not beneficial to the skin. You can make your own version very easily, using one of the recipes opposite.

3 Apply a **cleansing mask** to your face and throat, avoiding your eye area. Use any mask that is leftover on the backs of your hands. You can either buy a proprietary cleansing mask or make your own, according to skin type, using the recipes opposite.

To make an **eye compress**, soak two cotton wool pads in an eye compress solution (see opposite) and squeeze out any excess liquid. Place the pads over your eyes. Relax with the mask and compresses in place *for 10 minutes*. Remove the compresses and rinse the mask off with cool water.

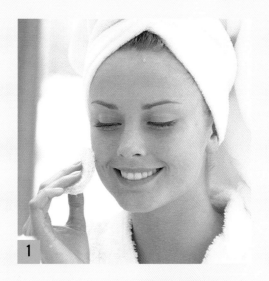

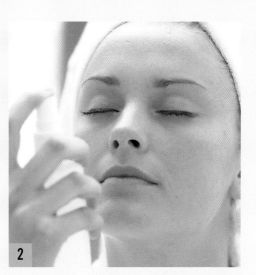

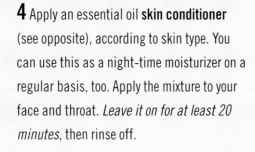

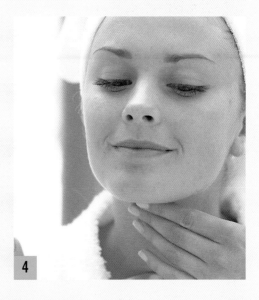

4 Apply an essential oil **skin conditioner** (see opposite), according to skin type. You can use this as a night-time moisturizer on a regular basis, too. Apply the mixture to your face and throat. *Leave it on for at least 20 minutes*, then rinse off.

SEE ALSO:

→ Healthy hair naturally, page 146

→ Aromatherapy, page 278

Exfoliation

Many skin problems can be prevented by regularly removing dead surface cells; exfoliation is a mechanical way of doing this. It smoothes wrinkles and rough skin and prevents pores from being clogged by dead skin debris.

Unlike cleansing, exfoliation is not a daily necessity, but an occasional treatment. It's like the dusting that precedes polishing when you clean furniture (in fact, most household dust is made up of human skin cells). If you do not get rid of those surface deposits first, they will get rubbed around with the polish, producing a smudge rather than a shine. Equally, no cleansing method will make your face glow if there is an accumulation of underlying detritus.

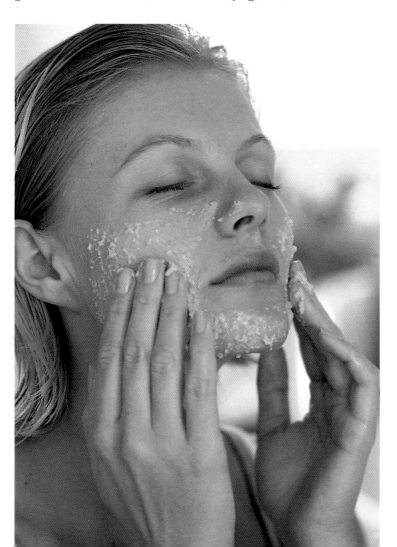

Exfoliation becomes more important with age, as skin cells are renewed more slowly and they have more creases to bury themselves in. Wrinkles packed with dead cells look deeper than those that are cleared out. Moreover, removing these cells speeds up the process of skin regeneration. That is probably why men's skin seems to age more slowly than women's: their daily shave removes not only stubble but also dead skin.

That said, the older your skin, the gentler a touch it needs. Unlike the rugged stuff on your knees that you can attack with a loofah, the delicate skin on your face is prone to thread veins, irritation or excessive dryness if rubbed too harshly. Some commercial scrubs, as exfoliators are often called, contain rough particles, which although natural can scratch the skin. Others, based on fruit acids, are too aggressive.

The epidermis may be largely made up of dead cells, but it is still metabolically active and if you remove too much of it, it will not serve its protective function of defusing dangerous free radicals (see Super scavengers, page 91) from the air or trapping moisture. You can use these harsh new tools when you are young to no apparent ill effect. But they can inflict superficial damage that becomes visible when the skin loses collagen and elastin. Fine oatmeal or ground almonds from the kitchen cupboard can remove dead cells more moderately and safely than a branded product claiming to do the ultimate scrape-and-shine.

Scrub ingredients

The four most traditional ingredients are salt, which is antibacterial, ground almonds and oatmeal, both traditional cleansers, and sugar. But other granular foodstuffs that are mildly abrasive will do the trick. They do not require special preparation to make them into

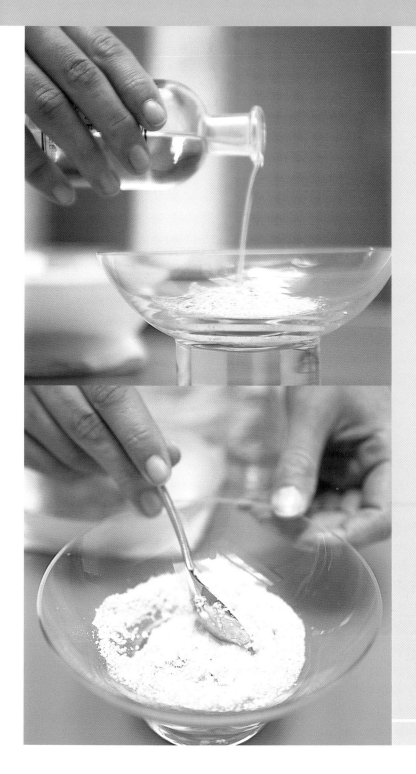

Facial scrubs

For any of these recipes mix all the ingredients into a smooth paste then leave for five minutes to bind. Gently massage into the face, avoiding the delicate skin under the eyes and rubbing up and out, against the direction of any wrinkles. Wipe off with a damp muslin cloth, rinse your face in warm water then pat gently dry with a towel.

OAT NUT SCRUB

2 teaspoons fine oatmeal
2 teaspoons ground almonds
orange flower water (**for oily skin**) or
cream (**for dry skin**), to blend

SUGAR CORN SCRUB

2 teaspoons cornflour
2 teaspoons raw brown sugar
1 teaspoon almond oil
apple juice (**for normal skin**) or
lemon juice (**for oily skin**), to blend

STICKY GRAPE SCRUB

2 teaspoons salt
1 dessertspoon grape juice
Greek yogurt, to blend

pastes and can be used just dampened with water for speed. Adding something like cream or yogurt makes them easier to apply, while grape juice will also take dead cells with it when rinsed off. Experiment with any of the three recipes provided in the above box to gain the confidence to invent your own.

SEE ALSO:

→ Why detox? page 90

→ Skincare basics, page 114

→ Improve your complexion, page 122

Face masks

Face masks, or facial feeds, are designed to bring about a quick improvement in the condition of your skin. The basic principle is that if you apply something to your skin that dries at room temperature, it will tighten the skin. If you include an acidic substance, it will exfoliate and tone. If the main ingredient is rich in natural oils, it will nourish and lubricate.

Home-made face packs can visibly improve your complexion by increasing local blood circulation, neutralizing bacteria, stimulating the elimination of wastes, trapping moisture on the surface, or firm up by closing the pores. The ingredients are readily available, inexpensive and are unlikely to cause allergic skin reactions.

Making up a face mask

The most important thing is to get the consistency right: too sloppy and you will be lying down to keep it in place; too firm and you risk damaging your skin as you scrape off the crust.

To produce a mask, you normally need some fluid, a binder and oil. The fluid may be ready-supplied in the fruit or vegetable you use; if not, you can add floral or plain spring or distilled water. If your chosen base is fruit or vegetables you will need a blender or liquidizer to pulp the flesh; use the blender to incorporate the remaining ingredients. If using plant foods or yogurt, or both, you will probably need some powdered clay or flour to bind it together.

When including oil, add it last and drip it in slowly so that it has a chance to emulsify. Adding a capsule of evening primrose or borage oil will give the mixture an anti-ageing edge as these help to kill free radicals (see Super scavengers, page 91) and to retain moisture. The oil most commonly used in traditional face masks is almond, but almost any will do. Choose yours according to your skin type (see What oil should I use? page 127).

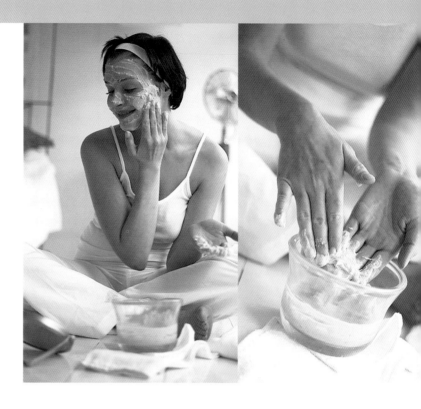

Applying the mask

First, make sure your skin is squeaky clean and if necessary exfoliate (see page 118). To enhance the effects of a face mask (see recipes, right) massage it into the face methodically, avoiding the areas around the eyes and lips, using some of the upward and outward movements from the massage routine on pages 128–131. The face mask needs to be left on for a minimum of 10 minutes. If it has not done its job after 20 minutes, it never will. Then rinse it off with warm water, using a clean flannel or muslin cloth if the mixture has solidified.

If you want the full treatment, then apply a toner afterwards. A flower water such as rose or orange is ideal and you can enhance its effect by adding an appropriate essential oil such as bergamot, cypress or juniper (see Facial toners, page 116).

Then leave it at that, and don't be tempted to put on make-up to complete the picture. If it can, skin uses 2–3 per cent of the body's total oxygen by direct absorption from the air and gets rid of at least as much carbon dioxide waste the same way. Both revitalize it. So just as you rest after a meal, after a good facial feed, give the skin a respite and let it breathe.

Face masks

AVOCADO AND HONEY NOURISHING MASK
A good feed for dry, ageing skin.

¼ ripe avocado

1 teaspoon runny honey

2 teaspoons Greek live yogurt

2 drops jasmine or rose otto essence

Mash the avocado very thoroughly with a fork, then stir in the remaining ingredients. Apply quite thickly to the face and leave on for at least 10 minutes. Wipe off with a dry muslin cloth, then rinse the cloth in warm water to remove the rest of the mask.

After such a rich mask, it is a good idea to refresh your skin with a toner, such as a rosewater toner.

CUCUMBER AND CLAY TONIC
A good tonic for normal-to-oily skin.

5 cm (2 in) piece of cucumber

4 teaspoons green clay

2 teaspoons brewer's yeast

Mix all the ingredients in a blender until smooth. If a little watery, add another 1–2 teaspoons of clay.

TURMERIC AND EGG FEED
A luxurious facial feed for tired and dry-to-normal skin.

1 egg yolk

2 teaspoons turmeric

2 teaspoons brewer's yeast

2 teaspoons pollen grains

2 dessertspoons jojoba essence

rosewater, to blend

Whisk the egg yolk and then add the remaining ingredients. This mask is easy to apply but rather sticky, so sponge off carefully and it will leave your skin beautifully smooth.

EGG FIRMING MASK
This mask can take years off your face – for an evening!

1 egg white

4–6 teaspoons kelp powder

1 drop geranium essence

Lightly whip the egg white until white and bubbly but not stiff. Thoroughly mix in the kelp powder and geranium essence. Smooth thinly over the face and wait for it to dry thoroughly before wiping, then rinsing, it off.

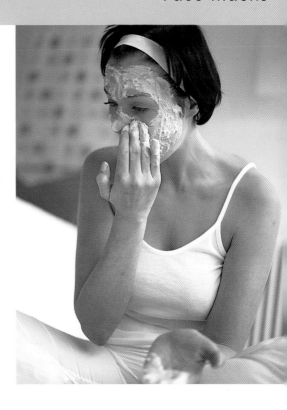

FULLER'S EARTH FACIAL MASK
Suitable for all skin types.

1 tablespoon Fuller's Earth

1½–2 tablespoons rosewater (for a medium-to-oily skin) or

a small quantity of a rich face lotion (for a dry skin)

Mix the ingredients thoroughly then apply with a natural bristle beauty brush. If you are using rosewater, keep the mask moist with thin slices of peeled cucumber. Leave for 10 minutes then remove with warm rosewater. Pat dry with a fine-textured towel.

SEE ALSO:

→ Skincare basics, page 114

→ Aromatherapy facial, page 116

→ Exfoliation, page 118

Improve your complexion

Most people think of cleaning their skin as a procedure involving cotton wool and something out of a bottle. However, cleansers simply address the issue of skincare from the outside in. Good skin depends on healthy blood getting to it and toxic wastes being filtered away. If this is not happening because the system is undernourished or overloaded it will show in skin problems.

They may just be blackheads or rough patches which disappear with a simple topical treatment, but they are signs that the skin is stressed and, like other organs, skin ages more quickly under stress.

Spring cleaning steps

1 First, the blood and lymph need to be cleared of the toxic sediment they are shifting around. This means avoiding toxins, giving the gut a break and stimulating the lymph to clear wastes efficiently. It is impossible to avoid ingesting all pollutants, but combining a detox diet (see page 98) with measures to boost your circulation is one way to get rid of many toxins. During detoxification toxins surface and your skin may become peppered with blemishes, but within a month at the most they should have made way for new, brighter, smoother skin.

2 Second, you need to boost your blood circulation. These first two processes are reciprocal, with blood and lymph function improving as toxins are cleared and vice versa.

3 Exfoliating (see page 118) to remove the dead cells and toxins on the surface is the finishing touch.

So if you have recurrent skin problems, or think your skin looks old, try the techniques below to increase circulation and detoxify your system.

Boost your circulation

There are many ways to increase the body's circulation. Do four or five of the following regularly and your skin should soon glow.

- **Dry skin brushing** Giving your body a firm brush all over has rapid internal as well as external benefits (see page 168).
- **Epsom salts bath** A bath in Epsom salts helps remove toxins at the same time as stimulating circulation (see page 152).
- **Essential oils** Certain essential oils help to increase circulation and detoxify. Apply during massage, which increases blood flow to the skin manually and aids absorption by creating heat (see page 278).
- **Lymphatic drainage** This is a form of massage that stimulates the lymph system into eliminating toxins (see page 106).
- **Herbal help** Many herbs help to stimulate circulation and detox the liver. Most can be taken as tinctures or tablets but some can be drunk as a tea or used in cooking. Ask a herbalist or healthfood shop.
- **Exercise** This is the single most effective way to boost circulation as it has immediate as well as long-term effects (see 'What aerobic exercise does for your skin', page 224).
- **Deep breathing** Mostly we breathe in a shallow, superficial way that uses only around one-third of our lung capacity (see Improve your breathing, page 240). Our circulation is compromised and cells do not receive sufficient oxygen to reproduce at their optimum rate — which leads, among other things, to lifeless skin.
- **Hydrotherapy** Having a cold bath has a remarkable effect on the circulation (see Hydrotherapy, page 170). Within three to five minutes of immersing yourself in a cold bath, your blood circulation increases fourfold and your lymph flow is equally boosted.

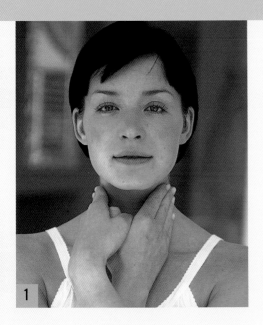

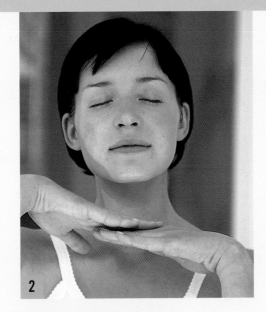

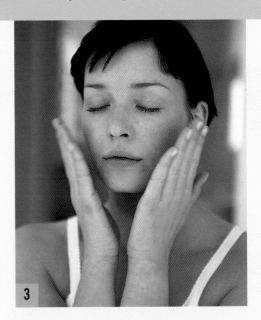

Increasing circulation to the face

This quick-fix circulation solution is a three-minute routine that involves gently hitting yourself on the face to get blood into it.

1 Cross your hands in front of the neck and, with the flat of your fingers, tap on the opposite sides of the neck, from the base up to the chin, avoiding the windpipe.

2 Hold the back of your left hand about 3.5 cm (1½ in) under the chin. With the back of your right hand, tap rapidly upwards on the area under the chin, using the back of the left hand as a 'stop'.

3 With the flat of the fingers and using both hands together, apply firm tapping movements all over the lower part of the face. Start lightly over the mouth and move outwards, covering each cheek and stopping

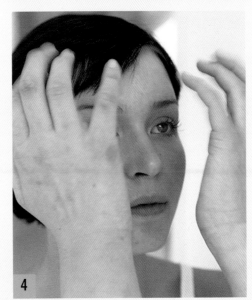

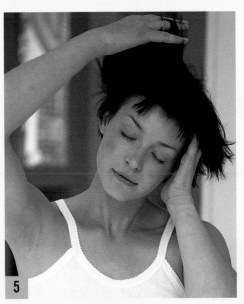

in front of the ears. If you are prone to thread veins, use only light 'piano' movements.

4 Using both hands together and the flats of the fingertips, apply firm tapping movements all over the forehead. Using the hands loosely clenched, 'knock' your head all over with a relaxed movement, varying the firmness of the movement depending on the sensitivity of each area.

5 Using the pads of your fingers, apply deep circular movements all over your scalp from the hairline to the crown, covering the whole head thoroughly. Using both your hands alternately, 'comb' through your hair from the hairline to the crown, using long, deep sliding movements.

Load up with water

Facial skin needs water more than anything else to flourish and the greatest benefits come from consuming the stuff directly (see Water, page 96) rather than applying it to your face. Unfortunately, modern living conditions encourage too much water to escape. Central heating, air conditioning, sunbathing, flying, smoking, drinking and dieting are all quick routes to wrinkles.

SUNSHINE

Problem Warm sun dramatically increases the rate of evaporation of water from the skin's surface. In addition, its rays spark the production of free radicals, the destructive oxygen molecules that accelerate the ageing process (see Super scavengers, page 91). Altogether, the sun causes 80 per cent of the changes associated with ageing.

Solution So, especially if you have dry-to-normal skin, seek out the shade. If you cannot avoid or resist being in the sun, apply creams containing the antioxidant vitamins A, C and E which have been shown to zap free radicals on contact. Sunscreens, creams, blocks and lotions do shield the skin from damaging ultraviolet rays, but they rely on synthetic chemicals. If you are exposed to moderate sunshine only and do not have very fair or excessively dry skin, apply a natural

vegetable oil with screening properties. The most effective are jojoba, which has a sun protection factor of 5–10; beeswax, whose high viscosity means it sticks to the skin; and shea butter, which is 50 per cent fat, including essential fatty acids, so provides a good protective seal and antioxidant protection.

SMOKING

Problem After the sun, smoking is the biggest wrinkler. It thins the skin by around 40 per cent, so that water escapes much more easily. Further damage is caused by the chemicals in cigarettes which accelerate normal ageing. Cigarette smoke destroys vitamin C, needed for collagen manufacture, and smoking also constricts the tiny capillaries that feed the skin, depriving it of nutrients and oxygen. Smoking can add 15 years to your skin's age.

Solution If you can't give up smoking then cutting back would be a positive step forward.

CENTRAL HEATING AND AIR CONDITIONING

Problem Both steal moisture from the air.

Solution At home, keep the heating moderate and use a humidifier – a bowl of water on top of a radiator can raise the moisture content of the air to around 80–85 per cent humidity, which is the optimum level for the skin.

DRINKING ALCOHOL

Problem Alcohol dries out the facial skin and it is diuretic, causing rapid water loss. Red blood cells stick together and capillaries gum up so that they can rupture and result in thread veins. Alcohol also ages the skin by robbing the body of oxygen and vitamin C.

Solution The recommended maximum amount is 21 units of alcohol per week.

DIETING

Problem The most common mistake when trying to lose weight is to cut down on all fats, but the skin relies on a regular supply of essential fatty acids to keep it moist and pliable (see opposite). Crash dieting causes loss of muscle and yo-yo dieting dries out and ages the skin in the long term.

Solution If you diet, do so at a sensible pace; include nuts, seeds and oily fish. Try to stick near your target weight once you reach it.

FLYING

Problem Recycling air in an enclosed cabin makes it excessively dry – there can be as little as 2 per cent humidity. Even a shortish flight can dry your skin significantly.

Solution Drink water before, during and after the flight, and avoid alcohol. On a long flight, spray your face once an hour (see opposite).

Feed your face

Like any other organ in the body, skin needs a complete supply of nutrients to regenerate, repair and defend itself. There is a vast array of nutritional creams, lotions and capsules containing assorted vitamins and phytochemicals, but it is more effective – and undoubtedly cheaper – to eat what the skin needs from your plate. In addition, many of the foods needed for healthy skin tissue are also those that benefit the circulation, digestion and elimination mechanisms. Two groups of nutrients that are crucial to keeping skin looking young are antioxidants and essential fats.

• **Antioxidants** Antioxidants (see Antioxidant foods, page 28) perform such a fundamental role in destroying the free radicals that are at the root of much age-related deterioration that they can effectively be defined as anti-ageing nutrients. Each of the major antioxidants benefits the skin, for example vitamin C is essential for the production of collagen, the elastic tissue in skin that declines with age, and vitamin E has the most powerful action against free-radical damage caused by the sun.

• **Essential fatty acids** EFAs, especially the omega-3 fats (see page 33), work as a sort of internal moisturizer by stemming the escape of fluids from the cells. A quick way of increasing your dietary intake of EFAs is to use sesame, rapeseed, walnut, soya bean or flax oils in the kitchen. At the same time, decrease your intake of saturated and processed fats as these compete with and cancel out EFAs in the body. A diet high in EFAs will result in softer, dewier skin and will defer, if not prevent completely, the appearance of wrinkles.

Spray away

Although only a small amount of fluid can be absorbed by the skin cells, the face benefits from external as well as internal watering. Splashing your face with water not only rehydrates the skin but also stimulates the circulation. You can enhance the effect by using cold water or alternating cold and warm. However, do not use iced water if you have very fair, sensitive skin as it may react by producing thread veins. After splashing your face, pat dry the drips and apply a water-in-oil moisturizer to control evaporation.

Away from the bathroom, a small plastic plant spray of distilled or bottled spring water combined with up to three drops of jasmine, rose otto or lavender essential oil makes an ideal portable irrigation system. Use the spray whenever the skin feels tight especially when flying or in very warm weather. Also spray your face before applying moisturizer which is designed to retain existing moisture in the skin rather than add it. Always remember to shut your eyes!

SEE ALSO:

→ Fats, page 22

→ Antioxidant foods, page 28

→ Why detox? page 90

→ 7-stage detox diet, page 98

→ Water, page 96

→ Exfoliation, page 118

→ Facial massage, page 126

→ Facial exercise, page 134

→ Skin brushing, page 168

→ Epsom salts bath, page 152

→ Hydrotherapy, page 170

→ Aerobic exercise, page 224

→ Improve your breathing, page 240

→ Aromatherapy, page 278

→ Healing herbs, page 288

Facial massage

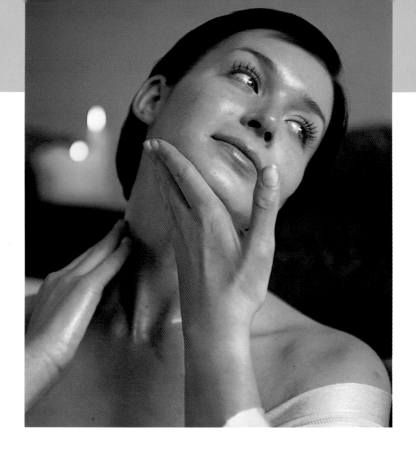

When you first get up in the morning your face probably looks paler, puffier and more creased than usual. You can blame some of the creases on the pillow you slept on, but the lack of colour and tone are the result of a nocturnal slow-down in circulation.

When the body is in a deep rest it puts the brakes on the systems that pump blood and lymph around the body. At night, when the lymph drainage of toxins from the tissues slows down, the waste builds up. Puffiness around the face, particularly the eyes, in the morning is just one of the most obvious signs of this; likewise, the relative pallor that follows the nocturnal slow down in blood circulation.

It is not only sleep that slows down circulation. During the day, lack of exercise, poor nutrition, shallow breathing and overexposure to pollution – all hazards of modern living – slow the drainage of lymph and flow of blood.

Facial massage jump-starts both (see page 128 for the exercises). A pinker glow is the obvious testament to improved blood flow. An acceleration in lymph action is less visible, but you can assume that if your face is a richer colour the lymph has also been stimulated, since its vessels run closer to the surface of the skin. In the longer term, a fluid lymph system shows in a resilient immune system and a bright complexion. Half of the lymph nodes in the body are in the neck, so unblocking them has an immediate effect on the facial skin.

A gentle touch

When you press or squeeze any part of your body, it increases circulation to that area. The face responds particularly well to touch as it is packed with small, sensitive muscles and so richly endowed with nerve endings.

Tension, and to a certain extent age, causes the connective tissue between the layers of the facial skin and the facial muscles to become less supple over time. As a result habitual expressions such as frown lines, rigid jaws, pursed lips and staring eyes tend to become set as part of the fabric of the face. The gentle pressure of a facial massage can loosen up the facial muscles and allow them to learn to slide back into place more readily after being tensed. The cumulative effect is such that with repeated treatment your face will be left looking relaxed, and therefore younger. Also, because massage stimulates circulation to the face, your complexion will be toned and glowing.

The muscles of the face are extremely delicate. Massage can be tremendously beneficial, but if given too deeply or frequently, it can encourage the muscles to lengthen. So the comparative fragility of older muscles and their adjacent tissues is important to bear in mind. The scalp is a different matter and can be massaged quite vigorously without any harm, with many benefits for the face.

Sensitive skin, which is typically fair and dry, should also be massaged with great care. It is more susceptible to the kind of surface damage that causes 'broken veins' (which are not actually broken, but simply closer than usual to the surface, so more

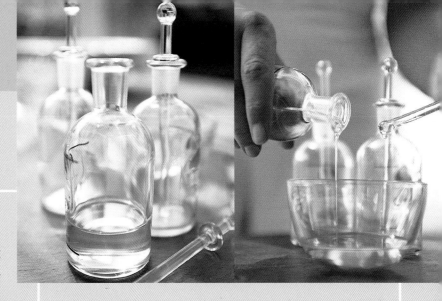

What oil should I use?

Oil is required to provide a fine, slippery surface for massage so that the skin is not pulled and stretched as you handle it. In principle, any pure vegetable or nut oil will do this. Such oils can nourish and lubricate the skin in a way that others cannot, as they are more efficiently absorbed and warm the skin to maximize absorption. Although any oil can block the pores of skin that is very fine or over-handled, pure vegetable oils do not spread a suffocating film over the skin or adversely affect its own oil production. In addition, vegetable oils contain fatty acids and fat-soluble vitamins. Many are absorbed relatively slowly by the skin, so take effect over time. Choose cold-pressed vegetable oils, which are usually sold in healthfood shops.

Some vegetable oils are better suited to certain skin types than others. Broadly speaking, the drier your skin the more it will benefit from an oil rich in saturated fatty acids. Being thicker and stickier, these are absorbed more slowly and curb water loss more effectively. Greasier skins require oils with a high percentage of polyunsaturated fats, which are thinner and quickly absorbed into the skin.

Try one of the following carrier oils according to your skin type and choose an essential oil to perfume it (see page 281), if liked.

DRY OR AGEING SKIN
Use **apricot**, **avocado**, **macadamia** or **wheatgerm oil**.

NORMAL SKIN
Use **almond**, **sunflower** or **sesame oil**. **Olive oil** is another option but is one of the thicker vegetable oils, so can be mixed with thinner oils for massage.

OILY SKIN
Use **hazelnut**, **peach kernel**, **thistle** or **hypericum oil** – the latter needs to be blended with one of the other carrier oils.

Borage and **evening primrose** are two oils with special anti-ageing properties. They are expensive so are normally blended with one of the above carrier oils, in a proportion of roughly one part to every seven of the main oil. They benefit all skin types.

---

visible). Also, if heavy oil is used for massaging sensitive skin it can penetrate the fine pores deeply, clogging them and leaving them open (see above).

Facial exercise

Despite all its proven benefits, massage alone will not rejuvenate your face. Like every other part of the body, to retain its youthful vigour, the face has to be exercised (see page 134).

SEE ALSO:

→ Skincare basics, page 114

→ Improve your complexion, page 122

→ Facial exercise, page 134

→ Self-help hair and head massage, page 147

4-minute massage

You can do this after removing make-up using a carrier oil or while applying your moisturizing cream. Once you have memorized the routine it should take no more than three to four minutes, so try to do it every day. If you have a specific area that you need to concentrate on, incorporate one of the massages from pages 131–133 into this routine.

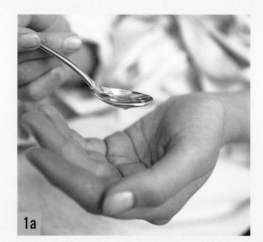
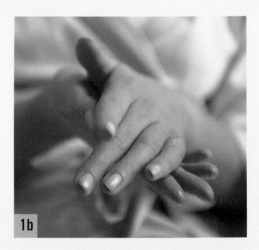

1a&b Pour just under a teaspoon of oil into one hand, rub it into both hands and apply the oil to your neck and face in long, upward and outward sweeping movements. Apply it very sparingly around your eyes, where the skin is most delicate, using the ring finger of both hands.

2 Using alternate hands, slide up your neck from the base to your jaw bone, turning the hands as necessary and working lightly over your windpipe. Cover your whole neck from ear to ear.

3 Using the first and middle fingers of each hand, slide firmly along your jaw line from your chin to the front of your ears. Your index finger should be on top of your jaw and the middle finger underneath.

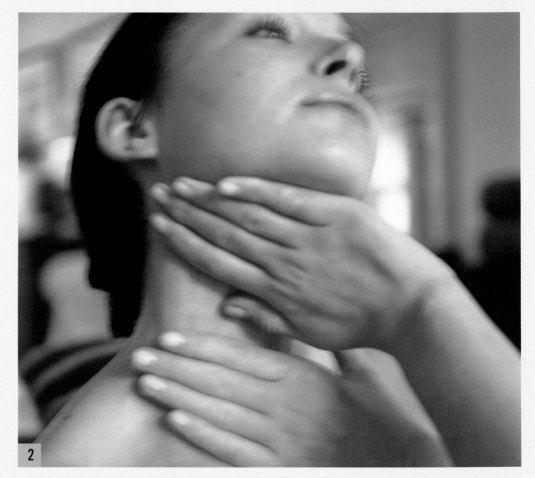

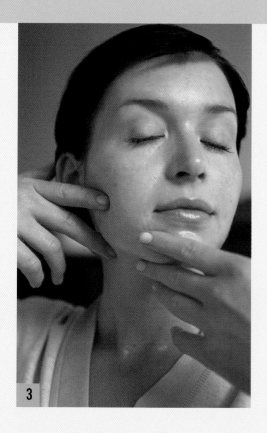

3

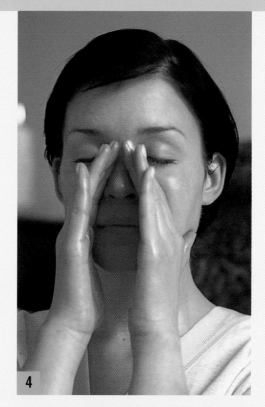

4

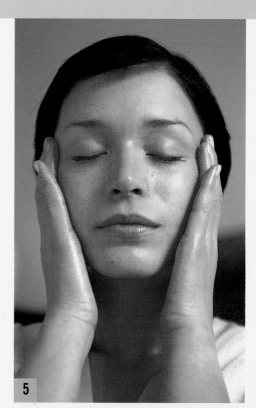

5

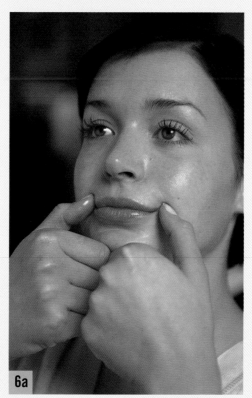

6a

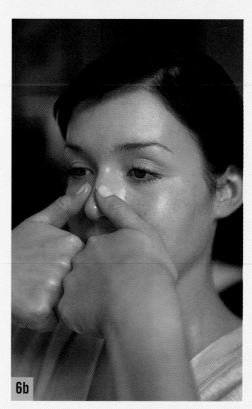

6b

4 With your fingers together and hands pointing up to your brow, holding the fingers straight, press firmly with the edge of your hands either side of your nose. **Hold for three to four seconds**.

5 Release the pressure slightly and, rolling your hands on to your cheeks, slide your hands outwards with your index fingers stopping in front of your ears and apply a firm pressure. **Hold for three to four seconds.** *Repeat.*

6a&b With your fingers held in loose fists underneath your chin, slide both thumbs upwards symmetrically around the corners of your mouth, in under your nose, around your nostrils and lightly off over the tip of your nose.

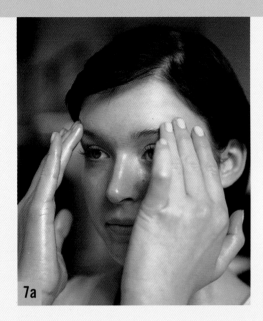

7a

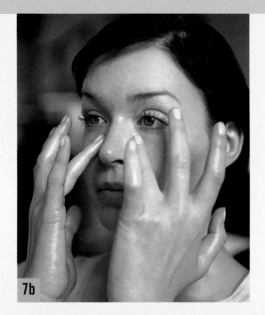

7b

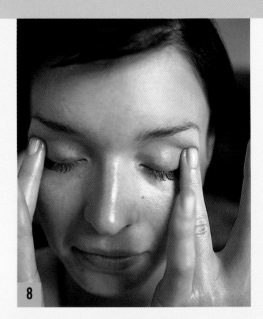

8

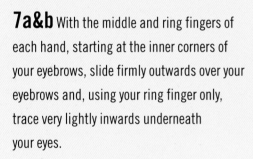

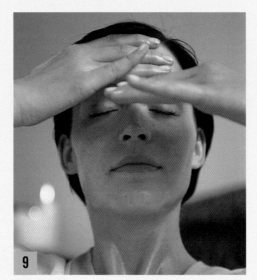

9

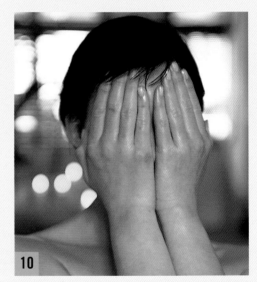

10

7a&b With the middle and ring fingers of each hand, starting at the inner corners of your eyebrows, slide firmly outwards over your eyebrows and, using your ring finger only, trace very lightly inwards underneath your eyes.

8 With the ring finger of each hand, slide lightly outwards over your closed eyelids and then lightly underneath each eye.

9 With your fingers together and the index fingers leading the way, alternately smooth your hands up to the hairline in a firm lifting movement, starting between the eyebrows and finishing at the hairline.

10 Close your eyes and, with the fingers together and using the whole of both hands slightly cupped to produce a gentle suction, apply a firm pressure to the face, holding for a second before releasing. Then, moving the hands outwards from the nose towards the

ears, cover the whole face, moving the hands up and down to cover the area between the chin and hairline.

11 With your fingers together and using the whole of the hand, apply pressure with the right hand to the left side of the neck, working from the base of the neck to the jaw but avoiding the windpipe. *Repeat with the left hand*, applying pressures to the right side of the neck.

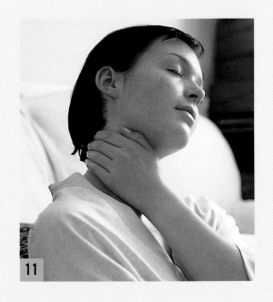

11

Massage for problem areas

You may have areas of your face that call for extra attention. The following massage exercises can remedy or prevent such problem areas, and can be fitted into the 4-minute massage routine on pages 128–130.

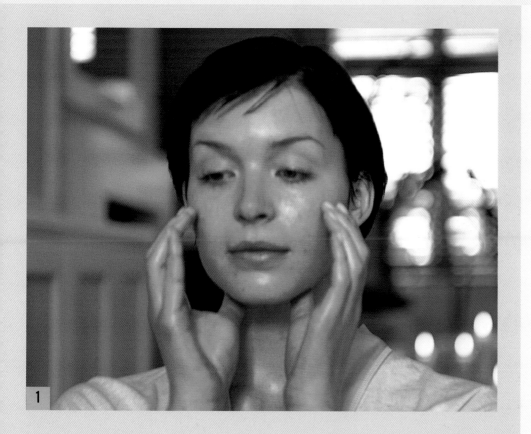

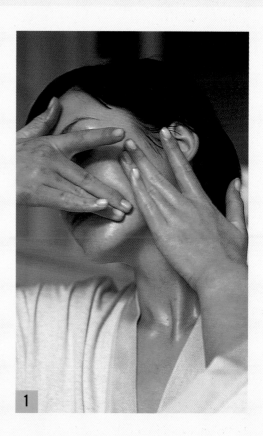

For a double chin

1 With the fingers relaxed, use the thumbs to press into the muscle underneath the jaw, starting in the centre of the chin and working outwards towards the angle of the jaw bone. **(This can be done after Step 2 of the 4-minute massage.)**

For jowls

1 Using the flat middle and ring fingers of both hands alternately and treating one side at a time, work on the muscles of the cheeks with a rolling, lifting movement, almost flicking the muscle upwards. **(Do this after Step 4 of the 4-minute massage.)**

For wrinkled lips

1&2 Smiling to stretch the lips taut, and anchoring the middle finger of your left hand on the left corner of the mouth, use the middle finger of the right hand to make small, circular movements all the way along the edge of the bottom lip. Then swap hands to use the middle finger of the left hand and repeat the circles on the edge of the upper lip. (**Do this after Step 6 of the 4-minute massage.**)

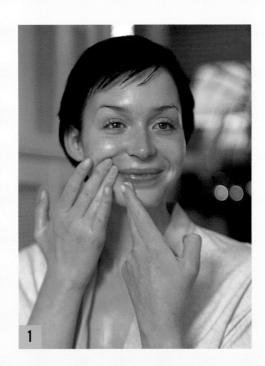
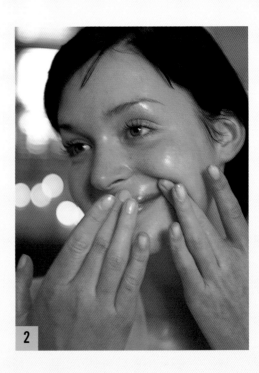

For frown lines between the eyes

1 With the index and middle fingers of your left hand supporting the skin in an upward V-shape, apply small circular movements with the ring finger of your right hand between the eyebrows. (**Do this after Step 8 of the 4-minute massage.**)

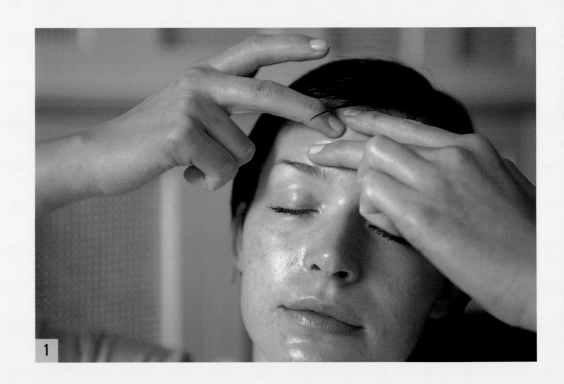

For open pores on the nose and between the eyes

1 With your middle or ring finger, make small circular movements all over and around your nose. Start by working around your nostrils, over the tip of your nose and up the sides of your nose, finishing on the bridge. (**Do this after Step 2 of the 4-minute massage.**)

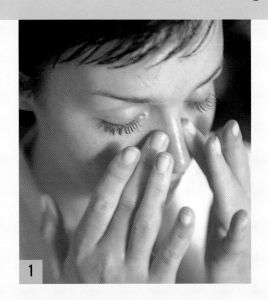

For crow's feet

1 With the middle or ring finger of each hand, make a crossroads shape where the crow's feet are emerging by tracing a horizontal then a vertical line, alternately working with the middle fingers of each hand, out from the corner of your eye and up towards the temple. (**Do this after Step 8 of the 4-minute massage.**)

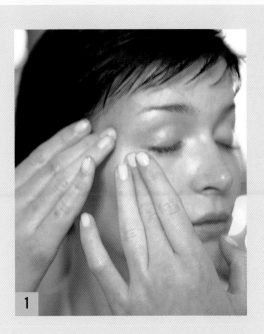

For brow lines on the forehead

1 Locate the brow lines across your forehead. Starting above your right eye, make small, circular, sliding movements along each line from right to left using the middle finger of your right hand. Use the index and middle fingers of your left hand to hold the skin firm on either side of the line. *Repeat the movement on each line.* (**Do this after Step 9 of the 4-minute massage.**)

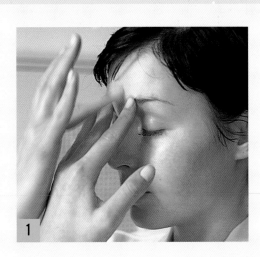

Facial exercise

Thanks to the prominence of aerobic exercise and body sculpting today most people are aware of the importance of muscle tone to general health and appearance. Yet it rarely occurs to even the most self-conscious individuals to keep the face toned. The facial muscles can, however, be trained just as easily as other muscles in the body.

Of course, the shape of your face is fundamentally determined by your bone structure. You can do little about the bulbous Roman nose or obtrusive ears you have inherited, without the help of a cosmetic surgeon. However, you can make your chin stronger, your eyes less hollow, your lips fuller or your cheeks more prominent by exercising the muscles there. You can also counteract the effects of the facial muscles being constantly pulled, contracted, tensed and stretched in unequal measures at different times, which results in the formation of corrugations deep in their structure and ultimately surface wrinkles.

Facial exercises require no special equipment or venue. You can do them virtually anytime, anywhere: in traffic jams, in queues, at your desk or in the bathroom. The younger you are when you start facial gymnastics, the better. However, it is never too late to start.

Three steps to a fit face

The facial exercises on the following pages all follow a similar three-part pattern, based on the following common principles:

1 FINDING Dormant muscles will not be very prominent and small ones may take practice to locate. At first, it will help to look in the mirror while doing the exercise.

2 RESISTING Providing resistance against which the muscle can exert its force limits blood flow to the muscle. The flow is then increased and the oxygen in the new rush of blood feeds and builds up the muscle.

3 RELAXING The exercised muscle needs to be consciously relaxed after it has been tensed. If this does not happen, then the sustained tension and tightness will interfere with the efficient circulation of blood and this may produce cramps.

Tips for facial exercise

- Always make sure your face is relaxed before you start.
- Apply a light cream or oil to help minimize stretching of the skin. Ensure your face is clean before you put on any lubricant.

- Warm up the muscles before you begin to exercise them, particularly if you are exercising a 'problem area' regularly.
- While you are getting used to these exercises, place a mirror at head height to comfortably follow the moves and watch your face as you exercise.

- If at any time you feel pain, stop. It is probably an indication that you are using the wrong muscles. Re-read the instructions, try to visualize the muscles you will be exercising, concentrate on them and attempt the exercise once more later on.

Before and after

When training any part of the body through exercise, it is important to warm up first and cool down after. A warm-up helps to relieve any tension in the muscles to be used and to increase circulation, while a quick cool-down routine helps to prevent cramp or aches developing. The face is no exception and will benefit most from the exercises on the following pages if the routines here are done before and after.

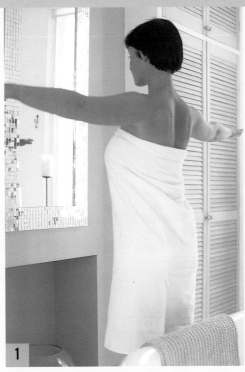

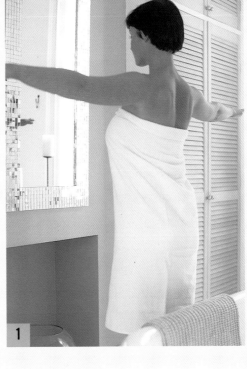

Warm-up

1 Standing or sitting upright, extend the arms out to the sides at shoulder height. Make 10 small circular movements forwards with the whole arm, rotating from the shoulder sockets. Do the same moving the arms backwards. *Repeat three to five times* each way, increasing the size of the circles with each repetition. This helps to loosen up the whole throat and neck area, improving blood flow.

Cool-down

1 *Repeat the procedure for the warm-up*, then slump forwards with your head almost touching your knees. The whole upper body should be limp, with the arms hanging like pendulums. **Breathe in** and **out deeply**. This helps to keep up the flow of lymph, which drains away any toxins that may have built up during exercise.

- Never pull the skin. The muscle is moved, not the skin in resistance exercises.
- In exercises for muscles that mirror each other on either side of your face, exercise each side equally. Symmetry is one of the fundamental principles of bodily beauty.

- Exercise your face every day if possible. As with other forms of bodily toning, a little regularly is more effective than a bumper session once in a while.
- Take time over each exercise. There is more benefit in doing one exercise properly than doing 10 in passing.

- Relax between exercises. The relaxation period should be as long as each exercise period.
- Focus on your breathing and do not hold your breath.
- Even if you feel tired or in a hurry, follow the 'cool-down' routine afterwards.

Exercise routines

Choose the exercises that work the areas you want to improve and spend no more than a minute on each. Starting with a mirror and bookstand at home, practise the moves until you can relinquish the prompts and props and exercise on the move, grabbing five minutes whenever and wherever you can.

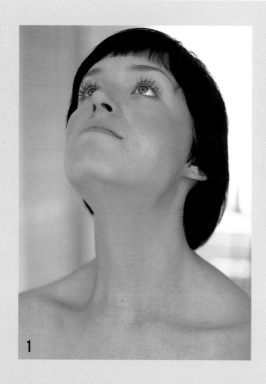

1

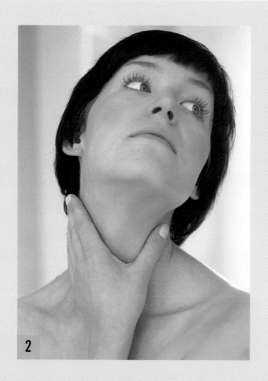

2

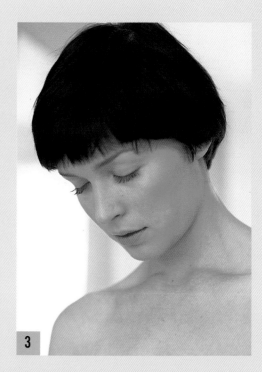

3

Neck

This exercise works on the four main muscles that run down the neck on either side of the Adam's apple. It helps to firm up the throat and lift the breast tissue, while increasing circulation to the whole face.

1 Tip your head back and jut out your bottom jaw. Pushing your chin forward so that the lower teeth overlap the upper ones, feel your neck muscles extend fully. Breathe the remaining air out of your chest.

2 Turn your head alternately to the right and left, attempting to look over each

shoulder. Holding the neck between your thumb and fingers, move your head from side to side again.

3 Let your head droop forwards and nod gently backwards and forwards then from right to left several times.

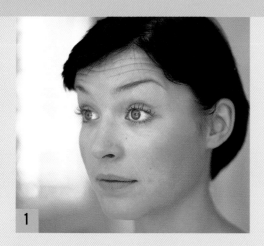

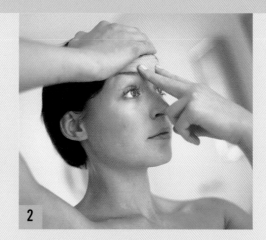

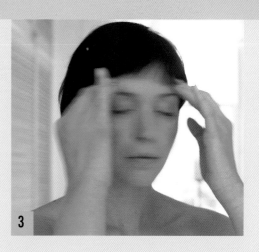

Brow lines

This works on the central part of the forehead muscles, helping to smooth out horizontal wrinkles of the forehead.

1 Raise your eyebrows, open your eyes wide and stare at a fixed point in front of you.

2 Place the tips of your index and middle or ring fingers just above the eyebrows and raise the eyebrows against their resistance.

3 Press three fingers of each hand above the eyebrows lightly and shake the head gently.

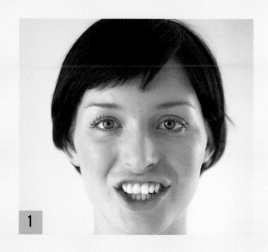

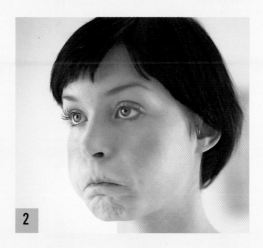

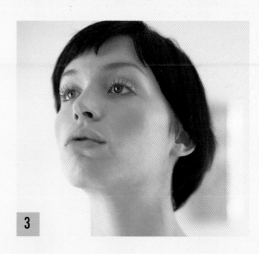

Laughter lines

This exercise works on the muscles of the upper lip by helping reduce the prominence of the lines running from the outer edge of the nostrils to the corners of the mouth.

1 Raise the corners of your mouth and upper lip, stretching the top lip over the top teeth while opening your mouth about 2 cm (1 in). Keep your mouth and neck muscles relaxed. You should feel a tension in the cheek pads.

2 Suck the air into one cheek then move it to the opposite cheek. Then suck air into both

cheeks and into the area above your top lip, in a way that no horizontal or vertical lines are visible. 'Chew' the air. *Repeat five to 10 times.*

3 Pursing the lips gently, open them about 1 cm (½ in) as if blowing bubbles and exhale the air gently.

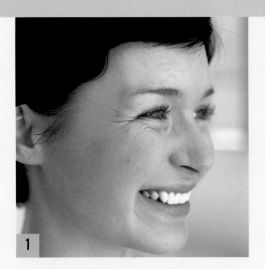
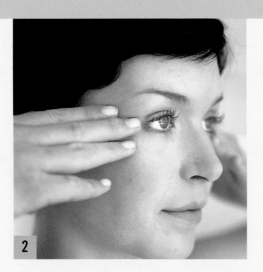
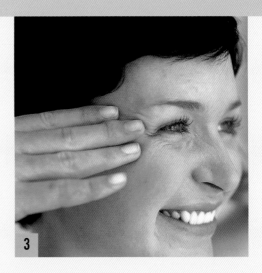

Crow's feet

This works on the outer edge of the eye ring muscle, which contracts when you laugh or smile.

1 Wrinkle your eyes so that you can clearly see the crows' feet on the outer corners of your eyes.

2 Put your three middle fingers horizontally facing inwards over the skin where the crow's feet emerge.

3 Try to create the crow's feet again against the pressure of the fingertips.

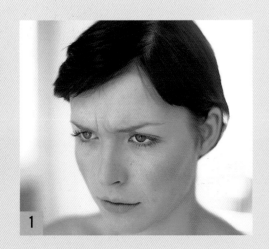
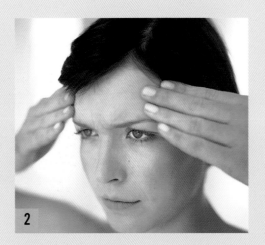
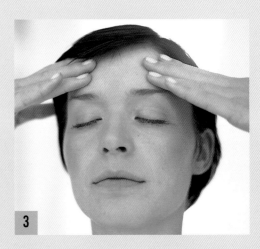

Frown lines

This exercise works on the muscles that create the vertical corrugations that form between the eyes when you frown.

1 Frown tightly, then relax the muscles.

2 Put your three middle fingers from each hand on the temple muscle, on the outer edge of each eyebrow, and frown again, feeling the pull on your fingers.

3 Close the eyes and loosely shake out the muscles by vibrating your fingertips over the muscle lightly.

Double chin

This works on the muscle that is connected to the breast bone and which tenses when you chew or stick your chin out.

1 Hold your head upright and tense the shoulder muscles. Roll your tongue back against the roof of the mouth, and press backwards towards your throat, as if swallowing the tongue. If you feel that this movement is overstretching your skin, open your mouth slightly.

2 Try to swallow. *Repeat four or five times.*

3 Bow your head, open your mouth slightly and slowly move your head from side to side, keeping your jaw loose.

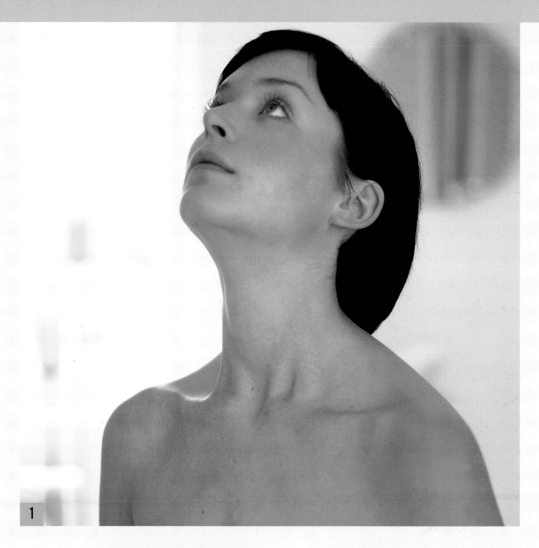

1

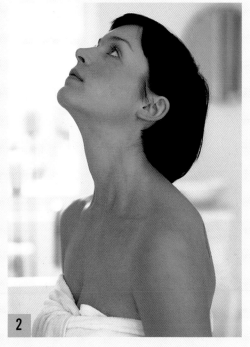

2

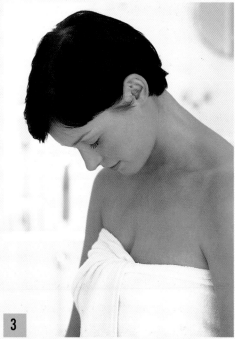

3

Sparkling eyes

Said to be the windows on the soul, your eyes are often the first thing people notice about you. Sparkling eyes are an indication of good health. The most effective way to maintain that inner sparkle is by resting your eyes with sufficient sleep and not overstraining them with inadequate lighting and overlong periods of close work or computer use.

Eyestrain

Tired eyes and eyestrain are common problems. The most obvious causes are long hours spent in artificial or bad light, reading and doing close work, especially in front of a computer screen; others include day-to-day stresses, incorrectly prescribed glasses and pollution. Feelings of tightness around the eyes, difficulties in focusing and headaches can all ensue.

Preventing eyestrain can be simple. Make sure you work or read in a good light, take brief breaks every hour from a computer screen or close work and focus on distant objects for a few seconds to alter your depth of vision. Have your eyes checked regularly and do not

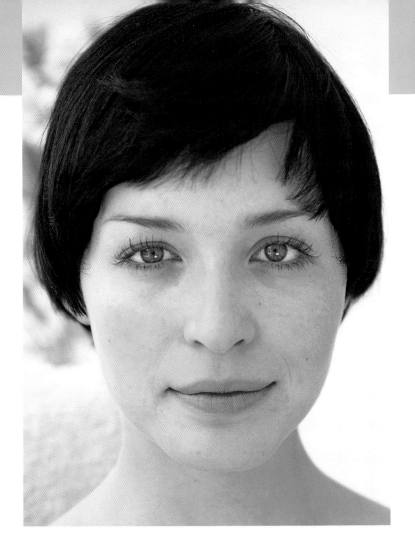

watch television in the dark. Closing your eyes and pressing very gently on the eyelids with your palms can also help (remove contact lenses first if you wear them). A simple remedy is to lie down in a darkened room, place slices of cucumber or cotton wool pads dipped in chilled milk over the eyelids and relax for 10 minutes.

Contact lens care

Spectacles have become a wonderful fashion accessory nowadays but you may prefer wearing contact lenses to glasses. Always wash your hands and dry them well before handling your lenses. Avoid perfumed or medicated soaps, and remember to apply make-up, hand creams and lotions after inserting your lenses to avoid getting particles in your eyes, which cause irritation.

Bags and circles

If you suffer from puffy bags or dark circles beneath your eyes they may be hereditary, in which case you cannot get rid of them although you can help them. Manual lymphatic drainage massage (see page 106) in conjunction with a good eye product may help reduce puffiness; drinking plenty of water and using an eye product that strengthens the under-eye area will help dark circles. Otherwise there is very little you can do about them, other than disguise them.

If the puffiness beneath your eyes is due to excessive alcohol, rich foods and little sleep, the following exercise is beneficial in

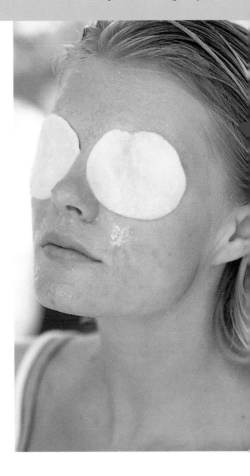

conjunction with an eye cream, but bear in mind that continual excesses will cause the delicate skin beneath the eyes to stretch and may result in a permanent problem. Using the ring finger of each hand, press firmly but gently for the count of three at small intervals along the eye socket, working from the inner corners out to the temples. Keep going until you reach the 'dip' just to the outside of your eye sockets. This is the point where the toxins you have moved along from the under-eye area will be released into your bloodstream.

Natural remedies

A number of herbs can help for soothing, toning and brightening eyes. Eyebright is a particularly helpful herb for various eye troubles and makes an effective eye compress. Make an infusion using 1 tablespoon of chopped eyebright and 150 ml (¼ pint) of boiling water. Leave until cold, strain into a screwtop bottle and use within 12 hours. To make a compress, soak two cotton wool pads in the cold eyebright infusion, squeeze slightly and place one over each eyelid. Rest for 10 minutes – an ideal time is while lying in the bath – replacing the soaked cotton wool once it becomes warm. Finally, dab the eyes with fresh cold water and pat dry with a soft clean towel.

An infusion of elderflower, made in the same way, is a mild stimulant and can be used in a compress for brightening the eyes. An infusion of camomile flowers makes a soothing compress and reduces inflammation.

Camomile or rosehip teabags, available from healthfood stores, can be used for puffiness and dark circles under the eyes. Steep two teabags for three minutes in boiling water, then remove and set aside. When they are sufficiently cooled, place one over each eye. Leave for 10 minutes and sip the tea while resting. Another remedy for puffy eyes is to apply the grated flesh of an unpeeled potato to closed eyelids for about 20 minutes. Cucumber juice applied to the area below your eyes every night at bed time may help if you have dark circles.

The sun and your eyes

Just as your body needs protection from the sun's rays (see page 154), so do your eyes and the sensitive skin around them. You should always wear sunglasses when you are exposed to solar radiation. Choose dark sunglasses with good-quality lenses that guarantee to block all or 95 per cent of UVB. Glasses that block less than this do not provide enough eye protection and are merely fashion accessories. Wraparound sunglasses are useful for hay fever sufferers as they help protect the eyes from pollen.

SEE ALSO:

→ Facial massage, page 126

→ Facial exercise, page 134

→ Sun safety, page 154

→ Peaceful slumber, page 238

→ Healing herbs, page 288

Mouth talk

There is little point in acquiring a smooth and glowing complexion if you don't have a smile to match. To avoid problems with your teeth and gums, have regular dental check-ups and treatment by a dental hygienist at least every six months – more frequently if you are a smoker and/or red wine drinker since both habits stain tooth enamel. If you are one of the many people with a dental phobia, try hypnotherapy to banish those anxieties.

Teething troubles

Clean your teeth morning and night, preferably using dental floss and an electric toothbrush. It takes only minutes for sugar to attack tooth enamel so also try to carry a travel toothbrush with you during the day so that you can scrub your teeth after eating anything sweet.

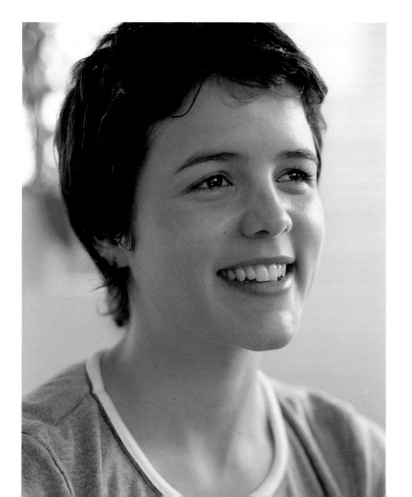

Toothache For emergency pain relief for toothache, add a few drops of oil of cloves to cotton wool and apply it to the gum. Apart from such obvious damage as a cracked filling or broken tooth, a more likely cause of sudden and severe tooth pain is an abscess or infection. This can often be associated with general feelings of being unwell or might follow a cold. Echinacea or garlic tablets are suitable herbal remedies that boost the immune system and counter infections. They can provide relief and may help disperse abscesses. Take three 200 mg capsules up to three times a day.

Bad breath Most bad breath (halitosis) originates from the mouth. It is caused by the bacteria present in the mouth acting on decomposing microscopic food particles to form plaque, which can produce smelly gases. Since saliva is the body's natural defence against bacteria, reduced saliva flow (a dry mouth) means more bacterial activity and therefore bad breath. Certain medication, alcohol and smoking can lead to a dry mouth, as can breathing through your mouth. A dry mouth on waking is normal and is remedied by rinsing, then consuming a couple of large glasses of water followed by a dry food such as bread to stimulate saliva.

Bad breath is largely prevented by keeping your mouth moist and by good dental hygiene. The former includes chewing sugar-free gum after meals to encourage saliva production, and drinking at least 1.8 litres (3 pints) of water daily. Good dental hygiene means keeping teeth and gums healthy with a daily, thorough removal of bacterial build-up. Using a toothbrush and dental floss, remove plaque from around and between teeth and use a toothbrush to clean your tongue of bacteria. Mouthwashes and mints can mask bad breath temporarily but they cannot prevent it. A mouthwash containing alcohol can in fact exacerbate the condition by making the mouth drier.

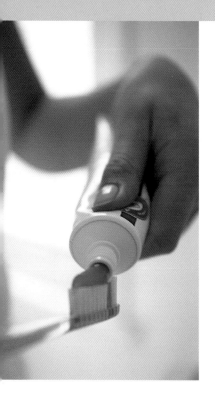

Dietary measures used to prevent bad breath include eating plenty of fresh fruit and vegetables and reducing your consumption of meat products, particularly red meat. Avoid snacking on foods packed with refined sugars, which can greatly increase the bacterial growth in the mouth.

If you do suffer from halitosis despite following the advice above, visit a dentist for advice on the state of your teeth and gums and on dental care.

Bad breath caused by foods such as garlic, onions, chillies or eggs is temporary and soon passes. Simply avoid these foodstuffs on the occasions that it matters.

Luscious lips

If you have continually chapped, cracked lips, it could be that you need to drink more water regularly to hydrate your body from the inside, and consume more vitamin B2 (riboflavin) – in the form of milk, dark green vegetables, wholegrains and cereals.

Using lipstick If you are prone to dry lips, apply a moisturizing cream before using lipstick. Lipstick applied with a small brush will last longest as it reaches inside all the lines of your lips, rather than being swept over the top of them.

Since the skin of your lips is very delicate, use a gentle moisturizing cream cleanser to remove lipstick. Smear it generously over your lips and gently wipe each lip in turn using a piece of cotton wool, ensuring you remove any colour left between the creases.

Home-made lip lotion

20 g (¾ oz) white beeswax
25 ml (1 fl oz) olive oil
1 teaspoon jojoba oil
1 capsule vitamin E
3 drops calendula essence

Heat up some water in a double boiler and, when the water is bubbling, put the beeswax and olive oil in the top compartment. When the beeswax is completely melted, remove from the heat and beat the ointment until it has started to thicken and cooled to around 40–45°C (104–113°F) – you can use a cooking thermometer to check. Add the remaining ingredients and beat thoroughly again. Leave to cool in a small jar. Lavender or geranium essential oils are also good for dry lips.

Use downward strokes for the upper lip and upward strokes for the lower lip, so as not to pull the skin in different directions and induce fine lines and wrinkles. Finally apply a layer of moisturizing lip treatment cream or a lip balm (see box above).

SEE ALSO:
→ Everyday toxins, page 94

→ Water, page 96

→ Skincare basics, page 114

→ Improve your complexion, page 122

→ Facial massage, page 126

→ Facial exercise, page 134

→ Aromatherapy, page 278

Haircare essentials

Your hair reflects the state of your inner health and wellbeing. An unhealthy diet and lifestyle, tiredness and stress all take their toll on your hair. However, the good news is that hair also has the ability to transform the way you look and feel – be it with a change of style or colour, or simply a cut or some new eyecatching accessory. Good haircare involves nourishing it and treating it well, and using the right products. The essential thing is to find a hairstyle that suits both you and your lifestyle.

Diet

Like the rest of your body, your scalp and hair require a balanced diet with vitamins, minerals and other nutrients. If your hair is looking dull and dry, it could be that that you are not drinking enough water (see page 96) or eating enough essential fatty acids (EFAs). EFAs aid the production of sebum, thereby naturally lubricating hair, so make sure you are eating plenty of nuts, sunflower seeds and sesame seeds.

Haircare products

There is a bewildering array of haircare products – containing various ingredients and making various claims. Choose those suitable for your hair type – normal, combination, greasy or dry – and experiment until you find the ones that suit you best. Your hair will benefit most from a four-step regime of care – rather like skincare – namely, shampoo, condition, protect and style. Such care on a regular basis will encourage your hair to become stronger and more resistant to damage.

Shampoos Shampoo cleanses the hair shaft, gently lifting away grime, dust and natural oil. Experiment with various good-quality pH-balanced shampoos until you find the one whose ingredients suit you best. Colour-treated hair has had its pH balance changed and needs a specially formulated shampoo that will gently cleanse while nourishing the colour.

Make sure you rinse thoroughly to remove all traces of shampoo from your hair until it feels 'squeaky' clean – the slightest residue of shampoo will leave the hair dull and sticky enough to attract dirt immediately. A final rinse in very cold water is beneficial for hair growth and shine as it stimulates the scalp.

Conditioners Just as face cream nourishes your skin, a conditioner is necessary to moisturize your hair and should be used each time you wash your hair. It coats each hair shaft protectively and helps repair weakened hair. If you have particularly dry hair, use a deep conditioning hair treatment or hair mask once a week. Since these conditioners are left on the hair longer, they have more time to penetrate the hair shaft and condition the hair. Similarly, colour-treated hair requires an intensive conditioner every third wash to help maintain moisture levels and enhance the richness of the colour.

Styling and finishing products These products protect hair from the heat and oxidation caused by ultraviolet light and everyday pollution. Again, you will have to experiment with the huge range of products available – sprays, serums, mousses, gels and waxes, which are variously designed to provide body and lift, to sculpt or hold styles, to control frizz or flyaway hair, to revitalize curls or to give shine. Avoid sticky products and don't drag your hair down by overusing products so that it looks lank and flat.

10 tips for top hair

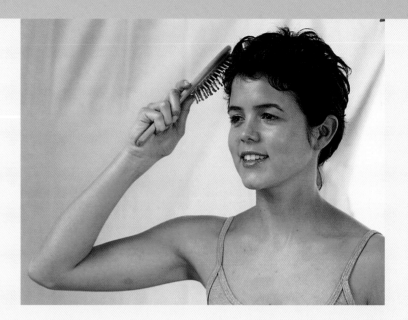

- **Banish split ends** by having your hair trimmed regularly. Use a wide-toothed comb rather than a brush on wet hair and don't overheat your hair when blow-drying — use a nozzle and direct the hot air parallel to the hair shaft rather than directly on the hair.

- **To treat dandruff** choose a naturally based product and avoid any that contain metal oxides. Rinse your hair well after a dandruff treatment and avoid touching the scalp as it may be more prone to picking up infection.

- Always use a **good-quality hairbrush**. Poor-quality brushes and combs will scratch the scalp and damage the hair shaft. Don't overbrush your hair since this will stimulate sebum production, encouraging oily hair, breakages and split ends.

- **Brush your hair before washing** it to massage the scalp and help loosen dead skin cells.

- **Never use hotter than a medium heat when blow-drying**. Finish blow-drying with a blast of cold air to close the cuticles — when cuticles lie flat, hair reflects the light and looks healthier and shinier.

- If you **colour your hair**, try to avoid non-organic dyes, especially peroxides. Temporary colours can be easily washed in and out at home — some lasting for just one shampoo, others for up to 12 washes.

- **Avoid overdrying colour-treated hair** with dryers, heated rollers or curling tongs. Let it dry naturally if possible.

- If you are of 'a certain age', why not forget about colorants and **consider letting your natural greying/silvering hair colour come through**? Perhaps make a fresh start and have your hair cut in a shorter style to remove all the damaged, discoloured and mistreated hair. Jump before you are pushed!

- **Try conditioning your hair** with inexpensive natural ingredients such as egg yolks (for normal to dry hair), egg whites (for oily or balanced hair), or a strong herbal infusion of camomile (for oily or balanced hair).

- **Protect colour-treated hair** against the effects of sun, sea and swimming pools. Wear a hat or scarf in hot sun, wear a swimming cap or apply a conditioner to act as a barrier against chlorine. Always shampoo hair immediately after swimming.

SEE ALSO:

→ A balanced diet, page 14

→ Fats, page 22

→ Top foods for health, page 28

→ Water, page 96

→ Healthy hair naturally, page 146

→ Living with stress, page 230

→ Aromatherapy, page 278

→ Healing herbs, page 288

Healthy hair naturally

Natural oiling means giving your hair a conditioning treatment by not washing it for several days. This will allow the hair's natural oils to imbue it with a rich cocktail of self-produced minerals and sebaceous fluids. It might sound a little off-putting in a culture obsessed with frequent cleansing and shampooing, but there are ways of minimizing the sense of your hair 'being dirty'.

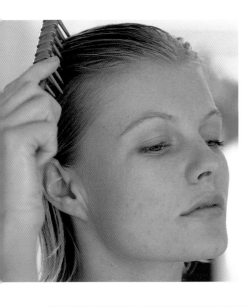

Pinning up or tying back longer hair is a useful cosmetic solution if you are concerned about how it looks during this period. Brush or comb through your hair twice daily and massage your scalp as often as you can to stimulate the production of the minerals that are your own natural bounty.

Hair growth stimulant

An aromatherapy hair growth stimulant can be a beneficial treatment if your hair seems very thin or if you have lost hair because of childbirth, stress or as a reaction to illness or drugs. Add 10 drops of rosemary oil, 10 drops of lavender oil and 5 drops of sandalwood oil to 50 ml (2 fl oz) of carrier oil and massage it into your scalp. Leave for a few hours or overnight before washing out.

Aromatherapy hair treatment

An alternative to natural oiling is to use essential oils to give your hair a deep cleansing treatment. Combine the hair treatment with an aromatherapy facial if you like (see page 116), applying it before you cleanse your face. It contains oily substances, so you will probably want to wash your hair once you have finished the facial. Alternatively, leave the treatment on your hair all night and wash it off when you shower in the morning.

Make up the treatment oil suitable for your hair type by adding the following essential oils to 50 ml (2 fl oz) of vegetable oil. For greasy hair, add 10 drops of cedarwood essence, 10 drops of lavender and 5 drops of grapefruit. For dry and damaged hair, add 10 drops of rosewood, 10 drops of lavender and 5 drops of sandalwood essence. Massage your chosen treatment in well, then wrap a towel around your head and leave for as long as possible.

Herbal help

Herbs can play a vital role in keeping hair looking healthy and lustrous, stimulating its growth and strengthening it. Good herbs for the hair are nettle, horsetail, camomile, rosemary, parsley and yarrow. A simple infusion made of any one of these herbs, and then rubbed daily into the scalp or used as a rinse after shampooing will stimulate hair growth and keep the scalp clean. Infusions of mixed herbs can be used for specific treatment. For example, combine camomile and yarrow flowers for use on blonde hair to highlight the colour, and use an infusion of sage and rosemary on dark hair to give it an impressive sheen.

Some herbs should be avoided in pregnancy or by those with very sensitive skin so do take advice from a herbalist or staff at your local healthfood shop before using them.

Self-help hair and head massage

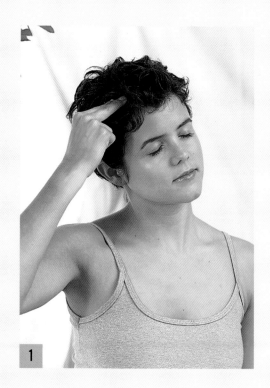

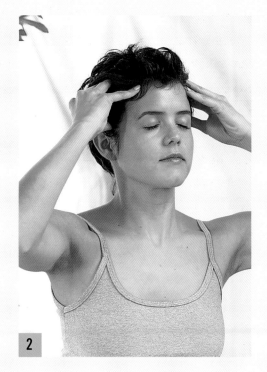

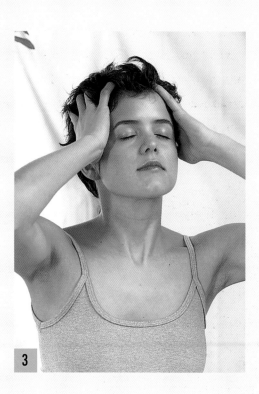

Experiencing a stressful day, becoming hot and bothered, grinding your teeth, squinting or even talking too much can all lead to pressure building up inside your head, contributing to tension headaches and lack of mental focus. The following sequence can help to relieve them.

1 Using your index and middle fingers, rub the scalp in circular spiral movements, lifting and lightening your hair. This simple technique helps to give the hair 'body' and invigorates the scalp. It will also recharge your batteries when you feel that your mental energies are flagging.

2 Using your fingertips, make small circular movements, moving the scalp away from the skull. *Repeat all over the head.* This can often bring almost instant relief from tension headaches, as does simply pulling tufts of hair close to the scalp.

3 Run your hands up over your face and rake your fingers through the hair. *Repeat from the nape of the neck through to the crown of the head.* This gives instant mental relief after a concentrated day.

SEE ALSO:

→ Haircare essentials, page 144

→ Stress in the workplace, page 236

→ Aromatherapy, page 278

→ Healing herbs, page 288

147

Pampering your body

Looking after your body entails the basics such as feeding and watering it, allowing it to rest, keeping it fit and clean and protecting it from a fierce sun and other harsh climatic conditions. However, there are many additional things you can do to pamper your body – not only for cosmetic reasons but for general good health, too. Not only will they make you feel good physically, they will also generate a sense of calm and wellbeing, and are the perfect antidote to stress.

4

Top-to-toe bodycare

Taking time out for yourself is an important aspect of general wellbeing. For many, there is no better way to spend such time than enjoying pampering, luxurious beauty treatments or products. It could be a visit to a health farm or beauty salon, a professional massage or manicure, or the pleasure of bathtime goodies in the comfort of one's own home. While some pampering treats have purely cosmetic results, others are for general good health, and all engender a sense of wellbeing. Some are luxuries to be experienced only once in a while, others are bodycare routines that should be regular rather than occasional.

Skincare

When it comes to skincare it is natural that your face steals the limelight, but you shouldn't neglect the rest of your skin. Nor should you consider skincare only a seasonal necessity – your skin needs attention all year round, not just in summer when you emerge from thick layers of winter clothing.

Just as with your face (see page 118), removing dead skin cells by exfoliation is important for overall skin health. It can be achieved using a gentle body scrub (see page 166) or using a special exfoliating sponge or body cloth with your favourite shower gel or body wash. The exfoliating action is also beneficial in stimulating circulation and lymph flow.

Moisturizing All skin is susceptible to dryness, flaking and blemishes so another key aspect of body skincare is moisturizing. Regular moisturizing helps prevent the skin from losing its moisture content and becoming dry and brittle, and protects it from harmful bacteria, harsh weather and the dry atmosphere of centrally heated or air-conditioned environments. Some modern fabrics also have a drying effect on skin, soaking up the protective layer of sebum and rubbing

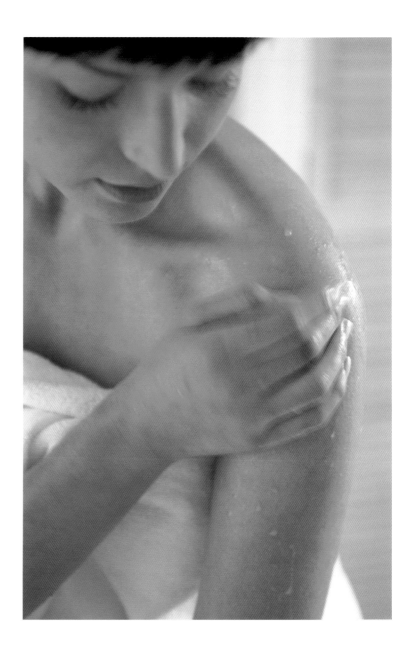

away the uppermost skin cells. The elbows and knees, where the skin is thinner than usual and invariably leant or kneeled on, are particularly prone to extreme dryness, which results in rough, dry or discoloured skin.

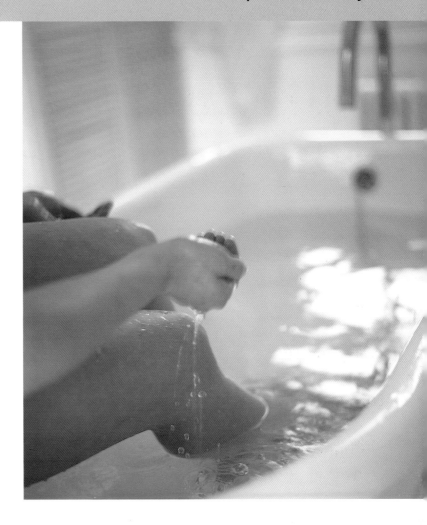

Some people naturally have drier skin than others. Your skin type (normal, oily, dry or sensitive), bathing habits, exercise routine and the season or climate in which you live will all determine how much moisturizer the skin on your body requires. If you have minimal moisturizing needs, a simple bath oil will lock in your body's moisture without oversaturating the skin. If you have particularly dry skin, however, apply a hand and body lotion while your skin is still damp from the bath or shower. Let your skin dry without towelling yourself to allow the moisture to be absorbed. Very dry skin will require an intensive body lotion for instant hydration – again apply it to wet skin and do not towel yourself dry afterwards.

As with facial moisturizing, your skin's response to moisturizing treatment is accumulative, so the more frequently you use your moisturizer, the better your skin will look and feel. Aim to apply it as often as possible.

Shaving tips

- It is essential to wash any area of unwanted hair with warm soapy water before shaving. The water softens the hair and makes it much easier to cut.
- Rinsing and shaking excess water off a razor blade rather than wiping it will help to preserve the blade's sharpness.
- Shaving under your arms reduces the bacteria in the armpits and therefore body odour.
- Do not apply deodorant or antiperspirant immediately after shaving under your arms.

Aromatherapy treats

Many of the latest bodycare products are mood specific, containing blends of certain essential oils to stimulate specific emotions, thoughts and feelings. Bath oils, shower gels, body washes, soaps and body lotions are just some of the bodycare products designed for pampering and for use on specific occasions – for example, relaxing for bedtime, calming for relieving stress, energizing for first thing in the morning, or sensual for a romantic evening. Discover the ones you like and pamper yourself!

SEE ALSO:

→ Skincare basics, page 114

→ Exfoliation, page 118

→ Bathing and showering, page 152

→ Salt body scrub, page 166

→ Skin brushing, page 168

→ Aromatherapy, page 278

Bathing and showering

Bathing and showering are a vital part of health and wellbeing since, besides the issue of cleanliness, in our increasingly hectic lives a long soak in the bath or an invigorating splash in the shower is often a welcome opportunity to relax. Treat yourself with pampering items from the huge range of bathing products available, and make this quiet time a refreshing and enjoyable experience that is just for you.

Luxurious baths

Although showers are quicker and often more convenient, soaking in a bath is a real treat. To maximize the quality time spent in this relaxed state, bathing should be a full pampering experience and not a rushed dip in and out. For the ultimate in relaxation, do some deep breathing exercises (see page 240), and make a conscious effort to relax all your muscles, one by one.

Comforting bubbles Add bubblebath or essential oils to your bath water (see pages 280–1 and 282), or make a sachet of therapeutic herbs using a small square of muslin. Place the herbs on top

of the muslin, knot the four corners together and tie the sachet under the tap so that the running water flows through it and the sachet is submerged when the bath is full. Use bay leaves or cinnamon bark for scent, camomile for sensitive skin, or ginger to improve your circulation.

Soothing scents Surrounding yourself with a favourite scent encourages complete relaxation. An alternative to using perfumed bath products is to fill the bathroom with scent by burning an essential oil in a burner or by burning aromatherapy candles.

Finishing touches Remain in the bath for at least 15 minutes to moisturize your skin but for no longer than half an hour. After soaking, sweep a sponge, flannel or loofah smeared with cleanser over your body with long smooth strokes, working from your extremities inwards towards your heart.

Use a pumice stone on any particularly tough skin on the bottom of your feet, knees or elbows. Finish by taking a quick shower to wash away any residual soap from the bath products, and apply a moisturizer, paying particular attention to overdry areas of skin, such as the feet, lower legs and elbows.

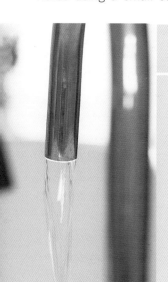

Temperature tip

Don't shower or bathe in water that is so hot that it makes you drowsy and robs you of energy – about 35°C (95°F) is ideal. If you have a tendency to develop spider veins, you should avoid very hot water.

Showertime

Even if you are stepping under the jet for only a few minutes, maximize the experience by using a luxury shower gel with a textured skin sponge to exfoliate your skin.

If your skin is dry or sensitive, choose an extra-moisturizing shower gel or a product that combines body lotion or oil with a foaming agent. If you have problem dry skin, use a specialist emollient shower product and avoid using a textured cloth or sponge. After showering or bathing, allow the skin to dry naturally, if possible, and apply a body lotion while it is still damp.

Epsom salts bath

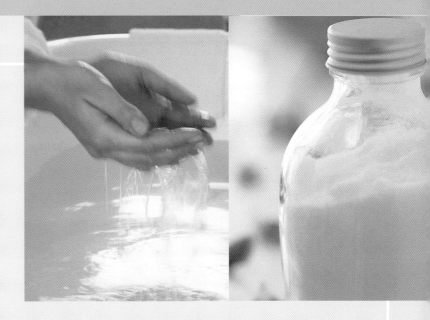

A bath in Epsom salts is a cleansing and relaxing, pampering treatment to be enjoyed just before bedtime. It helps remove toxins at the same time as stimulating circulation. The magnesium in the salts warms and soothes the body, so the joints and muscles relax. At the same time, you can expect to get hot – your temperature will rise and you will release toxins in the form of sweat.

Ensure the bathroom is warm and that you have plenty of towels handy. Run a deep, warm (but not hot) bath, tip in 1 kg (2 lb) of the salts – available from some chemist's and healthfood shops – and agitate the water until they are dissolved. It takes quite a lot of stirring to mix the salts into the water, but do make sure the entire contents have dissolved before you get in.

Soak yourself in the bath for at least five minutes. You will start to sweat copiously. However, don't worry, this is completely normal and is part of the process that detoxifies and relaxes your body.

Take up a loofah or bath mitt and, beginning with your feet, thoroughly massage them with circular movements. Don't try to go too fast or you may become overheated. Work your way up your legs, massaging as you go, then kneel up to work on your buttocks and your abdomen (go gently on the latter). Sit down and work gently over the lower half of your chest, avoiding your breasts, and working over as much as you can of your back.

Lie back and relax for another five minutes, if you can. If you are too hot, step out of the bath immediately. Wrap yourself in towels and pat your body dry very gently. Do not rub your skin. When you are dry, moisturize your face, then get into bed with a large glass of water by your side and prepare for a long, restful night.

This is good to do during a detox (see Chapter 2) but don't do it just before or during menstruation as it can increase blood flow.

CAUTION Do not use Epsom salts if you have eczema, psoriasis or broken skin.

Saunas and steam baths

A sauna is a real treat for your body – especially when detoxifying (see page 92) – and many sports centres now have one. The ideal way of taking a sauna is in short bursts interspersed with a cold shower or a swim. Go in the sauna for 5–10 minutes at a time, then shower and rest for 5 minutes or swim before returning. Do this three or four times, then lie down quietly for 30 minutes – you should feel completely invigorated.

Steam baths are also excellent, and many people find their heat gentler than the dry heat of the sauna. In both, try to wear as little as possible and rest afterwards. Don't use either if you feel unwell.

SEE ALSO:

→ The detox process, page 92

→ Detoxing weekend home health spa, page 102

→ Hydrotherapy, page 170

→ Moor mud treatment, page 172

→ Aromatherapy, page 278

Sun safety

Much of the sun's energy hits the earth as heat: part is visible light, part is ultraviolet light, which causes sunburn on brief intense exposure. Long-term modest exposure ages the skin and predisposes white-skinned people to skin cancer. Humidity and cloud partially protect us, otherwise we would burn even in winter.

The benefits of sunshine

Humans need daylight. Those who lack it can suffer from SAD (seasonal affective disorder): depression caused by lack of sun in winter. Sufferers may be treated with artificial daylight.

Vitamin D, necessary for calcium balance, is formed by the action of sunshine on the skin – just a few minutes exposure to the forearms a day is sufficient. Without this, people – especially dark-skinned people who have a poor intake of calcium and vitamin D – are at risk of rickets. Also, some skin conditions, for example psoriasis, acne and eczema, can be helped by sunlight.

The drawbacks

Sunburn is a true burn, causing tissue destruction a few hours after exposure to sun. Severe and repeated sunburn in childhood increases the risk of skin cancer. Many individuals also have a sensitivity to ultraviolet light and react with redness, rashes and itching. Unlike sunburn, this reaction occurs after just brief exposure to strong sunshine.

The risk of skin cancer is very high for white people living in high-sunshine areas. Fortunately, most cancers are relatively benign. Although comparatively few are aggressive, it is important to inspect your skin regularly, concentrating on exposed parts – your face, ears, chest, back and limbs. Look for moles or patches that change in appearance, becoming darker, itching or bleeding.

In addition, relentless exposure to radiation damages collagen and permanently alters skin cells. Eventually the skin is prematurely aged – dry, wrinkled and tough-looking and with colour variations.

The fashionable tan

The skin tans in response to sunlight or artificial ultraviolet light. Cells called melanocytes produce increased amounts of a pigment called melanin, which protects against burning from the sun's rays, but does not abolish the risks of long-term damage from sunlight.

Until the 20th century it was unfashionable to have a tan: being pale implied you were wealthy enough not to have to work in the sun. These days, a tan suggests you can lounge in the sun anytime. Foreign travel and a gradual increase in average temperatures means that many white-skinned people are increasingly exposed to more sun than they can handle (black- and brown-skinned people are protected by their natural melanin). Now, most of us are aware of the dangers involved; and you can fake it quite convincingly!

Sun creams

Sun creams containing titanium reflect or block ultraviolet light and do not allow tanning. The degree of protection is expressed as a factor number. For example, Factor 6 means you can be exposed for six times longer than the length of time in which unprotected skin would burn. In extreme sunlight you need Factor 25 or higher.

Ordinary sunscreens protect against medium-wavelength ultraviolet light (ultraviolet B), which causes sunburn. However, they don't protect against longer-wavelength ultraviolet light (ultraviolet A) which, while not causing sunburn, does cause long-term skin ageing and cancer. For complete protection, either cover up or use sunscreens that protect against both UVB and UVA.

Sun protection

DO...

- Cover up or use sunscreen with UVA and UVB protection

- Avoid the midday sun when ultraviolet radiation is greatest

- Wear cotton or silk; they are better barriers than looser weaves

- Encourage your children to enjoy being outdoors, but to wear protective clothing, sun hats and sunscreen; the greater their exposure to sun, the greater their risk of skin cancer 20 or more years later

- Be aware that altitude heightens damage: the higher you go the more you lose the protective effect of the ozone layer against ultraviolet light. A cool sunny day in the mountains carries more risk than a hot day at sea level

- Watch your skin and report unusual changes to a doctor

DON'T...

- Swim at midday, thinking water protects your skin; it does not

- Forget to renew your sunscreen after swimming and after every few hours

- Have short intensive sunbathing holidays, especially if you are fair-skinned or have more than 100 moles

- Use ultraviolet sunbeds all year long. Excessive use is more damaging to the skin than lying under the hottest sun

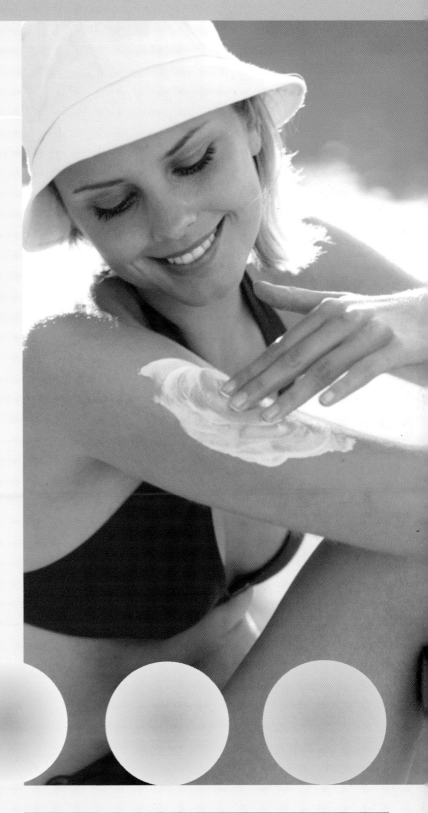

SEE ALSO:

→ Vitamins, page 24

→ Improve your complexion, page 122

Cellulite

Cellulite is the lumpy, chunky tissue, commonly seen in women of all sizes and ages. It is simply fat, which is packaged differently in women than in men because of the structure of female fat cells. Cellulite tends to appear where there is naturally more fat on the female figure – around the bottom, thighs and hips – and gives the skin the appearance of fleshy orange peel.

Formation of cellulite

Cellulite forms gradually as a result of water retention, bad circulation and an unbalanced diet. Although it originates beneath the skin, its unattractive appearance is very much on the surface. The dimpled look is due to the way in which the fat is stored in the fat cell compartments, surrounded by thickened dividers of connective collagen tissue.

Gender differences Female fat cells are tall and pointed and connected by vertical fibres to extend upwards, and are therefore more likely to be seen protruding against the skin. Male fat cells are smaller and flatter and are connected by horizontal fibres, which extend lengthways. These differences in male and female fat cell and tissue structure are accentuated with age. The fat cells are held together by a network of fibres that are nourished and cleansed by body fluids. Poor circulation can result in a slowing down of this cleansing process and an accumulation of waste materials that thicken and harden into immovable 'pockets' of fat. Drastic dieting can similarly slow the body's metabolism. In time the skin loses its elasticity and the cellulite becomes more prominent.

Does weight matter? Cellulite is not necessarily connected to being overweight; even the slimmest woman can have very noticeable cellulite. However, the fat cells of a woman who does gain weight enlarge and harden within their connective tissue sacs, making the skin surface appear lumpy and constricting blood and lymph flow so that metabolism is slowed. The result is a cycle of progressively worsening cellulite.

Combating cellulite

Cellulite can be very resistant to any form of treatment. The best way of dealing with it is to prevent it forming.

Home remedies A healthy diet and regular exercise are the main keys to fighting cellulite. However, skin brushing (see page 168), exfoliation (see Salt body scrub, page 166) and massage (see pages 158–165) can all help decrease cellulite, as well as improve the appearance of the skin. These three techniques improve circulation and lymph flow, which helps in the battle against cellulite.

Since vitamins C and E are both important in the modelling of collagen, they are believed to help fight cellulite by inhibiting the

5 ways to fight cellulite

1 **Improve your circulation** with massage, skin brushing, exfoliation and exercise

2 **Drink more water** to help reduce water retention and eliminate toxins

3 **Reduce your intake of salt** and chemical food additives

4 **Take plenty of exercise**: exercise helps improve circulation and eliminate toxins; improved muscle tone enhances the appearance of existing cellulite

5 **Take natural dietary supplements** to help improve circulation and detoxify your system

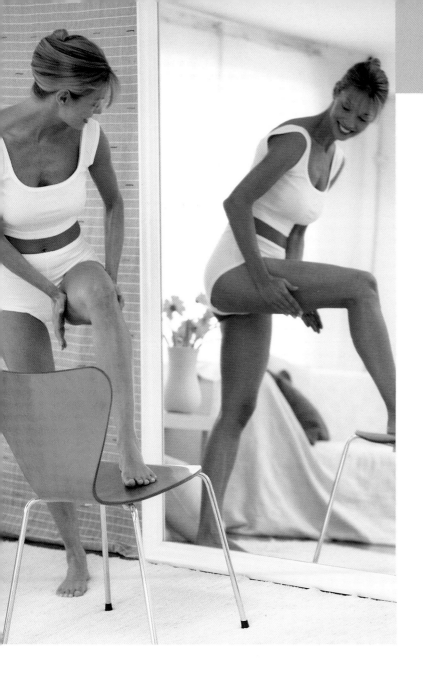

Massage for cellulite

Massaging areas of cellulite once or twice a day will improve circulation and lymph flow and minimize the appearance of the hard fatty lumps. You could visit a salon for an 'anti-cellulite' massage, although you can easily massage yourself at home, standing in front of a mirror to ensure you treat all the areas of your body that suffer from cellulite.

Apply a moisturizing cream or oil to the area to be massaged, so that your hands can glide smoothly over the skin. Massage firmly but not so hard that you hurt or bruise yourself, working in long, sweeping strokes towards the heart. Alternatively, try a special hand-held massager, which must be used with an oil or lotion to avoid friction and causing broken thread veins.

To make an aromatherapy cellulite massage oil, add 4 drops of fennel and 2 drops of geranium or juniper essential oil to 25 ml (1 fl oz) of a carrier oil.

thickening of the connective tissue sacs that package the fat cells in the cellulite. Less thickening inevitably means less cellulite. Including these two vitamins in a healthy, balanced diet will help combat cellulite.

Salon treatments Other remedies that claim fat-busting results include highly potent seaweed 'wraps' and all-over mud packs, both of which are salon treatments. Another salon treatment involves the use of a hand-held suction pump to massage the skin and stimulate lymphatic flow, encouraging drainage and removal of metabolic waste products. In addition, there are topically applied creams and lotions, as well as pills, which claim to help improve the skin's general texture and appearance by working on the sub-dermal layer of fat.

SEE ALSO:

→ The detox process, page 92

→ Water, page 96

→ Massage, page 158

→ Salt body scrub, page 166

→ Skin brushing, page 168

→ Hydrotherapy, page 170

→ Moor mud treatment, page 172

→ Trimmer thighs, page 210

→ Aerobic exercise, page 224

Massage

The ultimate treat is to have a professional massage – and it is particularly relaxing if aromatherapy oils are used (see page 278). Look for a qualified therapist – some therapists will even come to you, which means that after your massage you can simply relax at home. However, you don't need to find a professional. You can learn to give a massage very easily and, if you learn with a friend or partner, you can take turns to practise on each other. See the following pages to learn the basic stroke techniques, or you could even consider enrolling on a weekend course that will teach you the basics of massage.

The basics

Massage oils help your hands slide smoothly over the skin, but always take time to warm the oil in your hands before you start. It is important for the person being massaged to keep warm, so make sure the room is warmer than you would normally have it, and that there are plenty of towels to cover up any parts of the body not being massaged. Cold muscles become tense, which defeats the whole point of the massage.

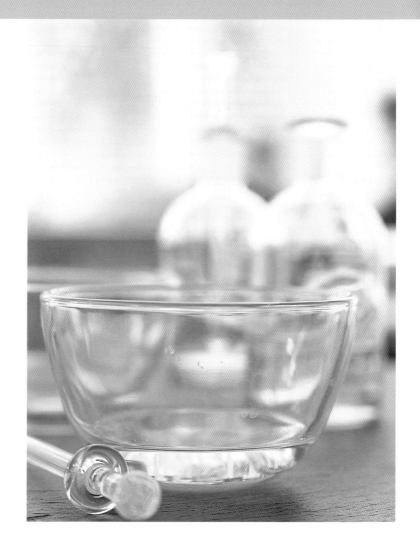

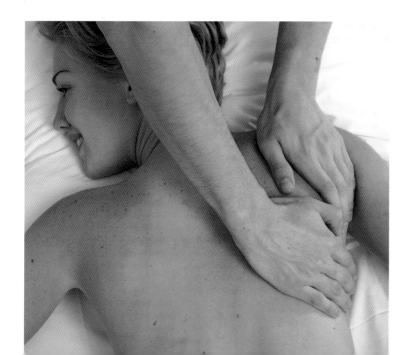

Make sure you aren't going to be disturbed and don't talk during the massage – unless it is to ask about the massage – as this is a disturbance in itself. When you give the massage, wear loose, comfortable clothes and take off any jewellery. You can either have a background of silence or play soothing music very quietly. Do the massage on the floor or a hard bed.

Try to trust your instincts when you give a massage and rely on your own sense of touch. You will soon get to know the feel of tense muscles that need to be released. Check at the start that you are using the right pressure for your massage partner – not so vigorous that it becomes painful or so light that it doesn't get to the root of the problem. If your massage partner finds that one area is very tense and needs more attention, or simply that a particular stroke feels good and brings a deeper relaxation, you can concentrate on that.

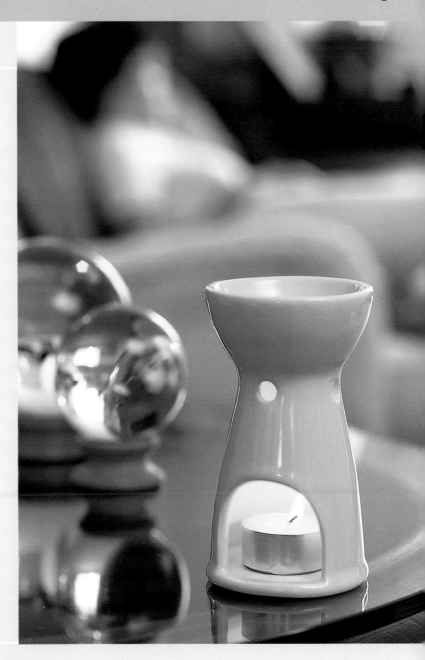

The massage environment

The effects of massage can be maximized by creating an environment that is conducive to emotional and physical relaxation. The surroundings need to be more sedating than stimulating so that your mind and body slow down.

- **LIGHTING** A gloomy light is a mild depressant and therefore necessary for relaxation. If you are doing your massage in the day, draw the curtains; if at night, have no more than a single side light on.
- **SOUND** Since noise is a powerful nervous stimulant and raises the levels of adrenaline in the blood, you should do your massage in the quietest room in the house. However, gentle music can be a powerful tranquillizer.
- **SMELL** Introducing an odour with tranquillizing properties can enhance the relaxing effects of a massage. The most effective method is to burn essential oil in the room. Those most popular for massage include **lavender**, **bergamot**, **petitgrain**, **sandalwood** and **ylang ylang** (see page 280).
- **TEMPERATURE** Cold muscles find it difficult to relax, so ensure the room is warmer than usual.

SEE ALSO:

→ Manual lymphatic drainage, page 106

→ Facial massage, page 126

→ Foot massage, page 177

→ Living with stress, page 230

→ 5-minute self-massage for sleep, page 239

→ Relaxing weekend home health spa, page 266

→ Aromatherapy, page 278

Basic massage strokes

Below are some of the basic strokes that will enable you to perform your first massage. As you practise you will soon discover the amount of pressure required – this will depend on the particular area of the body you are working on and will differ from one individual to another.

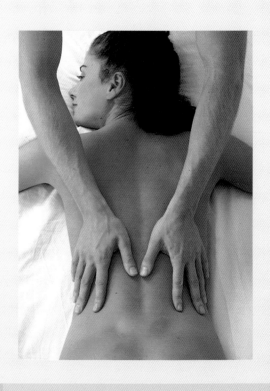

Effleurage

This is the first massage stroke. It involves making gentle, large, sweeping strokes over the area to be massaged in order to spread the massage oil and to soothe and relax the surface of the muscles. **Ensure your hands are warm and well oiled** and keep them relaxed, moulding them to the shape of your massage partner's muscles.

Squeezing

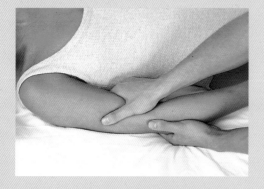

After effleurage, a squeezing technique is required to loosen tension in muscles before introducing further releasing strokes. When squeezing, always work up the body towards the heart. Work on the entire length of muscles for the best result and lessen the pressure as you approach joints.

Kneading

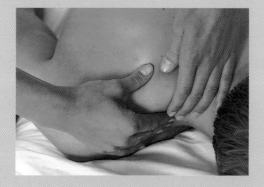

Kneading is a deep, releasing movement that effectively loosens and disperses tension. The technique involves the hands working alternately, firmly squeezing and rolling well-oiled muscles. It is best done over soft fleshy areas or smaller areas such as the shoulders. Use the thumbs to apply extra pressure and avoid kneading directly over bone.

Wringing

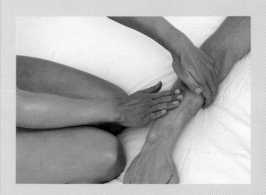

This is a good technique to do after squeezing and kneading. It involves pushing and pulling the hands in opposite directions, thereby twisting and pressing the muscles between the hands and releasing tension.

Opening

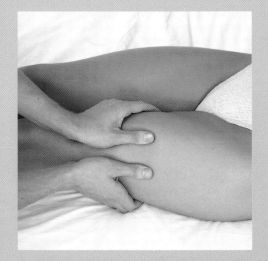

Opening strokes are made across the body rather than up or down, and help to disperse tension after deeper releasing strokes. The technique involves using a spreading movement of the thumbs or, over a larger muscle area, pressure with the heels of the hands. The movements are most effective if you cup your hands right around the muscles, and can be interchanged with wringing.

Raking

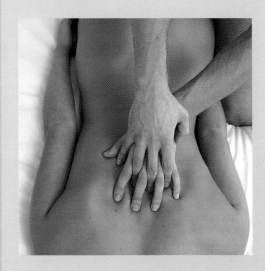

Raking involves forming your hand into a claw-like shape in order to rake down or across the body – usually the back, hips or tops of thighs – applying firm fingertip pressure. Do not rake too hard. Raking is best followed by soft feathering strokes.

Feathering

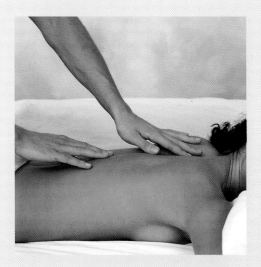

One of the lightest massage strokes, feathering is done with the fingertips of alternating hands to achieve a continuous rippling effect. It involves stroking downwards, finally lifting the hands so that the movement ends almost imperceptibly. It is ideal as the final stroke to bring a massage to a close.

Other massage strokes to try

- **Pulling** A releasing stroke done along the sides of the body – from just beneath the body to the top – to loosen up the whole area.
- **Circling** A soft, round movement over the body done with the hands circling in opposite directions or with one hand on top of the other.

- **Simple stretching** A gentle pulling movement of the limbs, possible only when the muscles are warm, that works on the fibrous tissue around joints and reduces muscle tension.

- **Pressing** A technique performed on soft, sensitive small areas, such as the forehead or soles of the feet, using the pads of the thumbs. The thumb pressure helps with general tension release.

Upper body massage

The person to be massaged should lie face down on the floor (with a towel underneath) or on a bed, and be covered with towels. Since it is the back, shoulders and neck that are usually the centres of tension, in this massage you will be concentrating on the upper body. However, you can continue and do a whole body massage if you wish. In this case, it is better if you start with the lower body and massage the legs first, then work up to the back, finishing, as here, with the neck and shoulders.

Since the aim during massage is to relax, it is probably most comfortable for the person being massaged to turn their head to one side when lying face down. They should turn their head to the other side half way through the massage or their neck may get tense on one side. Alternatively, a pillow under the forehead will raise their head off the floor while maintaining a straight spine.

CAUTION

Never massage anyone with:
- A heart condition
- Broken or infected skin
- Varicose veins
- Joints swollen by rheumatism or arthritis

1 Make sure your massage partner is lying comfortably face down, and uncover the back. Warm the oil in your hands and place them flat on the lower back, with your fingers pointing towards the neck. Leave your hands still for a moment to let your partner get used to your touch. With one hand on either side of the spine — **not on the spine itself** — gently glide up the back, spreading the oil as you go.

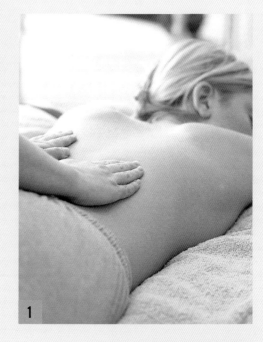

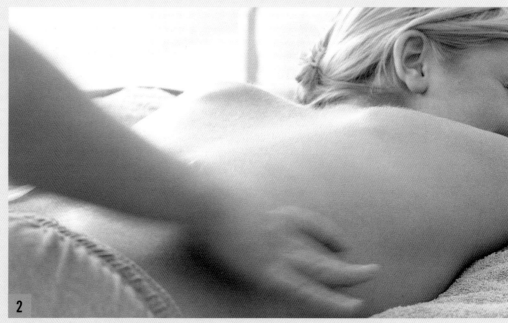

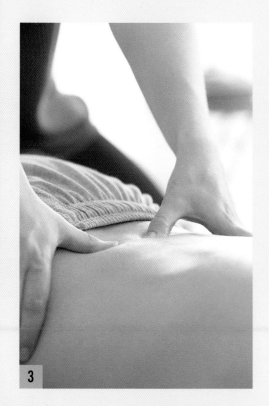

3

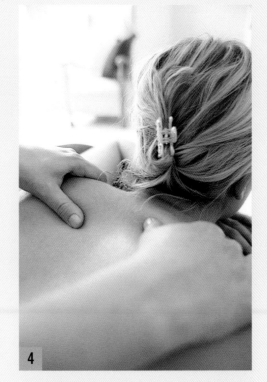

4

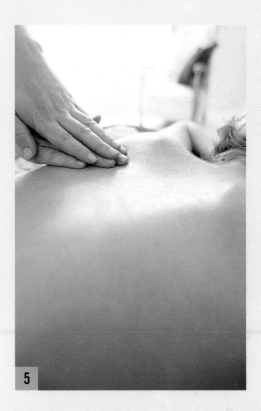

5

2 When you get to the top of the back, move out to the shoulders and then gently along the sides. *Repeat this several times,* keeping your hands flat throughout, in a slow stroking movement that is known as effleurage (see page 160).

3 Starting again at the base of the spine, work up the back, with the hands either side of the spine. This time, make little circles, using your thumbs only. You can apply more

pressure in this movement, and it is a very good way of releasing tension knots. However, check with your massage partner that you are **not using too much pressure**. It should not hurt. *Repeat several times.* **Never massage the spine itself.** Always work to the sides of it.

4 Knead the neck muscles, using both hands in the same way as you would knead bread. Knead gently here as these muscles can often be very tense.

5 Place one hand on top of the other at the neck. Make a figure of eight movement across the upper back, using the weight of your body to iron out the tension. Your hands circle the first shoulder, then move diagonally across the back to circle the opposite shoulder blade, returning to the centre of the back and circling the first shoulder again. *Repeat this several times.*

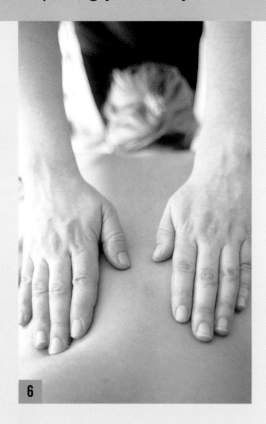

6

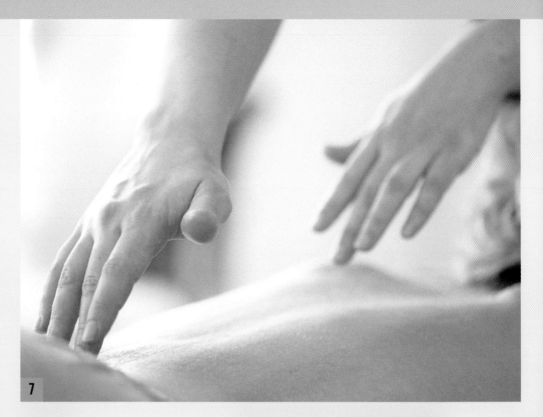

7

6 Move around to your massage partner's head and place your hands on either side of the spine, with your fingers pointing down the back. Make a long stroking movement all the way down the back, using your body weight to help release tense muscles. At the base of the spine, move your hands out across the tops of the buttocks, then up the sides back to the shoulders. *Repeat this step several times*, gradually lightening the pressure each time.

7 Starting at the base of the spine, and using the middle finger of each hand in turn, perform feathering strokes (see page 161) by stroking the whole length of the spine as far as the neck. Lift the finger off at the top and repeat with the middle finger of the other hand. *Each time*, make the pressure even lighter until it is as light as a feather.

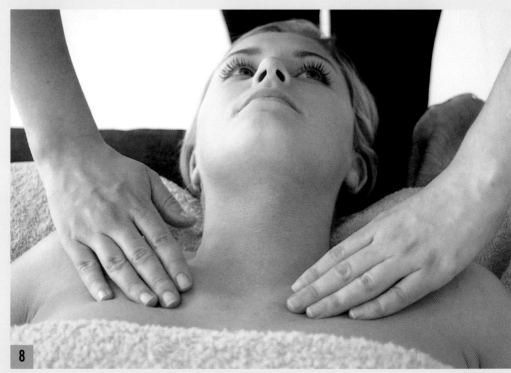

8

8 Ask your massage partner to turn over and cover her with towels, leaving the neck and shoulders uncovered. Warm some more of the oil in your hands. Lay them flat on each side of the upper chest and leave them there for a few moments.

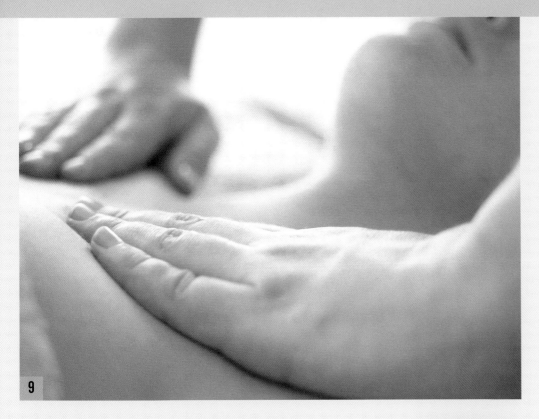

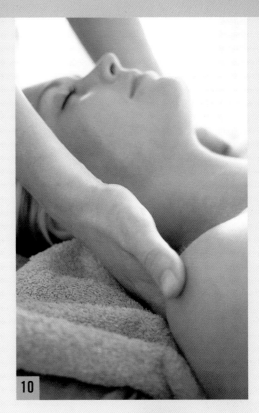

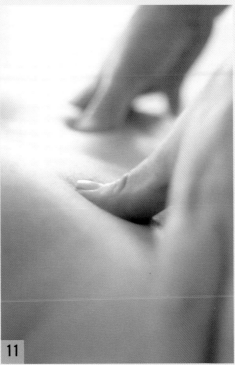

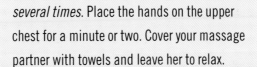

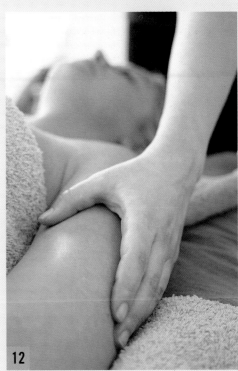

9 With a long, firm, stroking movement, take your hands to the centre of the chest, and then out to the sides.

10 Continue the stroking movements under the shoulders and back up to the neck, pulling out the muscles as you do so. This should help the back and neck to lie flatter.

11 Using the circular thumb movement you used in Step 3, move your hands across the upper chest. Start below the collarbone, working outwards from the centre. *Repeat this several times*, moving down gradually.

12 Place your hands, fingertips downwards, on the upper chest. Move them out smoothly across the chest, over the upper arms, and up over the shoulders back to the chest. *Repeat several times*. Place the hands on the upper chest for a minute or two. Cover your massage partner with towels and leave her to relax.

Salt body scrub

This is a gentler version of a treatment found in many European health spas, which is guaranteed to start your day with a boost of energy. A salt body scrub has a number of beneficial effects for the body, all of them stimulating:

- It clears the pores and sloughs away dead skin cells so that your skin is fresher and smoother.
- It stimulates the circulation and the elimination of toxins through the lymphatic system.
- It promotes cell renewal.
- It makes your skin tingle and glow with vital energy.

Preparing a salt scrub

There are many exfoliants on the market, yet one of the best is simple salt. For your body you should use rock salt in flakes, rather than fine salt which is suitable for use only on the face. You can apply it directly to your body in handfuls, but it is easier to work

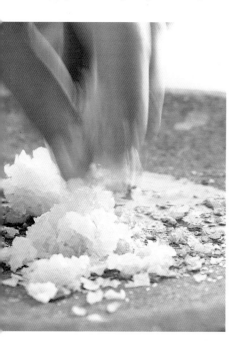

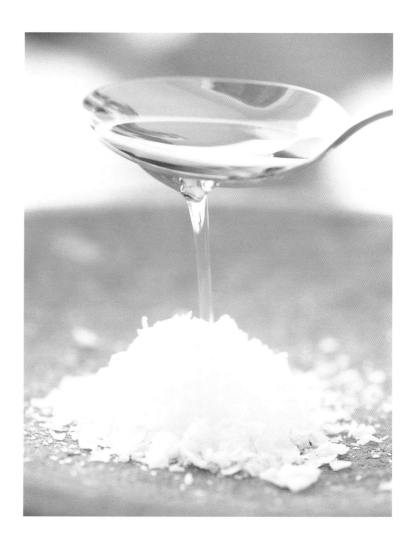

with if you mix it into a paste first with olive oil or sesame oil. This will have the added advantage of nourishing the skin at the same time. You will need a handful of coarse rock salt and two tablespoons of olive oil or sesame oil. If you would like a slightly less functional smell, add one drop only of rose or lavender essential oil. Mix all the ingredients together in a bowl and take this with you into the bathroom. Make sure that the bathroom is nice and warm and that you have plenty of warm towels and a towelling robe to hand.

If you wish, before you start your body scrub, exfoliate your face and neck using fine salt (rock salt is too coarse for the delicate skin found on the face) mixed with olive or sesame oil (use oil even if you have oily skin). You could use one of the facial scrub recipes on page 119 as an alternative.

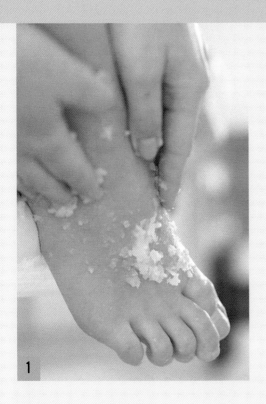

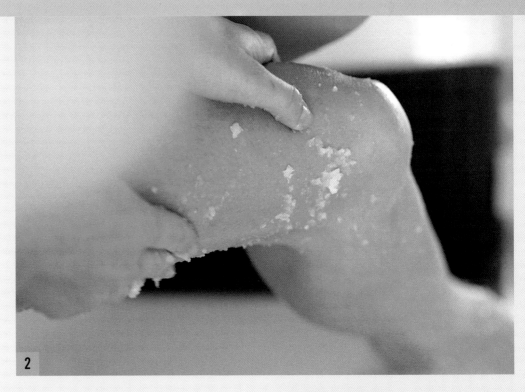

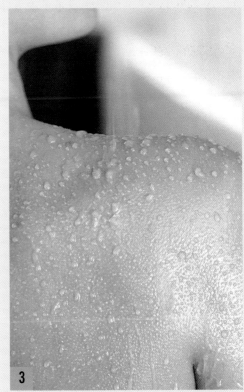

Body scrub

1 Stand under a warm shower for 1–2 minutes and make sure your whole body is wet. Step out from under the water, **scoop some of the scrub mixture into your hand** and, starting from your feet, **massage it well into your skin**, using circular movements with your whole hand. Make sure you scrub the soles of your feet, too.

2 Gradually move up your legs, using circular movements all the way. **Pay particular attention to your thighs** and **buttocks** as, when the circulatory system is sluggish, this is where **cellulite** is only too likely to appear. Reach as much of your back as you can and then very gently **massage your abdomen** and **chest**. Finally, **scrub your arms** and **shoulders**, as well as your **hands** themselves.

3 Step back under the shower and **massage the scrub into your skin** under the water until it has all been washed off. Turn the water temperature down to cold (cool, if you can't face it) and stay under the spray for a further minute, making sure that the water flows over your whole body.

Wrap up in a warm towel and dry yourself vigorously. Put on a warm dressing gown and lie down somewhere comfortable for five minutes. If you feel at all chilly, get under a duvet or blanket. **You should now feel a tingle all over your body and feel re-energized from head to toe.**

SEE ALSO:

→ The detox process, page 92

→ Exfoliation, page 118

Skin brushing

Giving your body a firm brush all over makes the skin glow by removing the top dull, dead layer of skin and encouraging new cells to regenerate. The gentle massaging motion of the bristles also has a beneficial effect on areas of cellulite, and it is an effective treatment for helping eliminate toxins from the body during a detox programme (see Chapter 2).

Technique

The technique is a simple one, and you need only a body brush with natural bristles, such as those of goat or boar, or a loofah. There are various types of brush, all widely available at chemist shops. You will need a brush with a handle – some have detachable handles – so that you can reach all the inaccessible parts of your back. There are also brushes mounted on long straps, which are ideal for the back and buttocks, and most loofahs are long enough to reach over the shoulders and down the back. You need a much softer brush, or a flannel, for the face.

Skin brushing is carried out on dry skin. Start at your feet and work upwards, brushing the legs, then buttocks, up the arms, then on to the chest and stomach and finally the face. Brush more gently where the skin is thinnest and always brush towards the heart.

Brushing your whole body in this way will take you between three and five minutes, depending on how many strokes you give to each area. Try to keep a rhythm going and brush for up to five minutes every day and preferably immediately before you have a bath or shower so that the dead cells are washed away. Skin brushing is best done in the morning as the acceleration of blood flow has quite an invigorating effect. You should be able to see the difference in your skin after just a few sessions – it will become very soft and develop an attractive rosy glow.

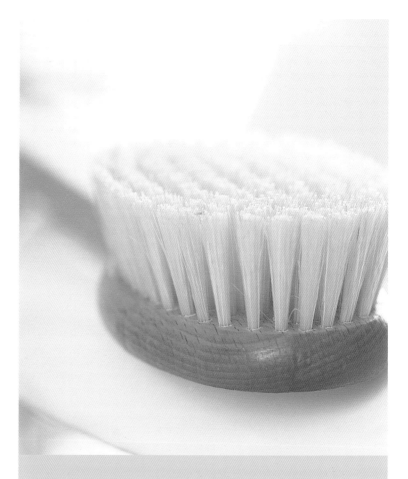

Good reasons for skin brushing

- Stimulates blood and lymph flow
- Helps eliminate toxins from the body
- Removes dead skin cells
- Encourages cells to regenerate
- Stimulates production of sebum
- Helps combat cellulite
- Results in smooth glowing skin

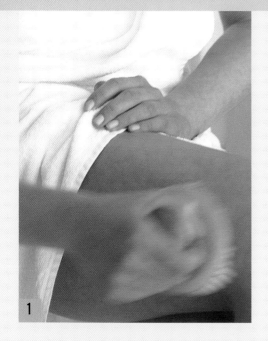
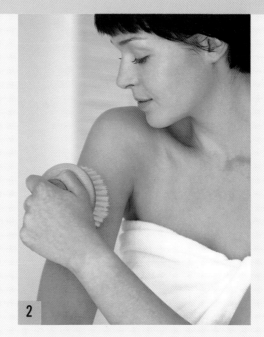
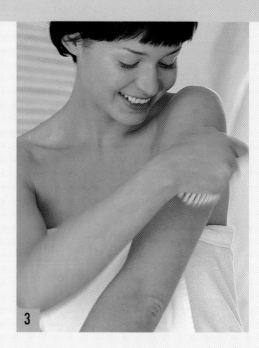

5-minute skin brushing routine

Make sure the room is warm and there are plenty of towels. Undress, and find somewhere comfortable to sit so that you can easily reach your feet and lower legs.

1 Take the brush and begin with the sole of your right foot. Use firm, rhythmic strokes to cover the sole several times. Next, brush the top of your foot, brushing up towards your ankle. Then go on to your lower leg, making sure you cover the whole surface – shin and calf. Always brush in an upward direction.

Stand up and brush the area from your knee to the top of your thigh. Make sure you cover the whole area several times, using long, rhythmic strokes. Brush your buttock area as far as your waist. Now repeat the whole procedure on your left leg, starting again with the sole of your foot.

Starting from the top of your buttocks, and always moving in an upward direction, brush the whole of your back several times all the way up to your shoulders.

2 Next, brush your right arm. Start with the palm of your hand, move on to the back of your hand and then brush from your wrist up to your elbow, always in an upward direction and ensuring that the whole surface of your skin is brushed. Brush your upper arm, working from your elbow towards your shoulder, again covering the whole surface of your upper arm.

3 *Repeat on your left side*, starting with your hand. Then, very gently, brush your abdomen, brushing in a circle, always in a clockwise direction. Cover the area several times but

with less pressure than on your arms and legs. If it feels uncomfortable, stop.

4 The neck and chest are also very sensitive areas, so, again, brush here very gently. Always work towards your heart. If the bristles are too hard on your neck, don't brush here. Lastly, work on your face. Use your soft brush or a dry flannel and soften and shorten your action, as brisk rubbing can stretch or otherwise damage the facial skin.

SEE ALSO:

→ The detox process, page 92

→ Detoxing weekend home health spa, page 102

→ Exfoliation, page 118

→ Improve your complexion, page 122

→ Hydrotherapy, page 170

Hydrotherapy

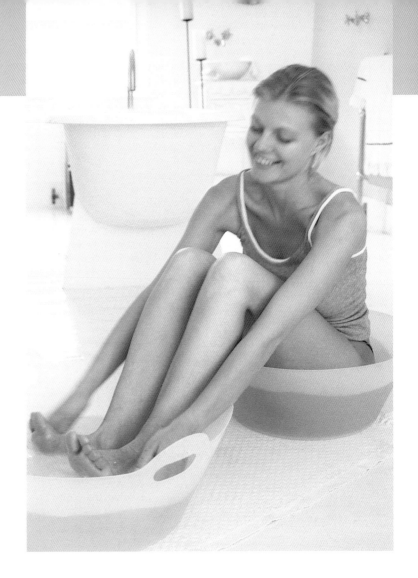

Hydrotherapy embraces a far-ranging collection of treatments using water and is one of the oldest of the natural therapies. It is extremely popular in the spas of Germany, Austria, Switzerland, Italy and France. As with skin brushing (see page 168), the effect of hydrotherapy is to jump-start the system, stimulating the circulation of the blood and lymph. This is often achieved by extremes of temperature and you quite quickly become accustomed to it. Saunas, steam baths and Epsom baths (see page 153) are all aspects of hydrotherapy.

Hydrotherapy shower

The bathroom must be warm while you have this shower and there should be plenty of warm towels to hand for when you finish. Begin by showering for two minutes in warm to hot water. Turn around under the shower to make sure your whole body is covered in the water. Now turn the tap to cold and, again, turn your body under the shower so it covers you all over for 30 seconds. (Try not to hold your breath as doing so will interfere with your body's adaptation to the cold.) Turn the water temperature back to hot for another two minutes, then to cold for a further 30 seconds. Repeat the whole process one more time, finishing with cold water. Turning your head so that the cold water pours on to your face is very beneficial for your complexion.

Get out and wrap yourself in warm towels. Pat yourself dry and put on a warm dressing gown. Sit or lie down for at least 10 minutes. You will find your whole body tingling with vitality – and your energy store will be increased throughout the day.

In the long term, hydrotherapy showers strengthen your immune system so you are less susceptible to every passing infection. They are even said to be an anti-ageing tonic!

Sitz bath

This treatment works on the same principle as the alternating of hot and cold water in the shower. Here, however, you are sitting in water. You need two bowls, large enough to sit in.

Fill one bowl with cold water; it should be very cold, so if you are feeling daring you could even put ice cubes in it. Fill the other with hot water – but test it first, you do not want it so hot that you scald yourself.

You can wear a top during this treatment to keep your upper body warm, but it should not be so long that it falls into the water and gets wet. Start with your bottom in the hot water and then place your feet in the cold. This will be quite a shock to the system at first, but after a minute or two, you will start to feel quite comfortable. After five minutes, change over bowls so that your bottom is in the cold water and your feet are in the hot. Dry yourself, wrap up in a dressing gown or get into bed and rest.

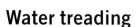

Water treading

This involves somewhat less of a shock to the system than the sitz bath as it involves only the feet. Wrap up to keep the body as warm as possible, but make sure your clothing does not extend beyond the knees. Your feet and lower legs should be bare.

Fill the bath with cold water, once again making it as cold as possible. Now, step into the bath and walk in the water on the spot, lifting the whole of each foot right out of the water after each step. (Take care that the surface of the bath is not slippery – put a rubber mat on the bottom if it is.) Tread water like this for one or two minutes. Get out of the bath, dry your feet well and put on a pair of warm socks.

Rest afterwards for at least 10 minutes.

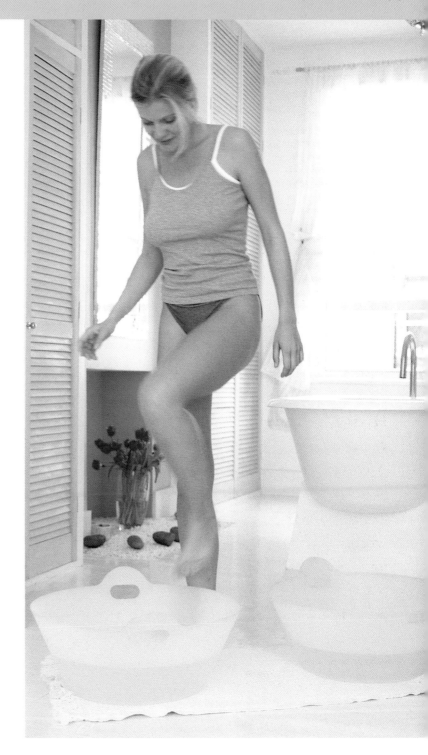

Benefits of cold bathing

Having a cold bath has a remarkable effect on the circulation. Within three to five minutes of immersing yourself in a cold bath, your blood circulation increases fourfold and your lymph flow is equally boosted. Apart from widening the arteries, cold bathing also boosts the body's production of white blood cells, destroying circulating toxins, and increases your metabolism so that you burn calories more quickly and feel more energetic.

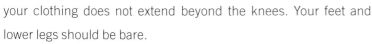

SEE ALSO:

→ The detox process, page 92

→ Detoxing weekend home health spa, page 102

→ Bathing and showering, page 152

→ Skin brushing, page 168

Moor mud treatment

Mud may not be one of the most glamorous forms of treatment in the world, but it is certainly one of the oldest. Mud packs and masks were used by the ancient Egyptians and Romans for various ailments as well as beauty treatments, and were often given with other spa treatments as part of a cure. Therapeutic mud often comes from areas around mineral springs, and the high mineral content of the mud is regarded as one of the main reasons for its beneficial effects.

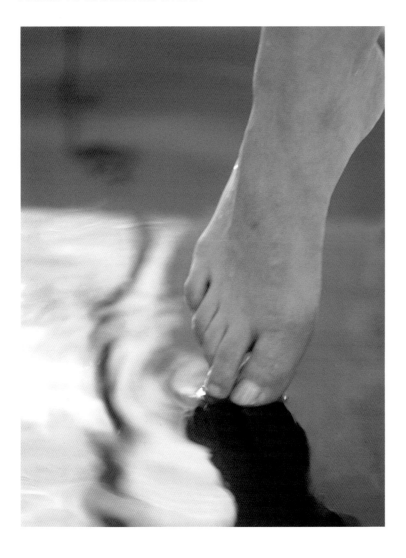

Therapeutic mud

Mud treatments, like spas, are particularly popular in continental Europe. Taking the waters – both drinking them and bathing in them – as well as all-over mud body wraps are frequently seen as important elements of a health regime and the annual spa 'cure' is very much a part of everyday life. People may take cures for specific problems, such as arthritis or psoriasis, or as a more general detoxification.

Although mud treatments are now enjoying something of a revival, people have known of their therapeutic powers for a long period of time. One of the most famous sources of therapeutic mud is the Neydharting Moor, about 60 km (37 miles) from Salzburg in Austria. Archaeological finds there have shown that it was in use from as early as 800BC by the Celts and, later, the Romans. Sick and injured animals were, and still are, drawn there by its healing powers. Paracelsus, the 15th-century Swiss alchemist and physician, thought that he had discovered the elixir of life in mud. Later visitors included Louis XIV, Napoleon and Josephine, all of whom took the cure.

Known just as 'Moor' or 'Moor-Life', the mud has been investigated and analysed by over 500 scientists, and has been found to be unique. Because the 20,000-year-old glacial valley basin in which it lies was first a lake, the waters of which have never drained away, the moor has retained all of its organic, mineral and trace elements. Other moors have dried out and lost such substances, but clinical analysis has shown that Neydharting Moor is uniquely rich in decomposed plant life, with over 1000 plant deposits: flowering herbs, seeds, leaves, flowers, tubers, fruit, roots and grasses. Three hundred of them have recognized medicinal properties, and many of them are extinct or even unique to this one site. Medical evidence shows that Moor mud is both anti-inflammatory and astringent. This means it

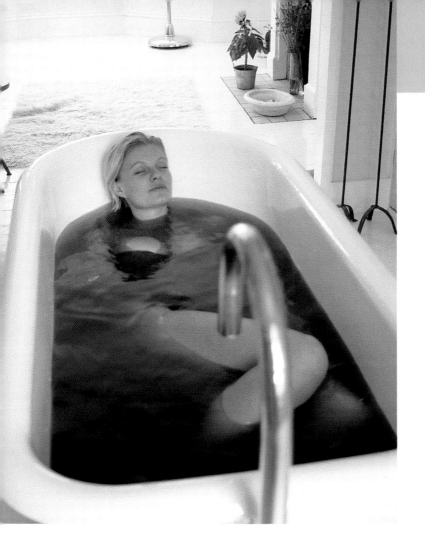

Dead Sea mud

This is probably even better known than Moor mud and has also been around for a long time. Cleopatra is said to have prized it so highly as a beauty treatment that she persuaded Mark Antony to conquer the region and present it to her as a gift. Dead Sea mud contains an extraordinary range of minerals – especially large quantities of potassium – that help to regulate the body's water balance. It is also a relaxing bath and is thought to promote cell renewal and detoxing. As well as these general properties, it is recommended in particular for people with **oedema**, **skin problems**, **sports injuries**, **rheumatism** and **arthritis**.

is particularly useful for detoxification, in treating skin disorders such as acne, eczema and psoriasis, and for rheumatism and arthritis. It is used, too, for beauty treatments, to remedy dry hair, and to reduce cellulite.

The mud comes in a variety of forms including body lotion and oil; the Moor mud bath and the Moor mud drink are particularly recommended. Many healthfood shops stock Moor Mud treatments and they are also available by mail order.

Moor drink and Moor mud bath

Drinking mud does not sound very appetizing and it does actually look like mud, which doesn't help. However, although a teaspoonful mixed in a glass of water or fruit juice may colour the liquid, it has neither taste nor odour. Take the drink about half an hour before you prepare for a Moor mud bath.

The best time for a Moor mud bath is immediately before bedtime. Make sure the bathroom is warm, and run a deep bath,

pouring in the Moor mud according to the instructions on the container. Mix it in well, or you will end up with muddy globules floating around in the water. Put some warm towels close to the bath to use when you come out.

Lie in the bath for 20–30 minutes. Splash the water on your face, too. You can also rinse it through your hair, if you don't mind having to dry it before you get into bed. Just try to relax in the bath, perhaps with some quiet music in the background. When you are ready to get out, pat yourself dry, but don't rub the towel over your skin. You want to leave as much residue from the bath on the surface of your skin as possible. Go to bed as soon as you are dry.

SEE ALSO:

→ The detox process, page 92

→ Detoxing weekend home health spa, page 102

→ Bathing and showering, page 152

Hands and nails

Various day-to-day activities take their toll on hands. Cold weather, the sun, detergents and too much hot water are all responsible for damaging our skin and weakening fingernails. Try to wear gloves for protection whenever possible, for example when gardening or doing housework, or smooth a barrier cream over your hands first. Wear rubber gloves for washing up and keep a bottle of hand cream near the sink for use afterwards.

Dry hands

If you do suffer from dry hands, avoid washing them too often. Use a mild cleanser or soap and avoid harsh commercial brands. Always apply a moisturizer after washing them. Ensure that you wear gloves in cold weather to protect them.

To give dry hands a quick fix, spread plenty of moisturizing cream or petroleum jelly over them. Put on cotton gloves, then snug-fitting latex surgical gloves. Leave the gloves in place for at least two hours, but preferably overnight. In the morning, remove the gloves and you will have beautifully smooth and supple, moisturized hands. Repeat when required.

Sun protection

Most people are now aware of the need to protect themselves from the sun by using creams and lotions with a high sun protection factor (SPF), but don't forget to look after your hands, too. The skin on your hands is very thin and often shows damage, in the form of sun spotting and loss of elasticity, before your face does. You should use sunscreen on your hands whenever they will be exposed, even when simply going about everyday activities.

Nailcare

There are plenty of chemically based commercial products for nailcare. If you prefer home-made treatments, dried dill and

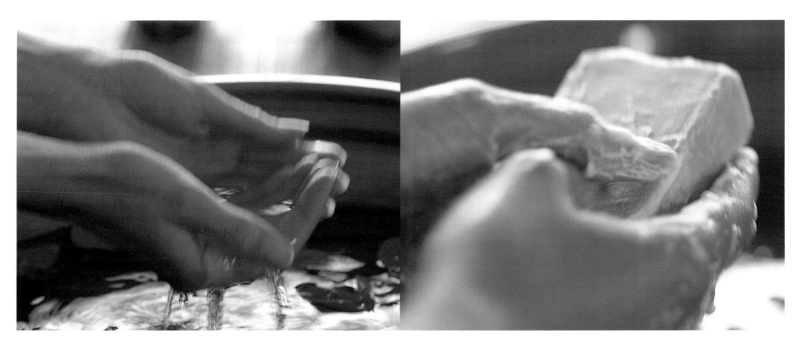

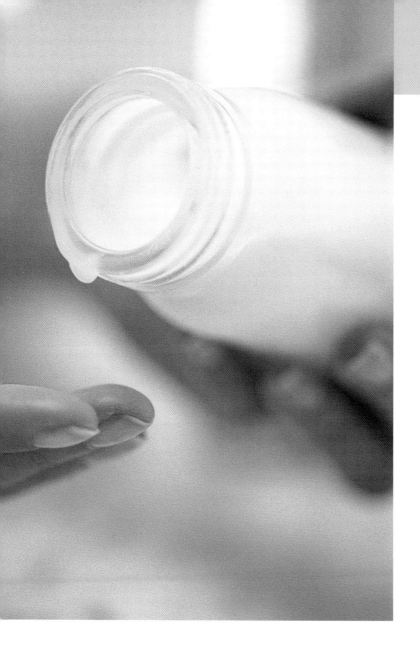

horsetail are particularly good for strengthening weak nails. Make an infusion of either herb by pouring 150 ml (¼ pint) of boiling water on to 2 tablespoons of chopped horsetail or dill. Leave to cool, then strain into a bottle. Use the infusion warm and soak the nails for 10 minutes every other day. On alternate days soak your nails in warm olive oil for five minutes.

Dietary supplements that will help your nails include brewer's yeast and vitamins A and D; chewing dill seeds will also help.

Manicure Soaking your fingernails in warm water before trimming softens them and makes them easier to cut. Use nail clippers if they are quite long and a large emery board rather than a metal file for shaping, as the latter can weaken and burn the nail. Don't rub back and forth, but use the emery board repeatedly in the same direction. Use orange sticks rather than metal implements for cleaning the nails and pushing back the cuticles. If you visit a salon for a manicure you may be offered a hand and arm massage, which is very relaxing. Hands, like feet, have many pressure points and reflex zones, and respond well to touch.

Nail polish Apply nail polish in just three brushstrokes – one down the centre of the nail, and one either side of it. Don't take the colour right to the sides of your nails – concentrating colour in the middle makes fingernails appear longer and slimmer.

Some brands of nail polish require just one coat; others require two or three and you must let the nail polish dry completely before applying another coat. The length of drying time will also vary from one brand to another. Applying a coat of topcoat daily will extend the life of your nail polish and keep its glossy look.

Remove nail polish as soon as it starts to split, chip and flake. Use ready-soaked nail polish removal pads or a ball of cotton wool soaked in nail polish remover (an oil-based remover is kinder to your nails). Firmly wipe the nail clean, working from base to tip. Wash your hands when all traces of polish have been removed and apply a good hand and nail cream.

If you tend to wear nail polish all the time, do give your nails a rest. Allow them to breathe by leaving them at least one day a week without nail polish.

SEE ALSO:

→ Top-to-toe bodycare, page 150

→ Sun safety, page 154

→ Footcare, page 176

→ Healing with herbs, page 288

Footcare

It has been calculated that, on average, we take about 8,000–10,000 steps a day. This adds up to about 185,000 km (115,000 miles) over a lifetime – enough to circle the earth four times! Our feet therefore deserve more care and attention than they usually receive. They are invariably forgotten in day-to-day bodycare until they start to give trouble. On the whole it is neglect and badly fitting shoes rather than any congenital condition that cause problems, and women are four times more likely than men to experience foot problems – high heels are partly to blame. Massage (see page 178), exercise and baths can all help to make life easier for your feet.

Healthy feet

Your feet mirror your general health; indeed, serious conditions such as arthritis and diabetes can show their initial symptoms in the feet. Some medical conditions can be treated with reflexology (see page 284), a pressure point practice that relies on treating the whole person via reflex points on the feet.

Walking is the best exercise for your feet. It also contributes to your general health by improving circulation, controlling weight and promoting general wellbeing.

Rough feet To soften rough, dry feet, apply a heavy moisturizer or petroleum jelly over your feet and wrap each one in kitchen cling film. (The plastic will trap your body heat, thereby increasing the moisturizer's penetration of the skin.) Wrap a warm towel around your plastic-encased feet and relax for 15–20 minutes or put on some woollen socks and leave them on overnight. In the morning your feet will be beautifully soft and smooth.

Smelly feet With 250,000 sweat glands in a pair of feet, they can sweat as much as 300 ml (½ pint) of moisture a day. If you suffer from smelly feet, you should wash them every day using a deodorant cleanser or antibacterial soap. Use a medicated antiperspirant or foot powder or baking soda to help absorb moisture and keep them dry. Soaking your feet regularly in a container of strong tea can help, as the tannin in the tea will eliminate foot odour. Always wear clean dry socks and avoid closed plastic and leather shoes.

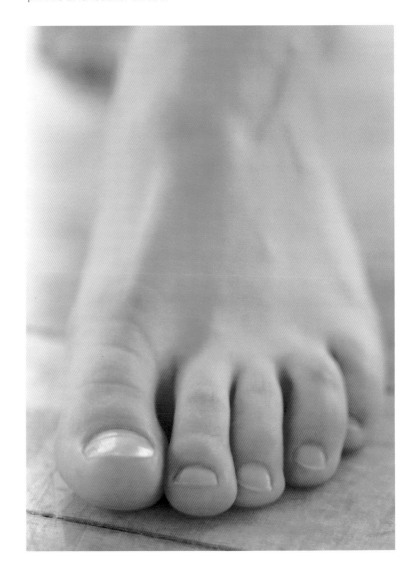

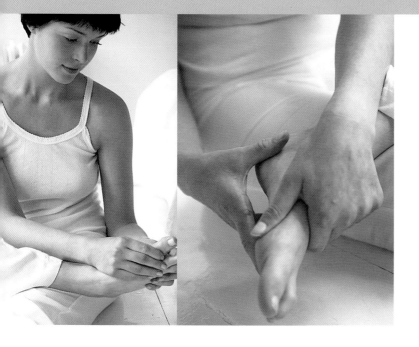

Sensible shoe shopping

Remember that shoes that feel tight in the shop will be even worse after a day on your feet. If your feet are different sizes, buy shoes for the larger one.

If you opt for a strappy pair of shoes, your feet need to look good – apply plenty of moisturizer, treat yourself to a pedicure and paint your nails.

Massage

After a long tiring day, try to spend 10 minutes lying down with your feet higher than your head. Using a massage oil, gently massage your feet (see page 178) to relieve stiffness, then gently massage each leg from the foot to the knee, working upwards to improve circulation. Combine lime, marigold or comfrey essential oils with sweet almond oil for a pleasant massage oil that will help reduce swollen, tired feet. Both marigold and cypress essences are also effective in combating smelly feet.

Foot baths

A foot bath can also be revitalizing after a long day on your feet, and can ease uncomfortable aches and pains. For a herbal foot bath, make an infusion by adding 1 tablespoon of chopped fresh rosemary or mint or juniper berries to 2.4 litres (4 pints) of boiling water. Leave to stand for 15 minutes then strain and use while still warm. Alternatively, add 6 drops of peppermint essence to a bowl of warm water and mix well; another option is a cup of sea salt and a few drops of lavender oil. Sit comfortably with both feet immersed in the water and simply relax or read for 20–30 minutes while the herbal infusion or essential oil soothes and tones your feet. Pat them dry and then apply a cooling and reviving moisturizer or a foot lotion, containing ingredients such as peppermint, aloe vera and comfrey, or gently massage the feet using a relaxing oil.

If you have the chance, try one of the small commercial foot spas available. These work by agitating the water, which adds to the overall enjoyment of a foot bath.

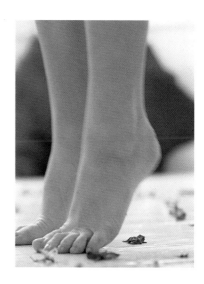

SEE ALSO:

→ Bathing and showering, page 152

→ Massage, page 178

→ Aromatherapy, page 278

→ Reflexology, page 284

→ Healing with herbs, page 288

Massaging your feet

The foot massage below uses some basic reflexology techniques (see page 284). Many people find that even a simple foot massage makes them so relaxed they fall asleep. Clearly, this will not happen if you are massaging your own feet but if you do feel tired afterwards, lie down for half an hour.

Wear loose, comfortable clothes and sit comfortably with your back supported. You will need to find the best position to access the sole of each foot. Some people can sit cross-legged with ease. Others prefer to have the foot they are massaging propped up by the other leg, which is extended in front of them. Use a firm touch throughout. Reflexology should not be practised if you are pregnant or if you suffer from a heart condition or varicose veins.

Foot massage

1 Start by relaxing your foot. Hold your foot so that one hand is on the sole and one on the top. Working from your ankle to your toes, massage it with long, firm strokes.

2 Holding your heel in one hand and your toes in the other, circle your foot five times clockwise then anticlockwise.

3 Starting with your big toe, stroke the length of each toe in turn and, when you reach the tip, pull gently to stretch it out. *Repeat this three times.*

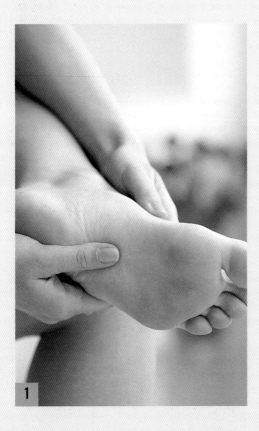

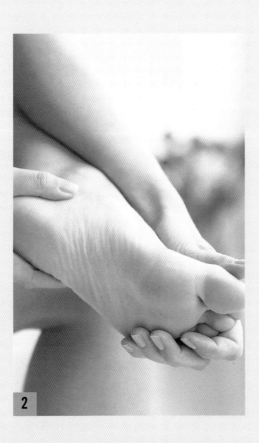

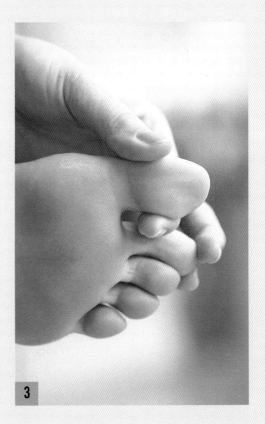

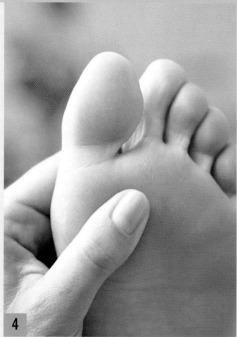

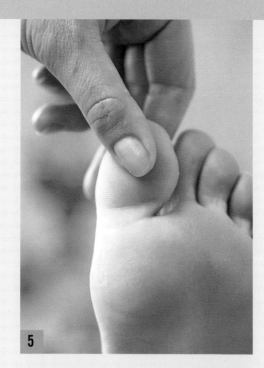

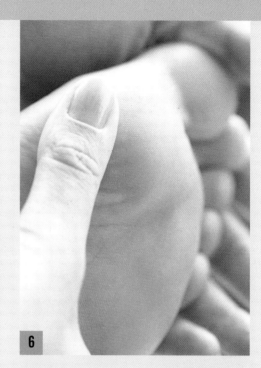

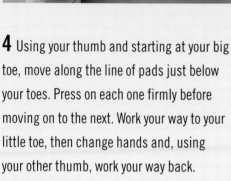

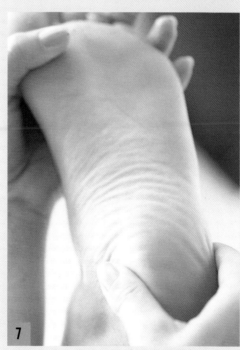

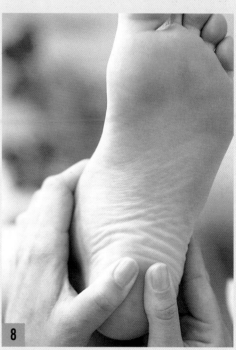

4 Using your thumb and starting at your big toe, move along the line of pads just below your toes. Press on each one firmly before moving on to the next. Work your way to your little toe, then change hands and, using your other thumb, work your way back. *Repeat twice.*

5 Use your thumb to press down gently from the top to the base of your big toe. *Repeat on all of your toes.* When you reach your little toe, change hands and use the other thumb to go back the other way. *Repeat twice.*

6 Holding your toes in one hand, use your thumb on the other hand to press along the sole, pressing in a line from the base of your big toe to the centre of your foot, following the line of the metatarsal. *Repeat on all your toes*, then repeat on the top of your foot following the same line.

7 Starting at your heel, use your thumb to press along the inside edge of your foot all the way up to your big toe. Press firmly and follow the line up over your instep. Then repeat on the outside edge of your foot, from your heel to your little toe.

8 Finally, massage the lower half of your sole, using firm pressure. Rotate your ankle, both clockwise and anticlockwise, as in Step 2. *Repeat Step 1*, using long, firm strokes from ankle to toes. Put on a cotton sock and *repeat the massage on the other foot.*

Posture and exercise

There isn't a wrong reason for wanting to get in shape
– but there is a wrong approach. Finding the time and
the discipline to starve, pummel and bully your body into
shape will be difficult. The Pilates techniques and the
gentle stretching exercises in this section are all aimed
towards increasing and improving awareness of the breath
and posture, while the stretching and toning exercises for
specific parts of the body are designed to improve its
shape, rather than build up bulky muscles.

Posture

Posture is of the utmost relevance when it comes to looking and feeling better. If you stop slouching, you automatically get a leaner, more pulled-up shape. Good posture is really just learning to use your body properly so that its moving parts – arms, neck, back, legs – are in alignment. It is so fundamental to the functioning of your body that it also means that you are breathing properly, too. If your shoulders are hunched or stooped or you slouch, your internal organs do not have sufficient room and you take less oxygen into the body, using it less efficiently – not to mention the effect on your digestion and circulation.

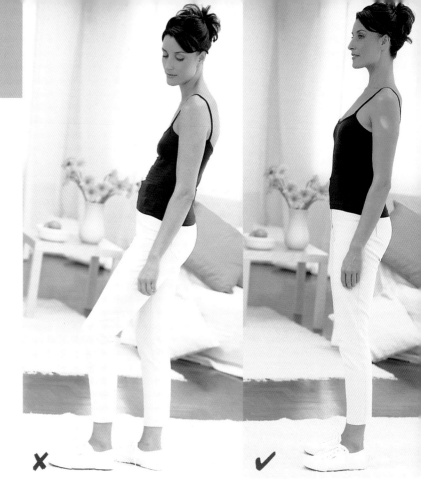

The roll down

The roll down is a deceptively simple exercise, devised to make you think about how your body connects together and then correct any postural problems. You start by putting your body into a good posture. Stand in front of a mirror and check from the top!

Head and neck Your neck is an integral part of your spine, so you should always keep it long and in alignment. In practical terms, this means that you should not allow your chin to jut out or tilt upwards – keep it down so that you are looking straight ahead. This position will help to release tension in the neck if you tend to store it there.

Shoulders Like the neck, the shoulders are a common seat of tension. This means they become hunched up, and one is often higher than the other as a result of carrying a shoulder bag. Check in the mirror that your shoulders are dropped down and relaxed; if you are not sure they are in the right position or if they feel stiff or tense, do some shoulder and head circles to help you become aware of them.

Arms You should move your arms from the centre of your back – not by lifting your shoulders. To learn how to move them, take your left arm behind your back so that the back of the hand rests on

your right shoulder blade. Now slowly lift your right arm up and out from the side, feeling the movement in the back and keeping the shoulder well down. Try the same movement lifting your arm in front of you, and with your arms reversed. Check in the mirror if you are lifting your shoulders; if they move, drop them back down.

Back Backs are a common problem. Many women have S-shaped backs, which make both their bottoms and their stomachs stick out. As you strengthen your stomach muscles your back will take less strain, so hold your stomach in and lengthen and straighten the line of your spine. Try to feel air between each vertebra. If you do this correctly, you should grow slightly in the mirror!

Stomach Hold your stomach muscles lightly and firmly to take the pressure off your back. During exercise do not put too much of a strain on them, though. If they bulge out during an exercise, you are pushing them too hard too soon; build up gradually by going back to a less taxing exercise.

Legs and buttocks Stretch out the muscles in the legs and buttocks when you are walking or exercising and try to feel them lengthening. This will improve their shape and tone.

Roll down

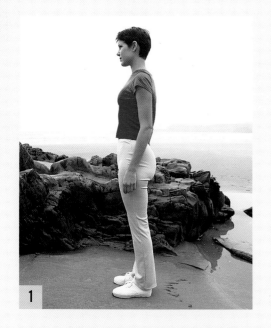

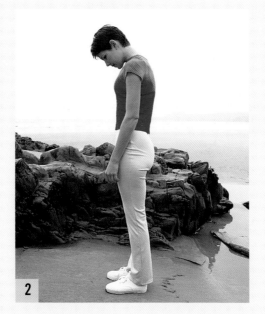

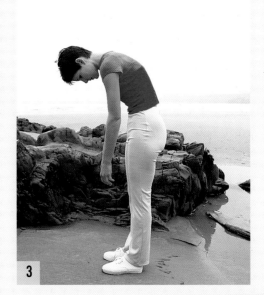

Once you have checked all the way through your posture (see opposite), the roll down will help you to feel your body in alignment. Always start with one before you exercise; it's a good way to start the day, too.

1 Stand with your feet about 45 cm (18 in) apart and slightly turned out, with shoulders dropped and relaxed, your head in line with your spine and stomach muscles held in lightly to stop your back arching. Your body should feel lifted, with space between the ribs.

2 Drop your head down on to your chest and, very slowly, let the curve continue into your shoulders and back.

3 Bending your knees slightly if you wish, continue the curve into the waist, letting your arms drop in front of you.

4 As you bend right over, extend your arms down and rest your hands on the floor in front of you. (If you cannot reach, allow your hands to dangle – do not strain to reach the floor if this is not comfortable.) Stay there for a few seconds and let the weight of your head stretch out your spine. Now, very slowly, roll the body back up. Feel your buttock muscles working to anchor the base of your spine and keep your stomach held in. As your knees straighten again, your legs lengthen and your back places itself vertebra by vertebra into a

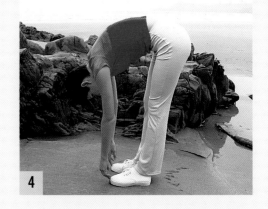

tall, elongated position. Your head comes up last, in line with your spine. Do this exercise several times so that you can really feel the placement of your body.

Pilates

The Pilates system was devised in Germany around 90 years ago, when a somewhat frail Joseph Pilates took up body building to increase his strength. His exercise programme, called 'muscle contrology', aims to bring about the complete coordination of the body, mind and spirit working with – not on, or against – the body's muscles. Pilates' philosophy has something to offer everyone, regardless of age and physical ability, particularly those who want to strengthen and tone without building huge muscles.

In summary, Pilates is about re-educating your body away from bad postural habits, which have become the norm, so that your muscles and joints function correctly. You might be unaware of the tension held in muscles, constantly pulling and twisting the skeleton, and tightening the muscles. This incorrect use of muscles and joints leads to a waste of energy and fatigue. Being aware of your posture adds synergy and control to otherwise unconscious movements. Thought is the key to Pilates; every movement is deliberate and demands concentration. By controlling our movements, we link mind and body, a concept that is fundamental to Pilates.

Key elements of Pilates

- Lengthens short muscles and strengthens weak ones
- Improves the quality of movement
- Focuses on the core postural muscles to stabilize the body
- Works to place the breath correctly
- Controls even the smallest movements
- Understands and improves good body mechanics
- Provides mental relaxation

Standing

Standing is an activity that many people find uncomfortable. Often when we stand still we do not know what to do with our bodies. We put our weight on one leg, bending the other, then we shift our weight to the other leg. We attempt to stand up straight, but we lock our knees and push the pelvis forward, creating an exaggerated hollow in the lower spine. At the same time, we do not know what to do with our arms. This unease tires us and it is as if we have no sense of the centre of gravity within the body, but if we can find it, it will hold us in a position of balance and ease.

Pilates teaches a way to stand that allows us to rest in the position with muscles relaxed and balance centred. It takes some practice before it becomes second nature, but once it is achieved it will mean you tire less easily, feel taller and are more relaxed.

Sitting

Like standing, sitting is something we often don't do very well. We sit balanced on one hip bone, then we shift to the other. We cross our legs or sit with one leg underneath us. We wriggle around in our seats, trying to find a position that feels comfortable. When we eventually find it, the comfort does not last long. We try to find external solutions to this, such as lumbar supports on chairs or car seats; but they are not suitable for most people.

When looking for a chair that will properly support your back and allow you to adopt good sitting posture, check for the following:

- You should be able to sit comfortably with your whole thigh supported by the seat of the chair.
- You should be able to place both of your feet flat on the floor.
- The back support should be as high as your shoulder blades (the backs of many office chairs are either lower or higher than this).

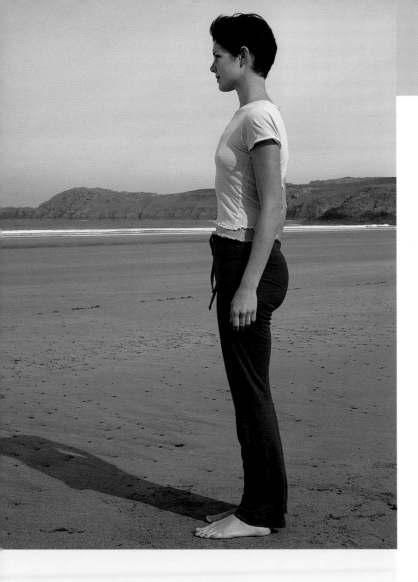

How to stand correctly

1 Stand with your feet hip-width apart.

2 Make sure that both your legs are facing forward.

3 Your legs should be straight but the knees should not be locked back into the joint.

4 Allow your arms to rest naturally at your sides, falling over the middle of your hips.

5 Feel your weight being supported in the middle of each foot.

6 Do not rock back, allowing the heels to take your weight, or place your weight on the balls of your feet.

Remember to sit with your weight evenly distributed, your knees slightly apart in order to support the weight, and your feet together, underneath the knees.

Lying

We spend approximately one-third of each day lying down. Lying down should be our ultimate position of rest, but still we manage to contort ourselves in various ways that put strain on our muscles and limit our blood circulation.

Many people sleep on their stomachs. This is not a good position as it does not support the spine. Also, people who sleep in this position usually bend one leg up, which twists the spine. To breathe properly while lying on the stomach, the head has to be turned to one side. This not only twists the neck but can also trap nerves in the neck, leading to a feeling of numbness or 'pins and needles' during sleep or on waking.

The best positions for sleeping are on your back or one of your sides. If you have a lower-back problem it can be helpful to sleep with pillows under your knees. This is also recommended if you are pregnant, when it can be extremely difficult to find a comfortable sleeping position and you are more likely to suffer from circulation problems.

Beds and pillows Extremely hard mattresses are not good – it is better to have a firm mattress that has some give in it, allowing some moulding to the body contours. The number of pillows you use depends on the density of the pillows, but one or two is the norm. It is important that the neck is fully supported by the pillow, and that there are no gaps between the neck and the pillow to put extra strain on the neck muscles.

Equipment and exercises

A Pilates studio uses some rather curious-looking pieces of equipment, with springs, pulleys, bars, handles and weights. They all tone and firm the body, and are designed, via gentle exercises that help release tension and stretch out the body into a graceful shape, to produce a beautiful, effortless posture with stomach and bottom pulled in, tension-free shoulders and the merest hollow in your back rather than a huge sway.

The exercises shown on the following pages are deliberately limited to those you can do at home with the minimum of equipment. Most exercises are done lying on the floor, and you will need an exercise mat, which you can get from most sports equipment shops. Alternatively, you can use a blanket folded lengthways, but it should also be wide enough to allow for some movement from side to side. Do not work on a carpet, as it is not sufficient to protect your spine from being bruised, and is uncomfortable anyway. Do not practise on a bed, as it is too soft.

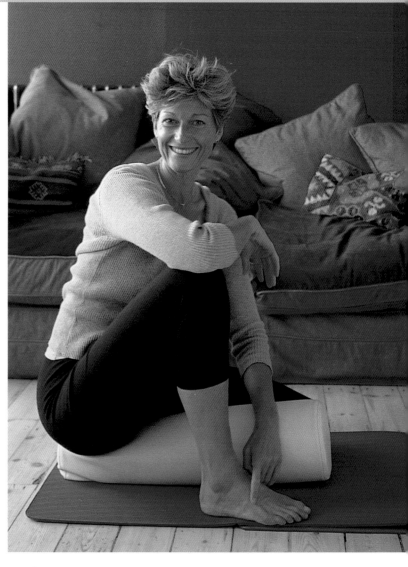

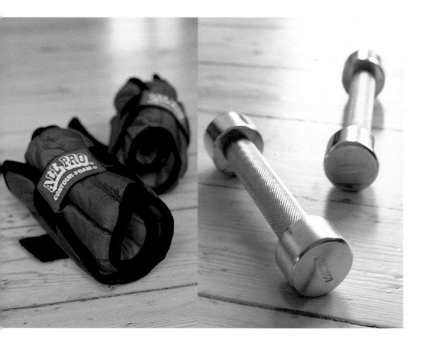

For some exercises you will need a pillow or cushion. People with neck problems might want to put a folded towel or small pillow under their neck for support. A few of the exercises require the use of light hand weights. These should be 1–1.5 kg (2–3 lb) a pair. Older people should choose the lighter weight first, whereas a younger, fitter person can use the 1.5 kg (3 lb) weight immediately. These, too, can be bought from a sports shop. Although you can substitute cans or bags of rice, you will find that it is better to use proper weights instead as improvised ones do not provide the same comfort or ease in performing the movements. You can also buy ankle weights, which will boost the effects of resistance in some of the leg exercises.

Pelvic tilt

Follow the WARM-UP routine on page 198 before you begin these exercises.

1 Begin by lying on the floor with your knees bent. Your feet and knees should be hip-width apart. **Breathe in** through your nose. Pull up your pelvic floor and pull in your lower stomach muscles.

2 Place a cushion between your thighs, just above your knees and rest your arms beside you, with the palms of your hands flat on the floor. Gently squeeze the cushion between your legs.

3 **Breathing out**, tilt the pelvis up, raising one vertebra at a time, until the lumbar spine is flat on the floor. Stay still, holding your pelvic floor and abdominals. Take a small **breath in**. **Breathing out**, slowly lower your spine down to the neutral spine position while still holding your pelvic floor and abdominal muscles. *Repeat six to 10 times.*

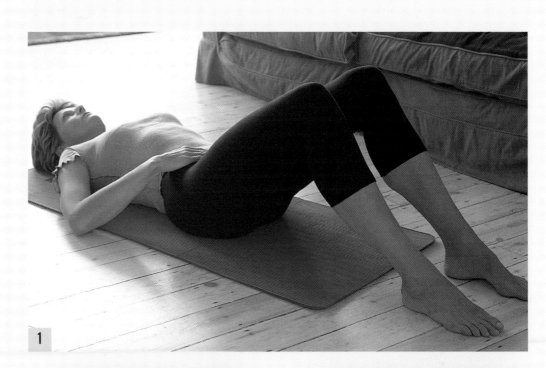

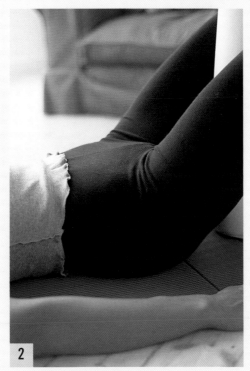

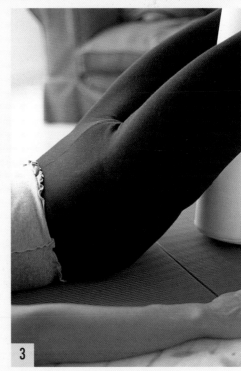

Pelvic lift

1 Repeat Steps 1–2 as for the Pelvic Tilt exercise. Then, **breathing out**, tilt your pelvis up, peeling each vertebra from the floor one at a time, until you are resting on your thoracic vertebrae, just below the shoulder blades. While holding this position, **breathe in** again.

2 **Breathing out**, lower your spine slowly back down to the floor, again taking care to lower one vertebra at a time. *Repeat six to 10 times.*

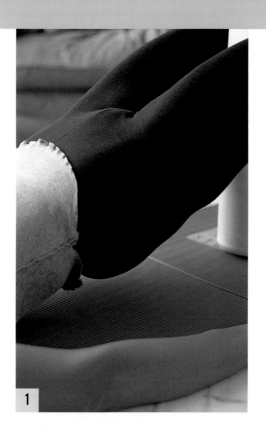
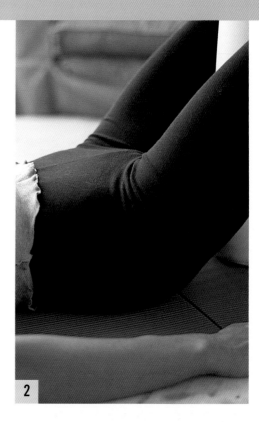

Small hip roll

1 Begin by lying down with your knees and feet together and your knees raised. Place your hands behind your head with your elbows pointing out to the sides. **Breathe in**, pull up your pelvic floor and pull in your stomach muscles:

2 **Breathing out**, bring your legs halfway towards one side. Once there, hold the position and **breathe in**. **Breathe out** and bring your legs back to the middle.

3 Repeat the movement to your other side. *Repeat three to six times each side.*

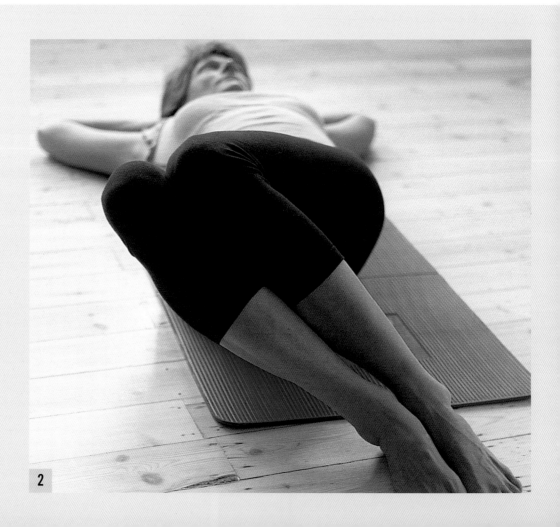

Single waist lift

1 Lie on one side, ensuring that your body is in a straight line. The arm of the side on which you are lying should be raised above your head, palm facing up. Rest your head on your arm. Your ear, the middle of your shoulder, and your hip and ankle should all be aligned. Allow your other arm to rest on your side with your hand on your thigh. Bend the leg nearest to the floor in front of you and flex your feet.

Once in the position, pull your shoulders down towards your hip and stretch your fingers towards your knee. Lengthen your waist by pushing your heels downwards slightly. **Breathe in**, pulling up your pelvic floor, pulling in your lower stomach muscles and tightening the muscles in your waist and buttocks.

2 **Breathing out**, lift your top, straight leg up to hip height. As you do this, reach with your fingers towards your knee.

3 **Breathe in** and bring your leg down, pulling the pelvic floor up and the stomach muscles in as you do so. *Repeat six to 10 times each side.*

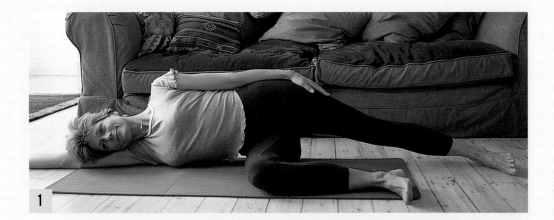

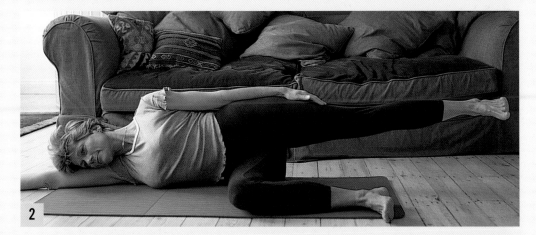

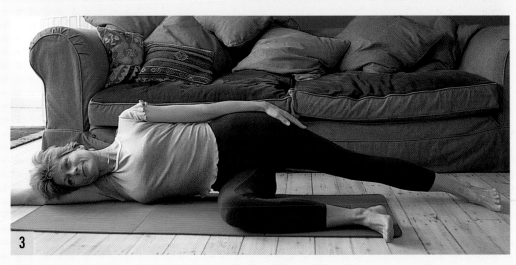

The cat

1 Start on your hands and knees with your knees hip-width apart. Ensure your hands are beneath your shoulders and your hips above your knees. Check that your back is flat, not tilted up or down and that your head and neck are in alignment with your back, parallel to the floor. **Breathe in**, sensing the breath coming in between your shoulder blades. Pull up your pelvic floor and pull in your stomach muscles.

2 **Breathing out**, curl your tailbone underneath you, push into the heel of your hands and lift your breastbone, tucking your chin and then your head underneath. Your back should now be rounded. Hold this position and **breathe in**.

3 **Breathe out** and lower yourself back into the starting position by reversing the sequence, bringing your head back up to its position parallel with the floor followed by your chin and then your tailbone. *Repeat three to six times.*

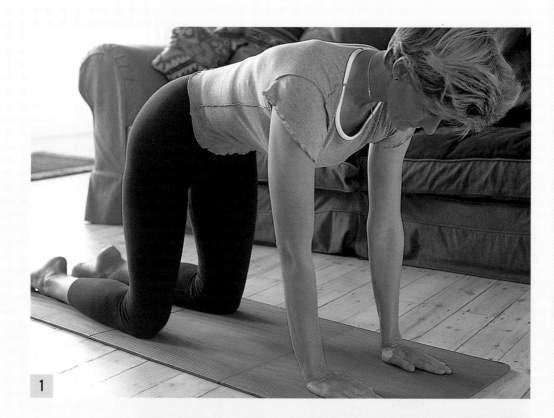

1

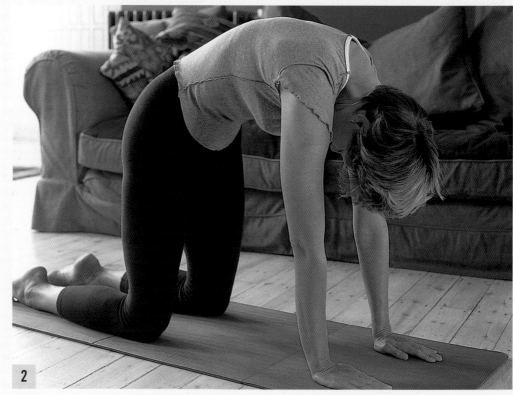

2

Sitting twist

1 Begin by sitting on the mat with your legs in front of you. Raise your right knee, and put your right hand behind your back. Rest your left elbow on your right knee. **Breathe in**, pulling up your pelvic floor, pulling in your stomach muscles and squeezing the buttocks, while lengthening the spine by pulling the vertebrae away from each other.

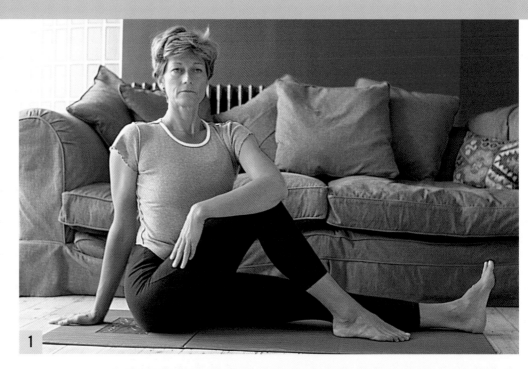

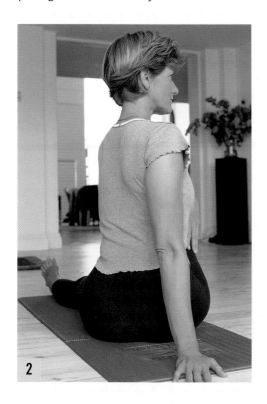

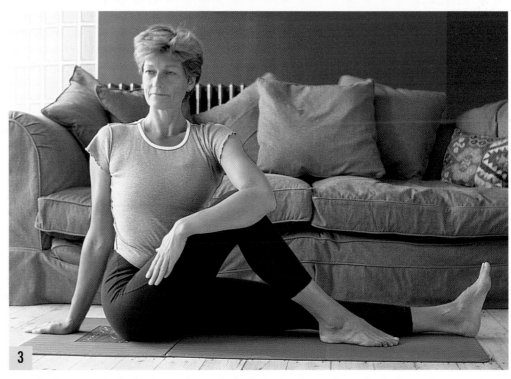

2 Breathing out, rotate your waist towards your raised leg, keeping your chin in line with your breastbone and your supporting arm straight. Take a **breath in** and lengthen the spine. **Breathe out** and rotate a little further.

3 Breathe in as you rotate back to the starting position. Repeat the sequence raising your left knee, placing your left hand behind your back and right hand on your left knee. *Repeat three times each side.*

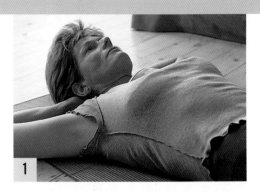

Abdominal lift

1 Begin by lying on the floor, knees bent and feet and knees hip-width apart, hands behind your head, elbows out to the side. **Breathe in**, pull up your pelvic floor, pull in your stomach muscles and squeeze your buttocks. (Do not move your pelvis or flatten your spine.)

2 As you **breathe out**, imagine a cord pulling you up from the centre of your chest.

3 Raise your head off the mat, support the weight of your head with your hands. Your shoulders will rise a little, but the bottom of your shoulder blades should still touch the mat. Your neck must not bend forwards. **Breathe in** as you lower your head again, keeping your stomach muscles working. *Repeat six to 10 times.*

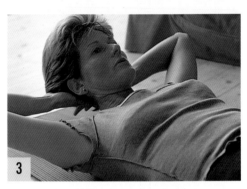

Abdominal twist

1 Begin by lying on your back with your knees bent, slightly squeezing a cushion. With one hand behind your head, cross your other arm over your body,, stretching it towards the opposite thigh. **Breathe in**, pull up your pelvic floor and pull in your stomach muscles.

2 **Breathing out**, imagine a cord pulling your breastbone forward and rotate your body. If you start with your right hand behind your head, rotate towards the right. (Do not let your hips lift off the floor and don't bend your neck.) **Breathe in** and return to the starting position, keeping your stomach muscles working. *Repeat three to six times each side.*

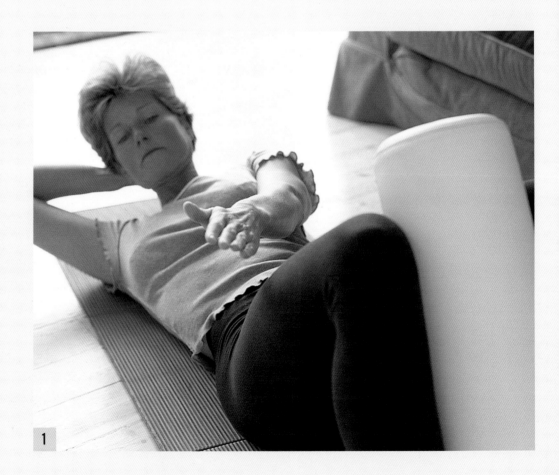

Chest opener

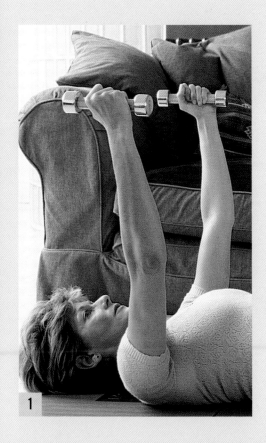

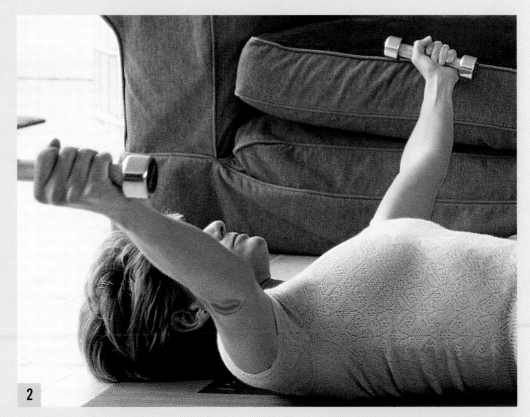

1 Begin by lying down with your knees bent, holding a weight of 0.5–1 kg (1–2 lb) in each hand, palms facing inward. Bring your arms up directly above you, keeping them straight but without locking your elbows. **Breathe in**, pull up your pelvic floor and pull in your stomach muscles.

2 Breathing out, lower your arms very slowly out to your sides. Hold the position and take a small **breath in**. (Do not allow your lower back to arch.)

3 Breathing out again, bring your arms back up slowly, using your chest muscles to do the movement. *Repeat six to 10 times.*

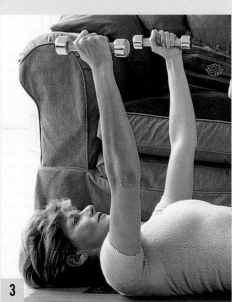

Arms over head

1 Begin by lying down with your knees bent and your arms raised, holding a weight between your hands. **Breathe in**, pull up your pelvic floor and pull in your stomach muscles.

2 **Breathing out**, slowly bring both your arms back over your head. Hold the position and **breathe in**. (Make sure your shoulders, your ribcage and your back do not lift off the mat as you bring your arms over your head. They must remain stable.)

3 **Breathing out**, pull the muscles that run down the side and back of the trunk towards your waist as you bring your arms back up. *Repeat six to 10 times.*

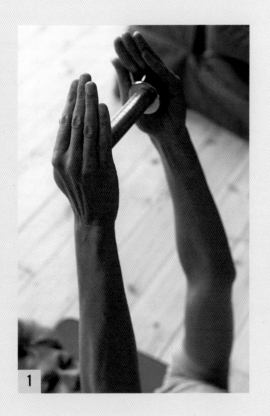

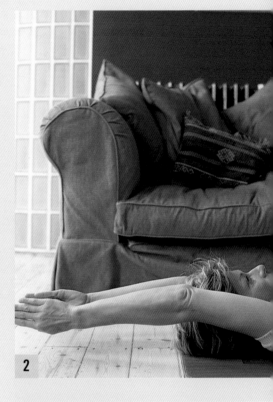

Arm circles

1 As in step 1 of the Chest Opener exercise (see previous page), begin by lying down with your knees bent, holding a weight of 0.5–1 kg (1–2 lb) in each hand, but this time rotate your hands so that the palms are facing downwards. Bring your arms up directly above you, keeping them straight but without locking your elbows. **Breathe in**, pull up your pelvic floor and pull in your stomach muscles.

2 **Breathe in** and bring your arms down beside your hips. Rotate your hands so your palms face upwards. **Breathing out**, circle both arms out to the sides horizontally, and up above your head, in line with your shoulders. **Breathing in**, bring your arms up and over, lowering them back beside your hips. *Repeat six to 10 times, then reverse the direction.*

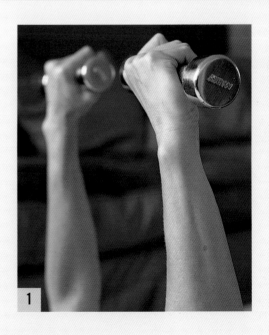

Outer thigh

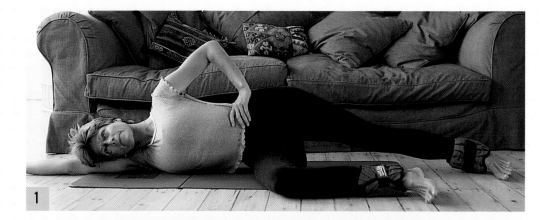

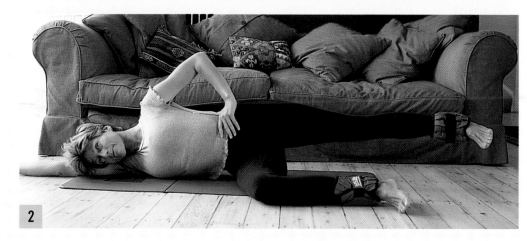

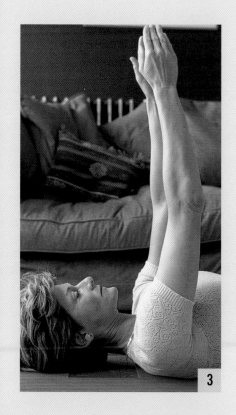

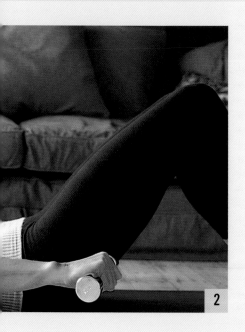

1 Begin by lying down on your right side. Bend your left arm and rest your hand on your hip bone. Bend your right leg in front of you. Raise your right arm above your head, palm facing up, and rest your head on your arm. Flex both your feet so they are at right angles to your legs, and lengthen your left leg without moving your hips. **Breathe in**, pull up your pelvic floor and pull in with your stomach muscles.

2 Breathing out, lift your left leg, feeling your buttock muscles squeezing together. (Do not arch your lower back or allow your waist to shorten. Do not allow your lower ribs to push forward.)

3 Breathe in and lower your leg to the starting position. *Repeat six to 10 times each side.*

Inner thigh

1 Begin by lying on one side again, but now bend your top leg and bring it in front of you. Put two pillows under this leg to support it and prevent you rolling your upper body forward. Place your hand on your uppermost hip and flex your feet as for the Outer Thigh exercise (see previous page). **Breathe in**, pull up your pelvic floor, pull in your stomach muscles and squeeze your buttocks together.

2 Breathing out, lengthen your lower leg without moving your hip and raise it 15 cm (6 in) off the floor. **Breathe in** and lower your leg. *Repeat six to 10 times each side.*

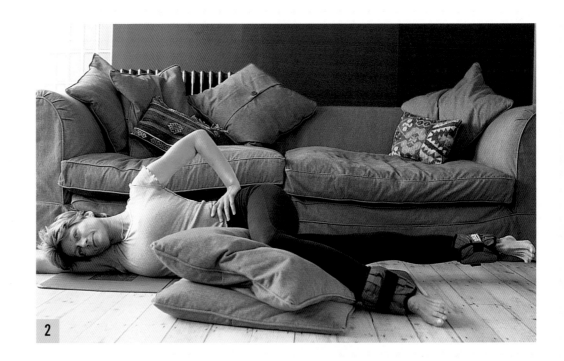

Buttock squeeze

1 Lie down on your stomach. Place a pillow or cushion between your thighs. Rest your forehead on your hands, elbows wide. **Breathe in**, pull up your pelvic floor and pull in your stomach muscles.

2 Breathing out, squeeze your thighs and buttocks together, and hold for a count of six. **Breathe in** and release your thigh and buttock muscles. *Repeat six to 10 times.*

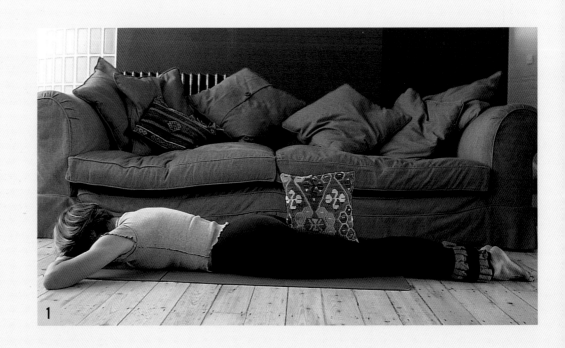

Hamstring lift

1 Begin by lying on your stomach with your forehead resting on your hands and your elbows wide. If you have a sensitive lower back, put a cushion under your stomach. **Breathe in**, pulling up your pelvic floor and pulling in with your stomach muscles.

2 **Breathing out**, raise one leg 10 cm (4 in) off the floor, keeping it straight as you do so. Feel your hamstring and buttock muscles working. (Do not arch your lower back or push out your stomach.)

3 **Breathing in**, slowly lower your leg to the floor. *Repeat six to 10 times with each leg.*

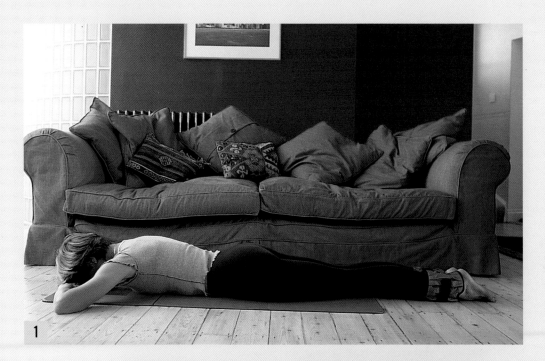
1

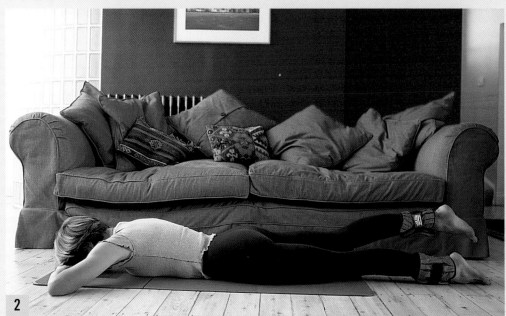
2

Warm-up exercises

Before you start working on any specific area of the body, be it to tone, shape or strengthen it or to play energetic sport, it is vital to warm up first. This prevents possible strains and injury, which are much more likely to occur when your muscles are cold. Warm-up exercises also loosen the shoulders, hips, ribs and the all-important spinal column. Do the exercises shown in the box, in the order given, as a full warm-up routine.

Roll down

Begin and end a warm-up routine by performing the **Roll Down** exercise on page 183 three times. By the end of the warm-up routine, your back should feel much looser.

Complete warm-up routine

EXERCISE	NUMBER OF REPEATS
1 **Roll down**	*3*
2 **Shoulder circles**	*3* in each direction
3 **Push me-pull yous**	*8* pushing, *8* pulling
4 **Arm stretches**	*16* upwards and *16* to the sides
5 **Leg swings**	*16* on each leg
6 **Pliés**	see text, page 200
7 **Roll down**	*3*

Shoulder circles

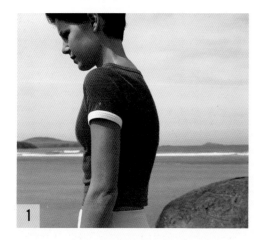
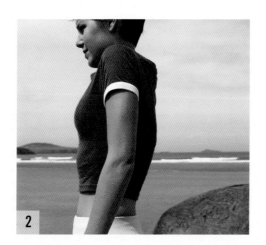
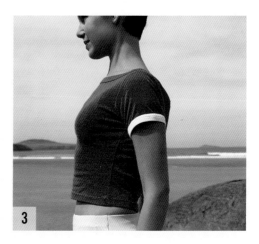

1 Stand with a good posture, your shoulders dropped and relaxed. Start to rotate the shoulders forwards. If you are doing it correctly, your arms will have turned so that your palms are facing towards you.

2 Continue the circle so that the shoulders lift up towards the ears then pull them down and back, so that your shoulder blades squeeze together. Make sure that at this point you don't arch the small of the back.

3 Finally, drop your shoulders right down. If you feel any tension in your neck, drop your head forwards on to your chest to relax the muscles. *Repeat three times, then reverse the direction,* rotating the shoulders back.

Push me-pull yous

1 Stand with good posture, your feet about 45 cm (18 in) apart. Clasp your fingers together in line with your chest, then pull them away from each other without actually letting go. You should feel the muscles of the upper arms working together with the pectorals as the chest opens. *Repeat eight times and then reverse the process*, pushing the hands together eight times.

Your head should be lifted throughout and your neck long. If you feel any tension in the area, drop your head forwards on to your chest to relax the muscles.

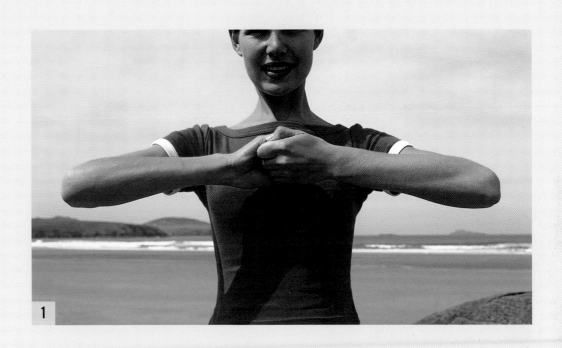

Arm stretches

1 Standing with your feet about 45 cm (18 in) apart, stretch alternate arms from the elbow upwards. Bend the knee on the same side as the arm you are stretching, shifting your body weight from side to side. The arm should stretch from the shoulder blade, shoulder well dropped down. This is not just an arm stretch – the top half of the body should be stretching up out of the waist. *Repeat 16 times.*

2 Now take alternate arms straight out to the side and *repeat this movement 16 times.*

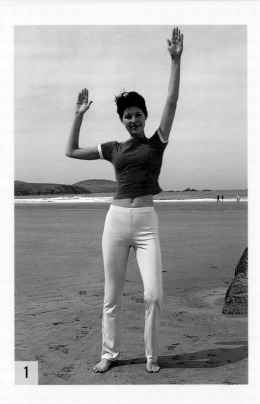
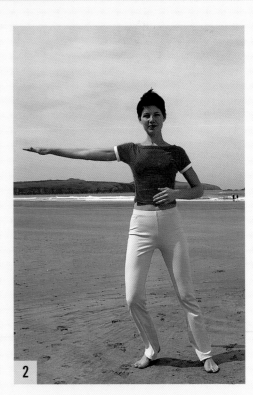

Leg swings

1 & 2 These exercises warm up the hip socket. Stand with a good posture, one hand resting on a suitable support, such as chair back. Take the outside leg straight back and then forwards in a gentle swing. *Repeat 16 times,* raising the leg a little higher each time. Change sides and *repeat with the other leg.*

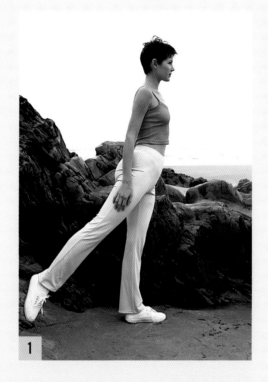
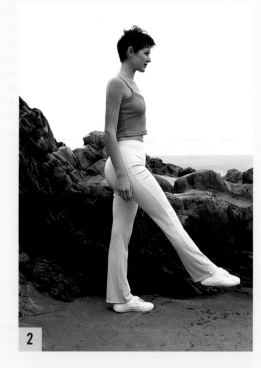

Pliés

1 & 2 Stand tall with your feet together, then bend your knees as much as you can without taking your heels off the floor. As you do this, feel your stomach muscles pushing back towards your spine and your spine growing longer – take care not to arch it. *Repeat eight times.*

3 & 4 Next, turn your feet out in a V-shape. Be sure to keep your knees over your feet at all times – don't allow them to roll in as this could damage them. Bend your knees, feeling your thigh muscles turn out and your buttock muscles pull under. *Repeat three times,* keeping your heels on the floor.

5 On the fourth bend, allow your heels to rise and go down as far as you can, keeping your back straight – you may want to hold on to a support to do this. *Repeat the sequence twice more.*

6 & 7 Finally, with your feet about 45 cm (18 in) apart, turn your legs out from the hip sockets so your knees are over your feet. Bend in the same way as the previous pliés, keeping your heels firmly on the ground, with your thigh muscles turning out. Do not lift your heels at all. *Repeat, slowly, four times.*

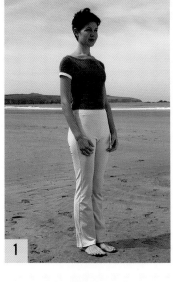

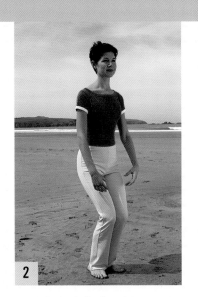

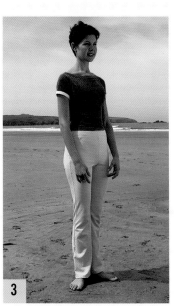

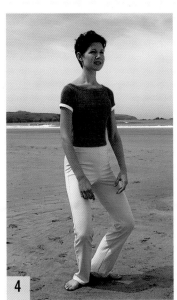

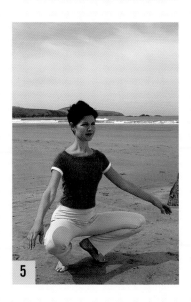

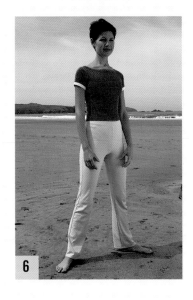

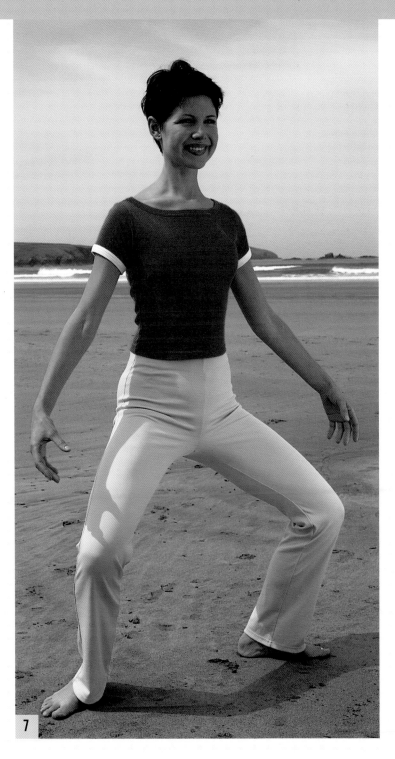

SEE ALSO:

→ Winding down, page 222

→ Aerobic exercise, page 224

Shaping and toning

The exercises on the following pages are gentle and aim to stretch and tone your whole body – not to build up bulky muscles. When you start to exercise regularly, you will be conditioning your body and at the same time discovering you have more vitality. This is due to a hormone called noradrenaline (or norepinephrine) which is released each time you exercise. It is nicknamed the 'kick' hormone because this is precisely what it does – it gives you a natural high that makes you more alert and increases your sense of wellbeing, as well as decreasing feelings of hunger. At the same time, exercise also raises the beta-endorphin levels in the body and these help you to relax and to sleep better. There's no doubt about it – our bodies deserve the benefits of exercise.

Flatter stomachs

The stomach muscles are often some of the weakest in a woman's body, and we can make up for this fact by letting the back take the strain. Our backs may end up hunched, tense and overarched as a result – doing us a double disservice: bad posture and possible permanent injury, too. Strengthening the stomach muscles takes pressure off the back, giving a flat tummy in the process.

If your stomach muscles start to bulge or quiver at any time during these exercises, you are attempting something that is as yet beyond them – so stop! When you are lying on your back, the lower your legs are towards the floor the more strain you will be putting on the stomach; lift them higher and the exercise will instantly become easier. When you are doing these exercises – and indeed all the time – try to think of the stomach muscles providing a natural girdle, keeping the body in a lifted, well-held posture.

Torso twists

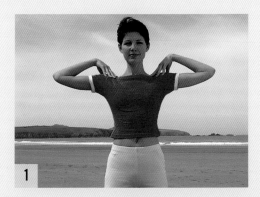

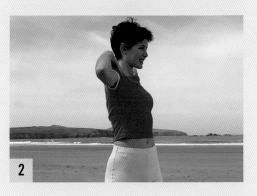

With these twists, it is important to remember that it is only the waist and upper body that turn – the hips stay absolutely still and facing the front.

1 Stand with your feet hip-width apart and slightly turned out, knees bent. Rest your hands lightly on your shoulders, elbows straight out. Feel your back straight and your tailbone dropping down towards the floor.

2 Turn from the waist to look over your left shoulder. *Repeat 16 times to left and right.*

Side stretches

1 With your feet hip-width apart and slightly turned out, clasp your hands together above your head, keeping your shoulders dropped.

2 In one smooth movement, looking straight ahead, drop down to the left, bending from the waist. Try to get low enough for your arms to be parallel with the floor. Come back to the centre and repeat on the right. *Repeat four to eight times each side.*

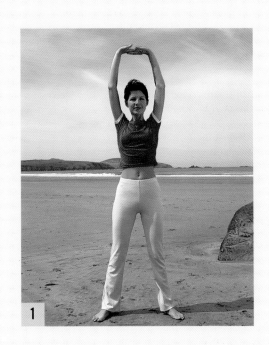

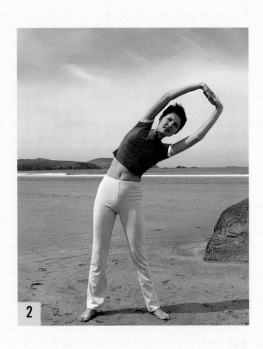

Upper body circles

This is a more complex version of the Torso Twists exercise.

1 Stand with your feet hip-width apart and slightly turned out, your arms raised, shoulders down and hands clasped.

2 Drop down to the left until your arms are parallel to the floor, feeling the stretch all the way up your right side.

3 Now turn so that you are looking down at the floor, keeping your back straight. This is a lot of work for the stomach muscles.

4 Turn back so you are facing sidewards again and then straighten up. *Build up to four times each side.*

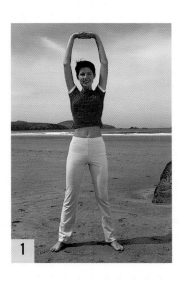

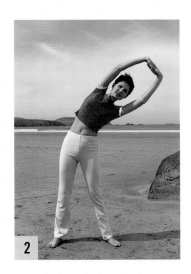

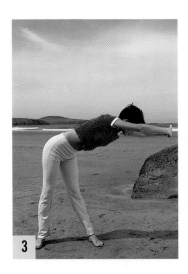

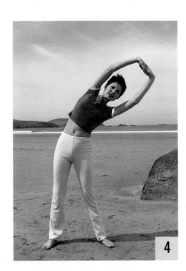

Roll-ups

This is a series of exercises that build up in difficulty, so start with the first one and only go on to the later ones as your muscles strengthen.

1 Lie on the floor with your legs stretched out and your arms at your sides, palms upwards. Pull your stomach muscles back into the floor, tightening your buttock muscles under you at the same time. This will cause your knees to bend slightly and your pelvis to tilt. *Repeat four times.*

2 In the second stage, repeat the pelvic tilt, this time moving your upper body off the floor, arms outstretched and parallel to the floor. Your head should come up last. Do not raise yourself far enough off the floor to make your stomach bulge or your shoulders tense. *Repeat four times.*

3 In the third stage, you begin as before and continue to raise your upper body until you are sitting straight up, arms stretched out in front, head and neck in a long line with your spine.

4 Now drop your head forward on to your chest and roll back down through the spine, holding on tight to the stomach muscles. Try to feel your back go down, vertebra by vertebra, lengthening out on the floor. *Repeat four times.*

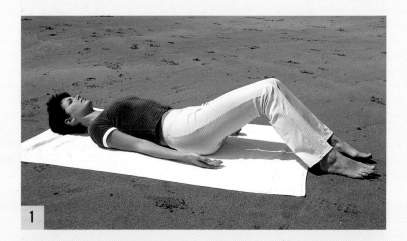

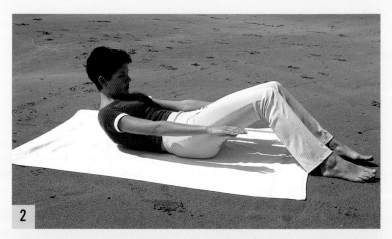

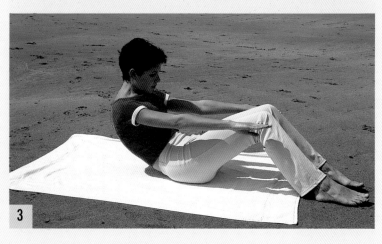

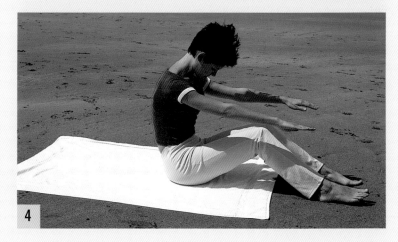

Rope climbing

This is quite tough for the abdominal muscles, so don't try it until you can do the first four stomach exercises comfortably.

1 Start by lying on your back on the floor. Contract your stomach muscles so that you start to roll up until you are about halfway to a sitting position, knees bent, arms stretched out in front of you. Loosely clench your fists, then raise one arm above your head. Lower it again and, as you do so, raise the other one. This movement looks as if you are pulling on a rope. If the stomach muscles start to bulge out or quiver, stop. *Repeat eight times.*

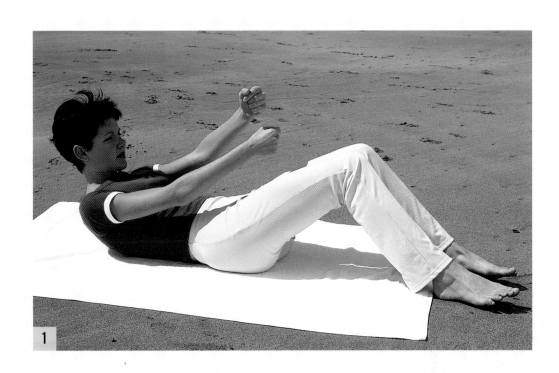

Scissors

If you're not ready to do this, the small of your back will come off the floor – stop if it does. The lower the legs, the harder it is.

1 Lie flat on the floor, arms by your sides. Bend your knees into your chest and stretch your legs upwards. With your fingers resting just behind your ears, lift your head and shoulders and look up at your legs. Pull your stomach well in (raise your legs higher if the exertion is too great). Scissor your legs, crossing them at the ankles. *Repeat 16 times.*

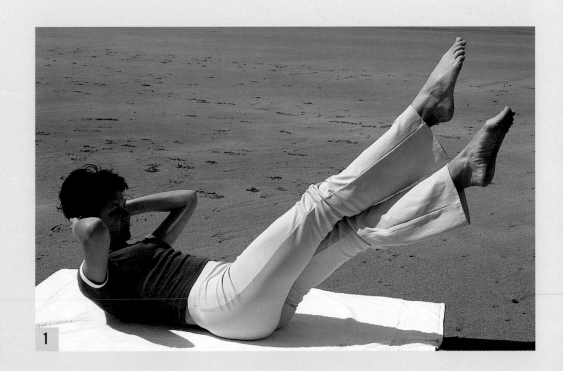

Beautiful bottoms

Many women are obsessed about their bottoms. One of the problems with bottoms is that their muscles don't get much use in everyday life. Improving your posture will be a good start at waking those muscles up, while the following exercises will strengthen them, thus lifting and firming the buttocks.

Back leg lifts

1 & 2 Lie on your front, resting on your elbows. Bend your right leg slightly and keep the foot flexed. Raise the left leg and stretch it to its full extent, pointing the foot. You should be able to feel the leg muscles working right into the buttocks. *Repeat 16 times each side, then repeat 16 more* with foot flexed.

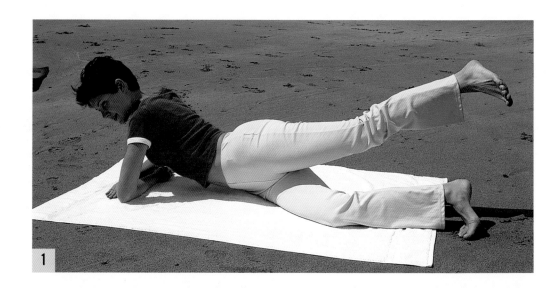

Leg circles

1 Lie flat on your front, your face on your arms. Raise one leg straight behind you and make little circles with your pointed foot, clockwise and then anti-clockwise. *Repeat 16 times with each leg.*

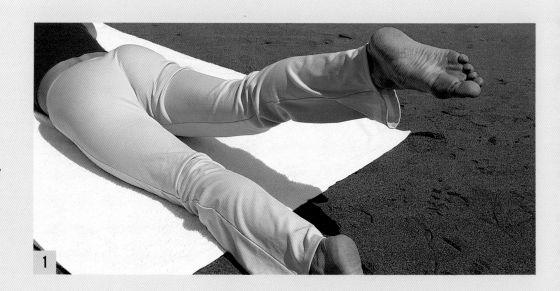

Buttock awareness

1 Sit on the floor, your legs stretched out in front, feet pointed. Your back should be perfectly straight, your arms beside you and hands on the ground. Pull your buttock muscles tight beneath you – you should find you are sitting about 5 cm (2 in) higher! *Repeat this clenching and releasing 16 times.*

2 & 3 With your buttocks clenched and your arms straight out in front, *point and flex your feet 16 times.* Point your feet again and, sitting tall, move each leg alternately from the hip as if you are walking on your buttocks. *Walk eight 'steps' forwards and eight back.*

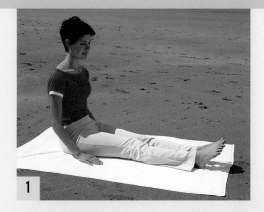
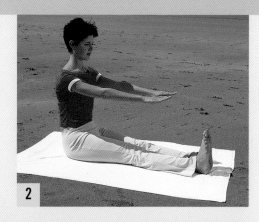
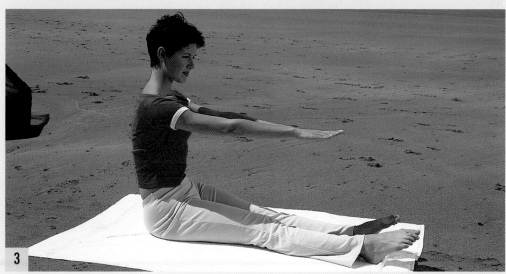

Leg stretches

1 Lie face down on the floor, arms and legs stretched, feet about hip-width apart. Pull up your stomach muscles. Stretch out your left arm and right leg simultaneously, feeling the stretch right through your body – it should lift your arm and leg about 15 cm (6 in) from the ground. *Repeat with the opposite arm and leg. Do the exercise eight times on each side.*

2 *Repeat eight times* with both arms and legs stretching at once.

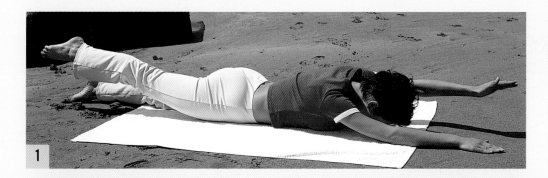
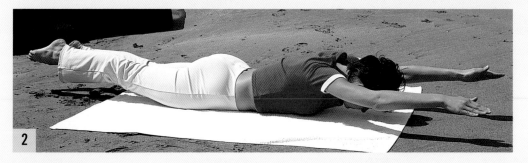

Foot tapping

1 & 2 Lie face down on the floor and stretch out your arms and legs, with your head and chest off the floor as well. Now tap the feet together, *working up to 50 taps.*

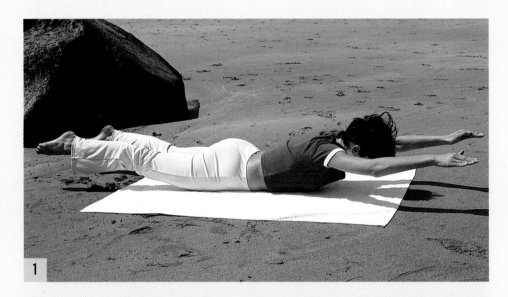

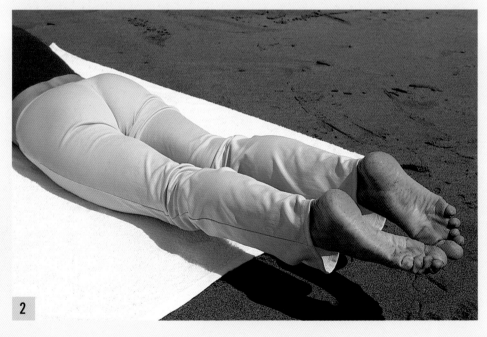

Turn-out

1 Stand up very tall, your upper body relaxed and your back absolutely straight. Turn out your legs from the hip sockets very slowly so that your feet form a 'V' shape. Don't take your feet too far – your knees should be over your feet at all times, not rolling inwards. At the same slow pace, draw your feet back to a parallel position. This exercise works the muscles of the buttocks and the inner and outer thighs. *Repeat for 16 complete movements.*

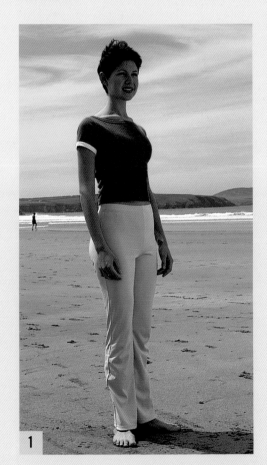

Deep pliés

The more slowly you do this exercise, the more effective it is. You may need to hold a support such as a chair back on one side to help you balance.

1 Stand tall with your feet about 45 cm (18 in) apart, your legs turned out from the hips without trying to over-extend the turn-out in the feet or ankles.

2 Keeping your back straight, drop your tailbone down towards the floor, bending your knees but without taking your heels off the floor, resting your hands on your thighs.

3 Squeeze your thighs together to straighten, pulling up the muscles in your buttocks and the backs of your thighs.

4 Keep on squeezing so hard that you rise up on to your toes. Come down in one slow, smooth movement and bend the knees into another deep plié. *Repeat the whole sequence four times in all*, changing sides if you are keeping your balance by holding a chair back.

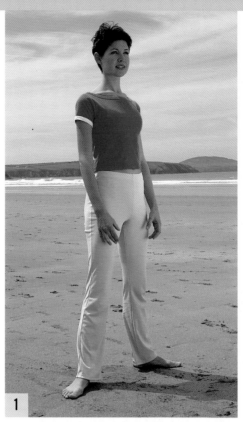

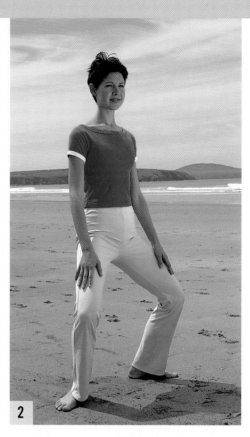

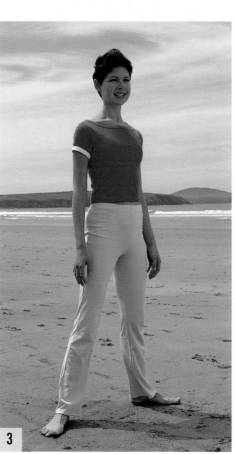

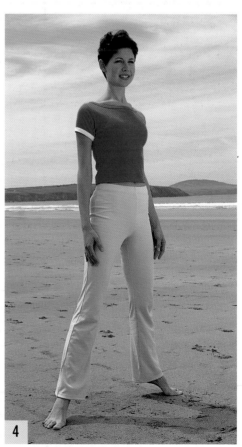

Trimmer thighs

Let's face it – nobody wants to be pear-shaped. That bulge over the hips and the jodhpur thighs are not exactly appealing. Unfortunately, for most women, this is exactly where fat is most likely to accumulate, often with the 'orange-peel' effect of cellulite. This needs to be attacked on two fronts, the first being diet and the second being exercises that lengthen and strengthen. The exercises that follow do not build up bulky muscle – they are designed to elongate the legs. Where the leg is to stretch in an exercise, you should feel it pulled out to its full extent all the way from the hip socket to the pointed toes.

Parallel pliés

These pliés strengthen the muscles at the front of the thighs, which not only gives your leg a firm, curved front but also protects the knees.

1 & 2 Stand tall with one hand resting on a chair back, feet together and facing forwards. Keeping your spine straight, bend your knees, dropping your tailbone directly down to the floor, completing it in one movement and only peeling your heels off the floor when you really have to.

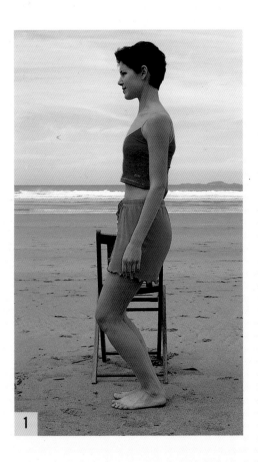
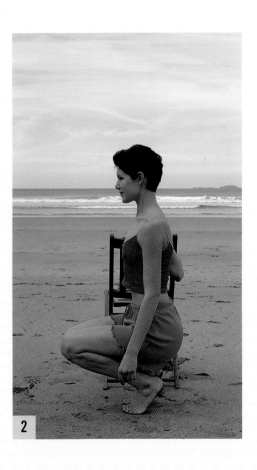
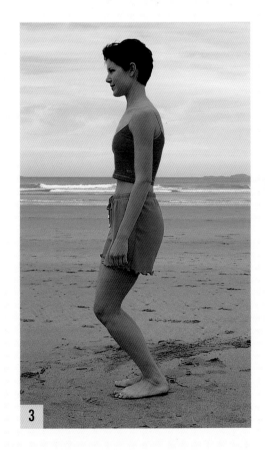

Come back to standing. *Repeat for four pliés and rises on each side.*

3 & 4 Move away from the chair but assume the same starting position. This time, as you bend, let your bottom stick out and aim to get your upper thighs parallel to the floor without lifting your heels. Swing your arms forward as you go down to help you balance. *Repeat 16 times.*

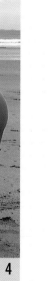

Inner thigh lifts

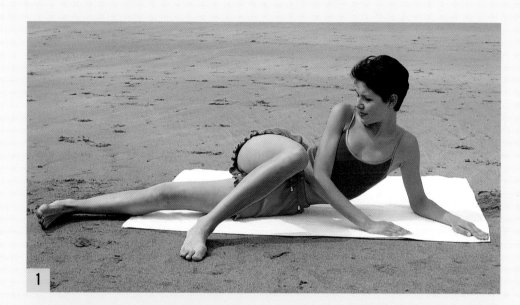

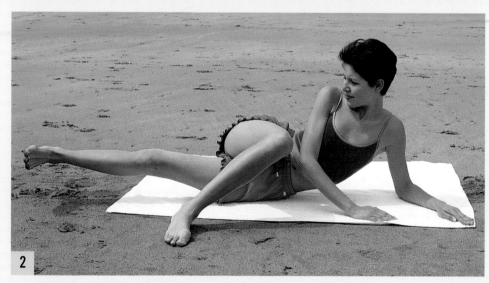

1 Lie on your side, propped up on one elbow or lying down flat along an outstretched arm. Bring your top leg over you, bending your knee, and place that foot on the floor. Extend your lower leg and flex the foot.

2 Lift your lower leg about 15 cm (6 in) off the floor. *Repeat 16 times. Now repeat for another 16 with your foot pointed. Repeat the whole exercise on the other side.*

Leg lifts

1 Lie on your side, propped up on one elbow or lying down flat along an outstretched arm, as you prefer. Bend your lower leg and flex your foot so your heel is raised slightly off the ground. Flex your upper foot and push your heel away hard so your leg feels as if it is pulling out of the hip socket all the way through the exercise. Keep your back straight and your stomach held in throughout.

2 Raise the leg and, from the raised position do a small lift. *Repeat 16 times.*

3 Lower your leg and take it forwards so that it is at a right angle to your body.

4 Keeping your foot flexed, *raise it 16 times.* Finally, in the raised position, make 16 small circles clockwise then 16 anti-clockwise. *Repeat the whole exercise on the other side.*

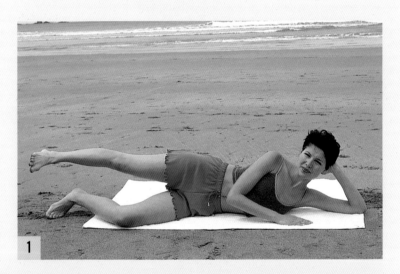

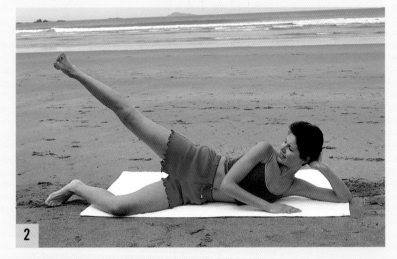

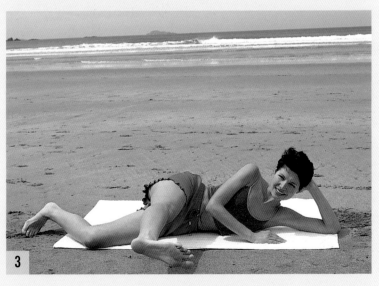

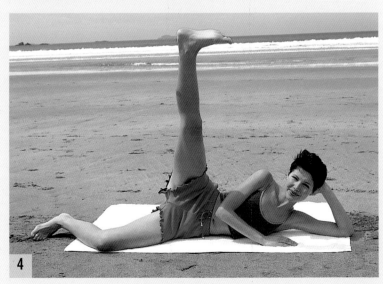

Double leg lifts

This exercise works the legs and the stomach very hard!

1 Lie flat on your side with your lower arm extended above your head. Point your feet to feel as if you are in one straight line from the tips of your fingers to the tips of your toes. Place your upper hand on the floor in front of you for balance. Slowly raise both legs at once, keeping them together. Lower and *repeat eight times.*

2 Now raise the upper body in a smooth, low curve, with your lower arm outstretched. Lower and *repeat eight times.*

3 Finally, lift your legs and your upper body and then lower them again *eight times.*

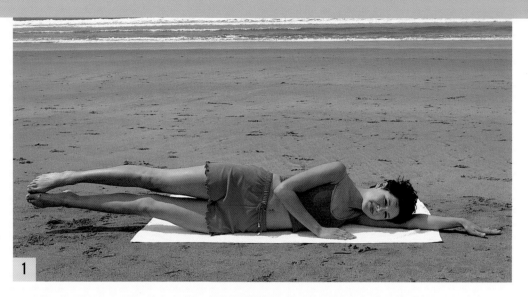

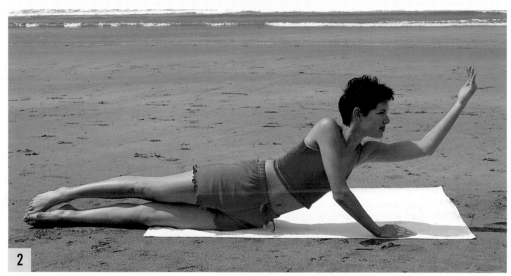

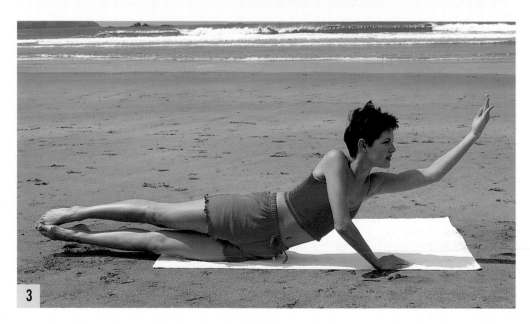

Leg sweeps

1 Lie flat on the floor on your back, with your knees and toes stretched and your stomach pressing back towards your spine.

2 Slowly lift your left leg straight upwards and then down towards your chest as far as it will go, keeping it straight.

3 Now let your extended leg cross your body and allow its weight to pull it down towards the floor.

4 Return your leg across your body and down to the floor in a smooth circle. Change legs and *repeat four times on each side.*

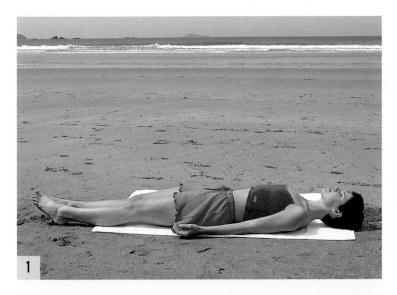

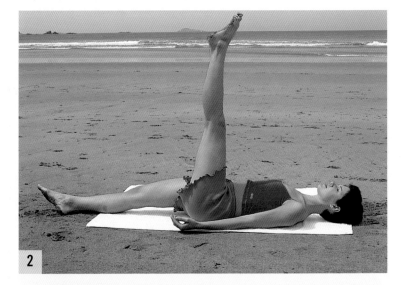

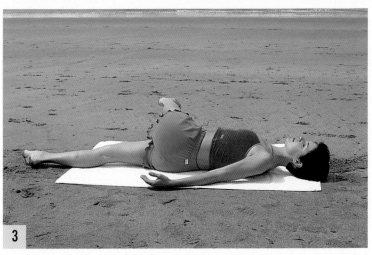

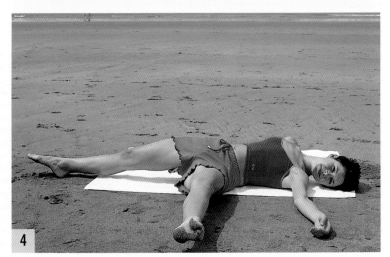

Leg kicks

1 Lie flat on the floor on your back, with your knees and toes stretched and your stomach pressing back towards your spine. Lift your left leg, placing it so that it crosses over your right at the ankle.

2 Lift it again very slightly and let it drop down on your right ankle to bounce straight upwards. Lower and place your right leg on top, bounce and kick. *Repeat, alternating, for eight kicks on each leg,* keeping the movement smooth and elongated and the small of your back on the floor.

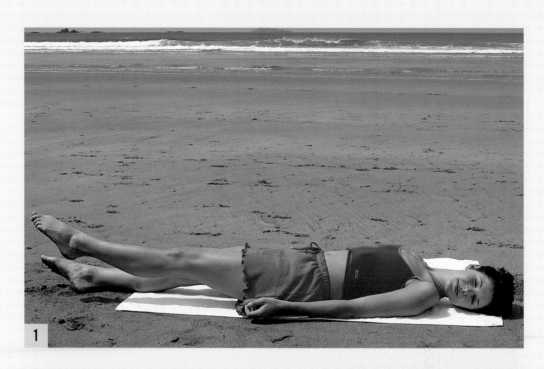

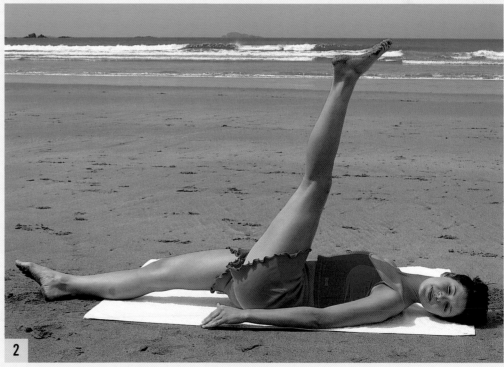

Ankle trimmer

This is a wonderful exercise for shaping both the calves and the ankles.

1 Sit on the edge of a chair, feet flat on the floor, hands resting on your thighs, upper body relaxed. Keep your knees and toes together but take your heels out so that they are about 15 cm (6 in) apart, still resting on the floor.

2 Now sweep the toes out so that they make a little semicircle, coming off the floor. *Repeat the sweep 16 times.*

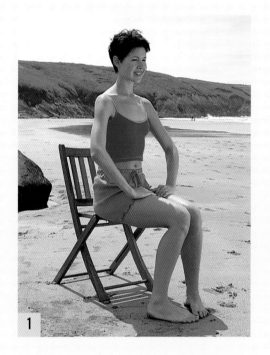 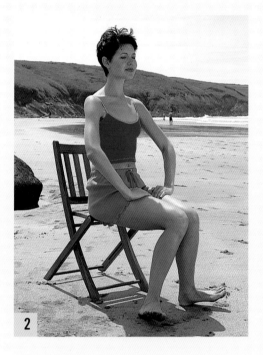

Double leg stretch

This exercise could have just as easily appeared as a stomach strengthener. It is a Pilates-based sequence (see page 184) and a good all-round exercise.

1 Lie on your back on the floor, legs outstretched and arms by your sides.

2 Raise your knees to your chest and rest your hands on your knees.

3 Keeping your stomach firmly held in, curve up your head and shoulders towards your knees, but without tensing up your shoulders or neck. Keeping the same curve in your back, pull your navel into your spine and extend your arms and legs so they are both pointing straight upwards.

4 In this position, turn out your legs from the hips and flex your feet (the more you flex, the better the exercise is for the thighs).

5 Keeping your feet and legs as they are, take your arms back towards your ears in the widest circle you can, up over your head and back to their previous position, stretching up.

6 When your arms are back to their starting point, point your toes and really stretch both arms and legs upwards. Bring your knees down to your chest and roll your back and head down to the floor. *Work up to repeating this exercise 10 times.*

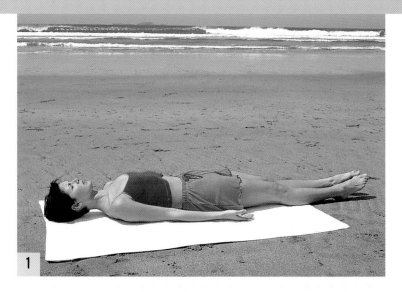

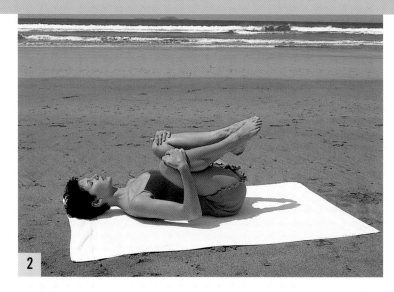

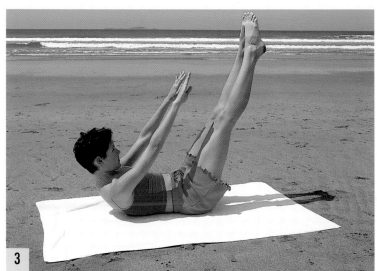

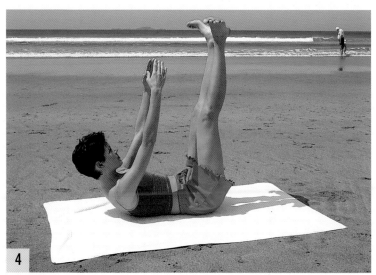

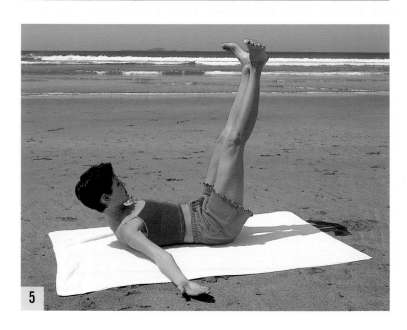

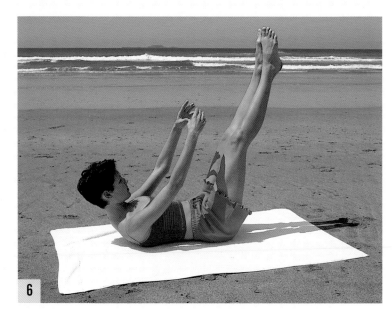

Head and shoulders

The following exercises are designed to remove tension in the neck and shoulders, improve posture and address particular problems such as flabby arms. Never let your shoulders hunch in tension or your spine slump; keep in front of you a mental picture of a lifted, elongated spine, a long neck and a gracefully held head. There will be an instant improvement in how you look.

Head rolls

1 Standing or sitting with a straight spine and dropped, relaxed shoulders, let your head fall forwards on to your chest.

2 & 3 Very slowly, roll it around to the left until it is parallel with your shoulder — make sure you don't draw your shoulder up to meet it. Return to the centre and repeat on the right. *Repeat the whole exercise six times.*

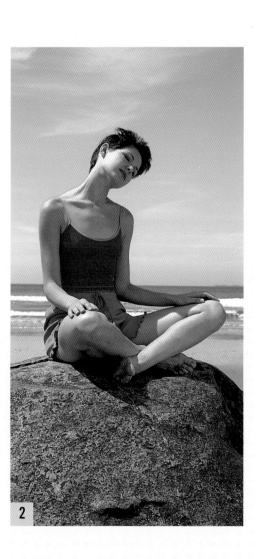

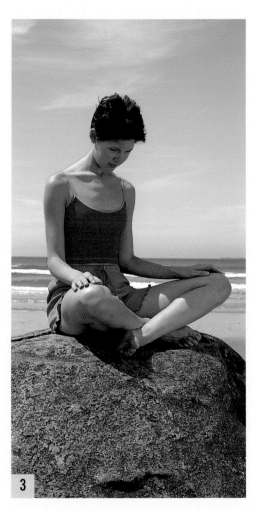

Shoulder lifts

1 Sitting or standing with a straight spine and a long neck, feel your shoulders dropped right down into your back.

2 Now lift them as high as you can – right up to your ears – then let them drop down. *Repeat eight times.*

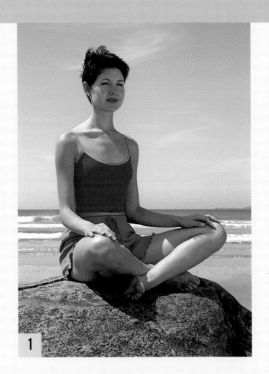

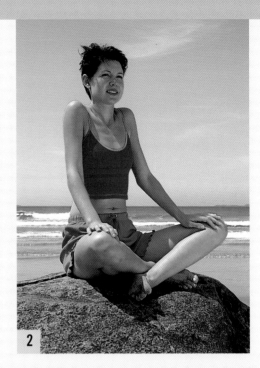

Clenching fists

1, 2 & 3 Sit cross-legged (or however you are most comfortable) with a straight back. Feel your body lifting up out of your waist and stretch your arms out low at your sides. Clench your hands into fists and then fling your fingers out, stretching them as far as they will go. *Repeat the clenching and stretching as you raise your arms*, taking eight flings to get your arms pointing straight up and another eight to get back down again. Build up to doing the whole exercise *four times.*

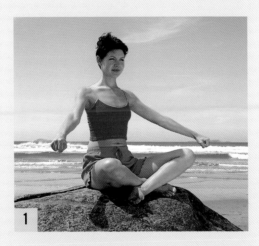

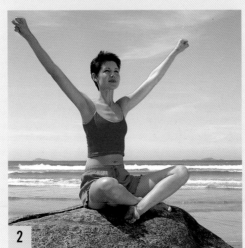

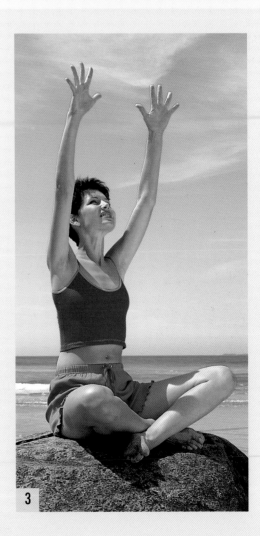

Bosom firmer

This works on the pectoral muscles that lie beneath the breast tissue – the breasts themselves have no muscles.

1 Sit cross-legged with your arms stretched out to the sides at shoulder level.

2 Raise your arms above your head until your palms meet, making sure your shoulders are dropped. Start to lower your hands in front of you, pressing them hard together as you do so. You should feel the pectorals working straight away, feeling almost as if they are pulling the arms down.

3 Bend your arms until your hands are in front of your breastbone, then take them straight out to the sides and *repeat the whole sequence four to eight times.*

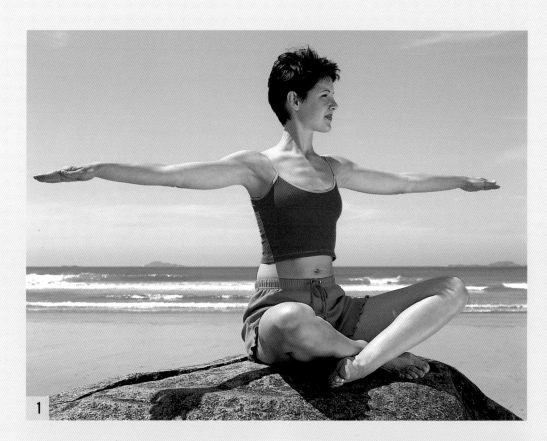

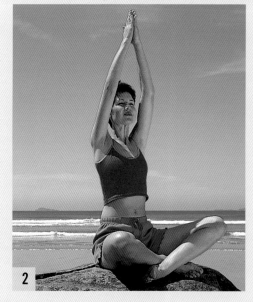

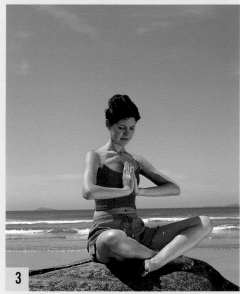

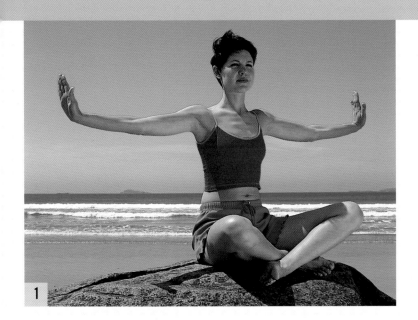
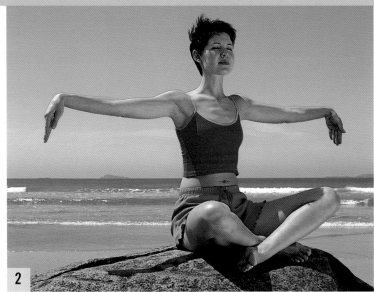

Flipper hands

This exercise is a really effective assault on flabby upper arms!

1 Sit cross-legged with your arms straight out to the side at shoulder level. Push away from the shoulders so that the arms are fully extended and flex the hands back, keeping the fingers straight so that you feel a stretch right along the underside of the arm.

2 Now drop the hands and curl them under as far as they will go. This time, you should feel a real pull along the backs of the hands, wrists and forearms. *Repeat the sequence 16 times*, keeping the shoulders dropped down throughout.

Arm crosses

This works on both the upper arms and the pectoral muscles.

1 Sit cross-legged with your arms stretched out in front of you, crossed at the wrists and pointing towards the floor.

2 From here, start to raise the arms, crossing and recrossing them, alternating which arm is on top. Take eight crosses to reach the top and another eight to come back down. Make sure you look straight ahead and keep your neck long. *Repeat four times.*

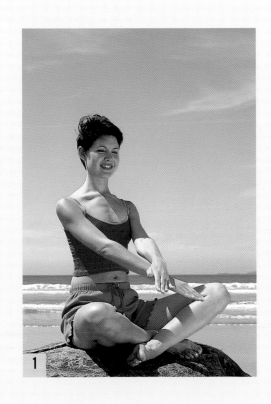
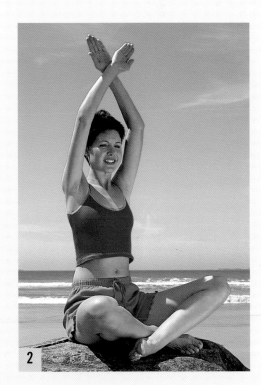

Winding down

The end of an exercise session is just as important as the beginning. This is when the muscles are fully warmed up and can be stretched out, and when you should feel both relaxed and energized. Besides the exercises given here, you can also use 'The Cat' exercise on page 190, the 'Child Pose' used in yoga on page 261 and the 'Roll Down' on page 183. You should find that your roll down is much more flexible by the end of a session and that your body feels generally looser. Any stiffness will disappear once you begin to exercise regularly.

Arm release

1 Sitting comfortably back on your heels or with crossed legs, raise one arm in the air.

2 Now fold it at the elbow so that your hand drops down towards the back of your neck.

3 With your other hand, push the raised elbow back and feel your hand drop further down your back. This is a gentle release – don't push too hard. *Repeat on the other side.*

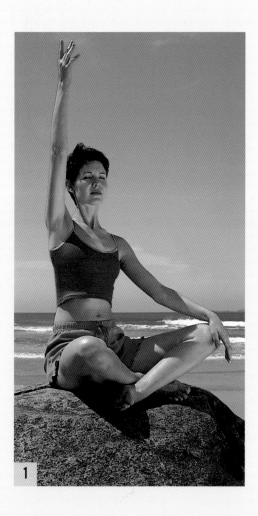
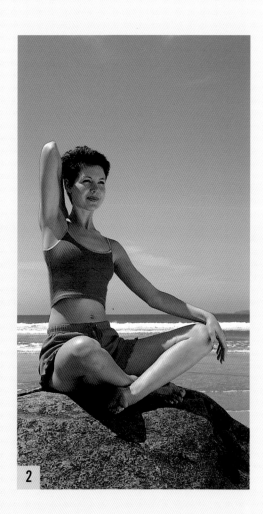
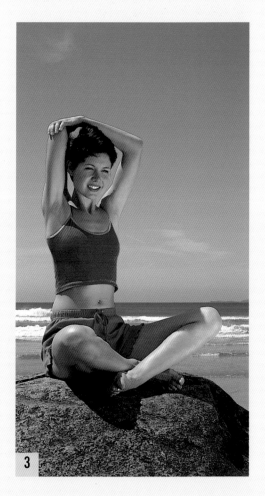

Revitalizing stretch

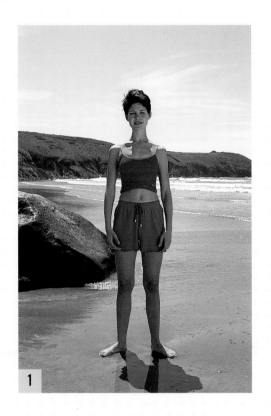

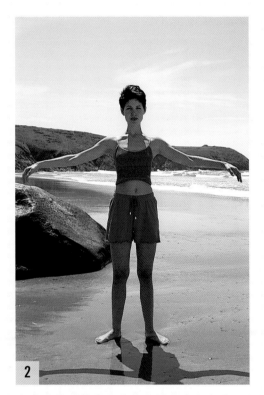

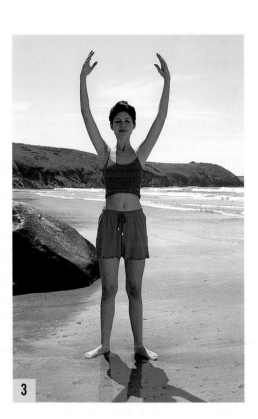

A revitalizing stretch at the end of the exercise session will leave you feeling full of energy and ready for anything.

1 Stand up straight, feet hip-width apart. Feel all your muscles pulled up.

2 Now let your **breath out** and, as you **breathe in** again, let the air fill your body and lift your arms out gently to the side. **Breathe out** as you lower them.

3 With **each breath**, lift the arms a little higher until they touch above your head. On the final intake of **breath** in the sequence, look up into your palms and bring the arms down again. The whole sequence should take around **eight breaths.**

4 Now **breathe normally** for a few moments and feel your spine straight, your knees, thighs and stomach muscles pulled up, and your shoulders dropped down and relaxed. Your head is lifted and in line with your spine and you should feel just full of oxygen!

SEE ALSO:

→ Warm-up exercises, page 198

→ Yoga, page 252

Aerobic exercise

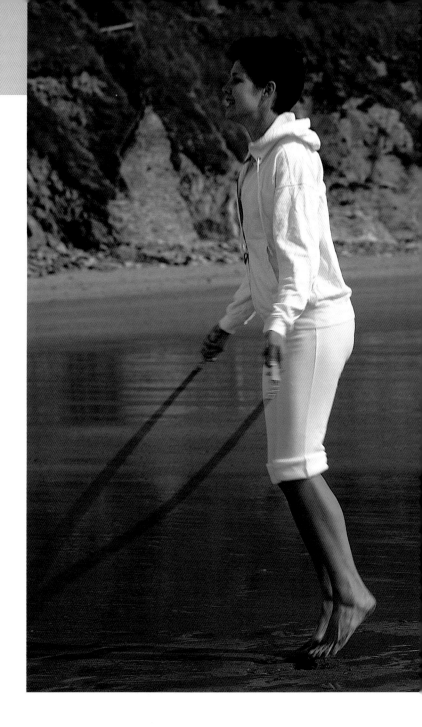

All of the exercises on the previous pages are for body toning and shaping. While these are excellent for defining and sculpting your figure, you do also need to do aerobic exercise. This type of exercise makes you slightly breathless and increases your pulse rate. It does not necessarily mean 'aerobics' – there are plenty of other forms of aerobic exercise, such as swimming, cycling and running. However, aerobic exercise of some sort is vital for several reasons. First, and most importantly, it increases cardiovascular fitness.

What aerobic exercise does for your skin

Regular exercise improves your circulation, which in turn benefits your skin. Minutes after starting to exercise, many of us turn an embarrassingly beetroot tone. That may be bad for our self-esteem, but it is generally good for our skin. In the first moments of an exercise session, blood supply to the skin actually decreases, as the body feeds the working muscles. But as soon as you start to warm up, it sends more blood to the skin surface, in order to cool the body core down. The whole process is impressively efficient: within a few minutes of starting to exercise, the heart rate triples, blood volume increases sevenfold and the amount of oxygen multiplies by 20, feeding the smallest capillaries in the skin.

Exercise also helps to clean the body out by increasing the elimination of toxins through the lungs in air and through the skin in sweat. Sweating also helps to lubricate the skin – a particularly valuable function as it ages and dries.

Cardiovascular fitness means that your heart muscle actually becomes stronger and pumps the blood around your body more efficiently. Lymph flow, too, benefits from exercise – the lymph has no internal pump so relies on bodily movement to keep it flowing. Aerobic exercise also protects against certain diseases – including coronary heart disease and, it is now thought, some types of cancer – and increases the mineral content of your bones, making problems such as osteoporosis less likely. It gives more flexibility to the joints, preventing stiffness and lack of mobility and, very importantly, burns fat while building muscle.

How many calories are you burning?

The chart on the right is a very rough guide to some everyday activities, together with the number of calories you would burn on average if you undertook the activity for 20 minutes. Some of these activities are definitely more work than pleasure, but the figures prove that simply increasing your overall daily activity can significantly improve overall fitness and energy levels. Simple ways to do this include using the stairs instead of lifts or escalators and parking further from your destination than usual – or getting off the bus a stop or two earlier – and walking the rest of the way.

Aerobic options

Build new aerobic exercise into your lifestyle gradually. If you start flat out for a fortnight, it's likely that you will go off it and never do it again. Try aerobic dance classes to see if they suit you. Many people find the discipline of going to a class to exercise helps them to stick to it, and there is also the advantage of drawing support from the other people exercising along with you. If this doesn't appeal to you, though, there are plenty of other choices.

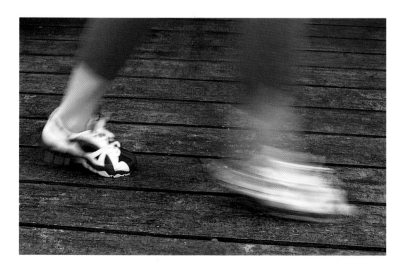

How many calories are you burning?

ACTIVITY	CALORIES/20 MINUTES
Running	300
Circuit training	260
Rowing	200
Jogging	170
Cycling	160
Horseriding	150
Aerobics	140
Swimming	140
Weight training	140
Mowing the lawn	130
Skiing	130
Gardening	120
Tennis	120
Washing windows	120
Skipping	100
Scrubbing floors	90
Bowling	80
Golf	80
Ironing	80
Walking leisurely	80
Housework	60

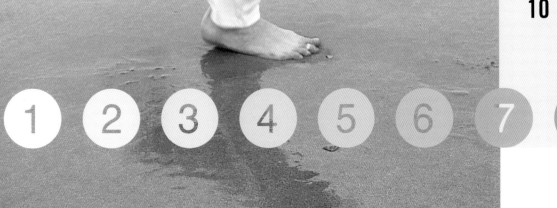

10 good reasons to do aerobic exercise

1 Increases cardiovascular fitness

2 Strengthens bones and makes joints more flexible

3 Increases the basal metabolic rate (BMR) – your body burns more calories, even at rest

4 Burns up stored fat

5 Suppresses your appetite

6 Enhances your skin

7 Relaxes you and makes you sleep better

8 Improves body tone and definition

9 Reduces blood pressure and cholesterol

10 Increases your vitality and wellbeing – exercise is a natural anti-depressant

1 2 3 4 5 6 7 8 9 10

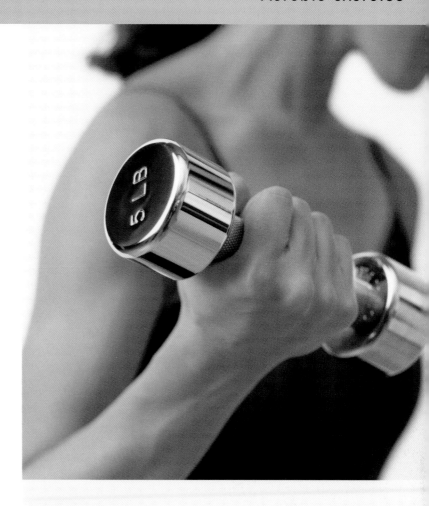

Walking This is one of the easiest and best ways to exercise aerobically, but you do need to walk at a pace that will have an effect. Walk briskly with a long stride and breathe deeply. Wear sensible shoes and work right through the foot with each step – from heel to toe – to exercise the leg muscles and increase your speed as you get fitter. Try to do this for 20 minutes every day. The great advantage about walking as exercise is that you do not have to set aside a special time – you can do this on your way to work or to the shops.

Jogging Although jogging is very popular and will certainly raise the heart rate, it does bring with it the possibility of damage to the joints – especially the knees – because of the impact of running on a street surface. (Breathing in traffic fumes is another disadvantage.) Try to jog on grass or on a treadmill in the gym and always wear good-quality supportive trainers. Three times a week for 20–30 minutes is ideal.

Swimming This is one of the best forms of aerobic exercise: with your body supported in water the chances of injuring yourself due to stress on the joints is virtually nil. Again, 20–30 minutes three times a week is ideal. There are also aqua-aerobics classes in many swimming pools now and these are good ways of exercising, too, as working against the water increases resistance and makes you work harder.

Cycling Riding a bicycle is another excellent form of aerobic exercise – cycle to work if you can or go with a friend at weekends. As with all aerobic exercise, little and often is best (20–30 minutes three times a week), building up speed gradually.

Other activities Only those sports with a prolonged period where the heart rate is increased make good aerobic exercise – short spurts of activity don't count since the increase in the metabolic rate is not sustained. Consequently, the best sports for aerobics are enduring ones such as rowing. Dancing (provided it is non-stop) is good, too, as are activities such as skipping or trampolining.

Weight training

Weight training (often called resistance training) is a good supplement to aerobic exercise. It focuses on the size, strength and stamina of specific muscles. Regular weight training firms and tones the body; it can stimulate and strengthen bones (a good counter-measure against osteoporosis), improve posture and help prevent lower back problems. Research shows that it can slow and even reverse the declines in strength, bone density and muscle mass associated with ageing.

SEE ALSO:

→ Warming-up exercises, page 198

→ Winding down, page 222

→ Living with stress, page 230

Rest and Relaxation

6

In addition to a healthy diet, plenty of water and exercise, other requirements for our bodies are sleep and rest. An undisturbed night's sleep facilitates physical and mental renewal and repair. Periods of rest in which to unwind are just as important. This section is largely concerned with 'switching off' – relaxing by getting rid of stress, and calming the mind by practising techniques such as meditation and relaxation on a regular basis.

6

Living with stress

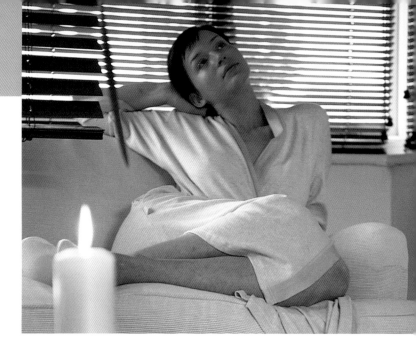

Human beings were not designed for life in the 21st century. We have not evolved anything like quickly enough to deal with the demands of a fast-paced, information-rich, stressful environment.

The adrenaline rush

Modern life exposes us to myriad pressures, producing a stress response from our endocrine system, including the release of adrenaline which prepares the body for physical or mental exertion but puts us under actual physical pressure. Our bodies have hardly changed since prehistoric times when, as hunters, we would be exposed to extreme short-term dangers. Then, the body needed adrenaline to fight or flee from the danger. However, while adrenaline is highly effective in helping us escape from short-term danger, it is less so when faced with ongoing, long-term stress. In fact, adrenaline and the other chemicals our bodies produce in reaction to stress cause the body to produce toxic substances, free radicals (see page 28). They are implicated in most human diseases, including cancer, heart disease, Alzheimer's disease and degenerative diseases.

The immediate chemical effect of stress is to reduce the immune system's ability to function, making us more susceptible to disease. Sustained stress may develop into depression, raising corticosteroid levels and putting further pressure on the immune system. A growing body of research links depression with an inability to fight cancer.

Ageing effects of stress

Many of us live a stressful lifestyle without really being aware of it. Life in the fast lane often means we eat quick fixes of carbohydrates, fats, salt and sugar, and rely on alcohol and caffeine, followed by drugs to get back on track. This hard living will soon show in our bodies.

The face is the first place to register emotional or physical distress, as furrows and creases between the hairline and neck. Everyone responds in a similar way, but unlike a child or teenager, whose skin bounces smoothly back into place once the problem has passed, adult skin, short on springy tissues, hangs on to the stress, embedding it deep in the dermis. The deceleration in blood flow and lymph drainage caused by repeated stress shows not just in pallor and puffiness, but in the slower regeneration of skin cells.

This, and other long-term consequences of stress – increased blood pressure and cholesterol, lowered metabolism and immunity, blood sugar imbalance and depression – adds years to your body.

Insomnia

One of the most common manifestations of stress is insomnia, which can mean not being able to get to sleep to begin with, or waking in the night and not being able to fall asleep again. Even if you do not suffer from insomnia, you may have a problem with light, restless sleep, which leaves you still feeling tired the next morning. This, in turn, can lead to tension headaches or general aches and pains. There are several options that may help you sleep that you can try before resorting to medication, for example aromatherapy and self-massage (see page 278).

How stressed are you?

While few, if any of us, can hope for a totally stress-free life, there's no doubt that too much stress is bad for your health and wellbeing. Try our quiz to check whether life is getting to you and what you can do to change things for the better.

	YES	NO
1 Have you recently experienced the death of someone close to you?	☐	☐
2 Have you recently been through a divorce or the break-up of a serious relationship?	☐	☐
3 Do you feel under pressure in the work you do and feel that you aren't meeting your own and others' expectations?	☐	☐
4 Do you spend more time at work or thinking about your job than you really want to?	☐	☐
5 Do you have trouble getting to sleep or wake frequently at night?	☐	☐
6 Do you ever feel that family and friends ask too much of you?	☐	☐
7 Do you ever feel that life is out of your control and that others are pulling all the strings?	☐	☐
8 Have you lost touch with close friends and family or do you see them less than you used to?	☐	☐
9 Do you regularly have symptoms such as an upset stomach, backache and headaches and catch one cold after another?	☐	☐
10 Do you lose your temper or cry easily when things go wrong?	☐	☐
11 Are you too busy or tired to take regular exercise?	☐	☐

	YES	NO
12 Do you find it almost impossible to relax and 'switch off' in your free time?	☐	☐
13 Do you find it hard to take time out just for yourself or feel guilty when you do?	☐	☐
14 Do other people ever comment that you seem stressed or tense?	☐	☐

HOW YOU SCORED

0–4 YES ANSWERS

Your stress is within manageable limits and unlikely to have any effect on your health. Maybe you haven't been completely honest? Pretending all is well when it isn't doesn't pay in the long term, and if you don't deal with any sources of stress in your life they will simply get worse.

5–9 YES ANSWERS

You can probably just about cope most of the time, but it is worth taking a closer look at what's causing the stress. Consider what you can change and what steps you can take to help you live with what you can do nothing about for now. It is bound to take time to recover from a bereavement or the end of a relationship, for example, and you can't always reduce work-related stress overnight. However, you can make up your mind to take more exercise, say no to unreasonable demands from others and put more effort into cultivating a circle of supportive friends and relatives with whom you can share your worries.

10–14 YES ANSWERS

If you go on like this, your mental and physical health is likely to be badly affected, if it isn't already. You may be feeling too bad to tackle the situation on your own: if you don't have a supportive and practical friend or relative to turn to, consider making an appointment with your doctor or with a professional counsellor. Make sorting out your life top priority, even if it means taking time from your other responsibilities.

What's the solution?

If the consequences of stress are complex, the solution is simple: relax. But how? It sounds so easy, yet true relaxation eludes many of us. We slump in an armchair, straining our backs; we watch television, stressing our eyes; we drink coffee, increasing our blood pressure.

Trying to relax, in any sense, is of course a contradiction in terms. What we need are techniques to help us release tension at will when the pressure starts to show. Full relaxation is only achieved when the mind – which leads the body – is also relaxed in a meditative state. Many long-established and effective techniques, such as yoga (see page 252) and meditation (see page 244), can be practised at home as long-term, daily routines that soothe your mind and control your emotions rather than letting them control you. Often, all you need is a simple aid – a pillow, incense, meditative music – and peace and quiet. Other techniques require a professional therapist. So help yourself at home or put yourself in the calming hands of an experienced therapist. Either way, learn to relax, revive – and rejuvenate.

Herbal remedies

If it is proving impossible to cope with ongoing stress, then a major reassessment of lifestyle may be necessary. For minor peaks, however, herbs can provide relief – especially in advance. If a stressful time is looming, such as exams, the school holidays or a heavy work period, then it is worth taking tonic herbs (see page 288) before the event to provide an energy boost, rather than depending on short-term stimulants once the stresses mount.

- **Siberian ginseng** is ideal at helping the body to cope more efficiently with stress and improve performance: take up to 600 mg a day for 10–14 days before the stresses are due to peak. (Do not exceed the standard dose or take for prolonged periods.)
- **Withania** is similarly effective: make a decoction of the root or take up to 600 mg daily in capsules.

Reducing stress

Everyday stress is a fact of life and most people cope. But coping does not reduce the sources of stress, so the effects are merely postponed. The answer is to manage it. Before embarking on any specialist techniques, try to reduce the stress in your life with some simple and commonsense measures.

Unresolved dilemmas, reinforced by lack of energy, are the major causes of stress in our lives. Start by listing everything that is causing you stress and work out how to resolve each problem. There is always an answer, though you may need help to identify it.

In our 24-hour society, in which the division of labour between the genders is breaking down, lack of time is an increasingly common source of stress. How do you take the children to the swings when you have to cook supper? How do you find time to buy the food for supper when you need to talk about paying the bills with your partner?

To limit, if not eliminate, the stress caused by such conflicts of interest, take these as your watchwords: **prioritize, delegate, eliminate**. Work out what is really important to you and what you really must (or want to) do. What tasks on your list can you get someone else to do? Cross out those things that aren't essential. Leave the sheets unironed, buy a ready-cooked meal or two, decline an unwelcome invitation to give yourself time and space for positive relaxation.

Top strategies for combating stress

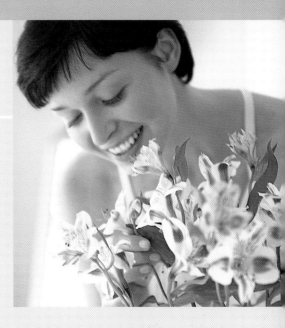

EXERCISE

Working out seems diametrically opposed to relaxation, but it is a short-cut to it. Exercise doesn't only boost your circulation, it also burns up the residue of stress chemicals in the body while generating the production of feel-good hormones, such as endorphins, which induce relaxation.

Aerobic activities not only build heart and limb muscle, they also increase your oxygen supply, feeding your skin and making you feel more awake, whatever you did last night. All you need to do is 30 minutes three to five times a week to make a difference.

So take regular exercise, preferably in the fresh air, but don't overdo it otherwise you will be inclined to give it up and put your feet up. You don't have to don trainers or even leave your house for beneficial exercise. Two good forms of exercise that are often overlooked are laughter and sex.

LAUGHING AND SEX

It quickens your breathing, enhances the absorption of oxygen from the blood, makes your eyes sparkle by stimulating the tear glands, exercises the stomach muscles and works the facial muscles in a way that increases blood flow to the brain – all while using up 10 calories a minute. Ten seconds of a good belly laugh can raise your heart rate to the level achieved by 10 minutes of rowing. In a similar way, sex boosts the circulation and triggers the release of opiates in the brain. Although they exert their effects by radically different means, sex and laughing both kick the parasympathetic nervous system into play, triggering the release of relaxant hormones and inducing tranquillity afterwards.

RELAXING MASSAGE

Massage is a delightful experience and can be deeply relaxing for both body and mind. One of the most pleasant forms of massage is

aromatherapy massage (see page 282); the scents are in themselves both beneficial and uplifting, and the oils can help benefit dry, damaged or problem skin.

POSITIVE ATTITUDE

Worry and anxiety are a curse, especially to a person with lowered vitality and a gloomy outlook. From this moment onwards, determine that you are going to kick the worry habit. It only weakens the willpower, saps the nerves, unsteadies the thought patterns and ages the body. When life threatens to overwhelm you, try and see the funny side of things and put the situation into the context of the 'bigger picture'. Replace frowns with smiles and, even if this is done with some effort of will, it will affect the release of mood-enhancing brain chemicals such as endorphins and serotonin. If you have a ton of work to do and a deadline that looks impossible, smiling isn't easy, but even releasing your frown can help.

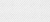

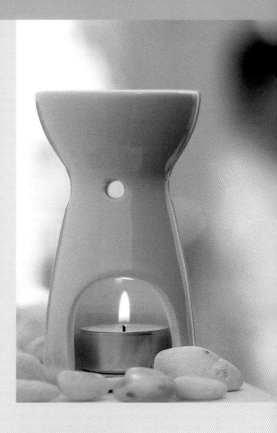

RELAXATION AND MEDITATION

These thoroughly proven methods of switching off from chronic stress allow our systems to calm down and recuperate (see pages 242–249). Consider taking up a yoga class (see page 252) at least once a week. Alternatively, take advantage of some of the wonderful relaxation tapes and CDs on the market. Regular use of these techniques will create helpful patterns of behaviour and you will find fewer things irritate you or cause the stressed condition in the first place.

CO-LISTENING

Shared listening is a well-recognized psychological tool. Having an outlet to express your thoughts, feelings and frustrations, and knowing that you are being heard is a most wonderful tonic.

DETOX

Regular or even occasional detoxification of the digestive and alimentary system is another traditionally recognized way of de-stressing an overworked and overloaded body (see page 92). Therapies such as colonics (see page 277) and enemas can make the world of difference to one's energy levels and ability to deal with stress, and can prevent debilitating illness.

HEALTHIER DIET

Eat more seasonal, fresh produce, preferably organic. Start your day with a cup of hot, boiled water. Make sure your fluid intake is sufficient (see Water, page 96) and does not consist solely of toxin-laden, caffeine-rich drinks such as tea and coffee (see Everyday toxins, page 94).

BREATHING CONTROL

Controlling your breathing (see breathing exercises, page 240–1) by slowing it down and focusing on it will help you deal with stress. Regularly take several deep breaths, which fill the lower part of your lungs and expel stale air. Chair-bound office workers are often in danger of decreased oxygen levels due to restricted seated positions and lack of exercise.

WATER THERAPY

Wash away your worries at the beginning and end of the day. Try skin brushing (see page 168), hydrotherapy (see page 170) and aromatherapy baths (see page 282).

AROMATHERAPY

Inhale and/or absorb essential oils via burners and candles, bathing or massage to improve emotional, spiritual and physical wellbeing (see Aromatherapy, page 278).

SPACE CLEARING

Clearing away the clutter (see page 265) is the best way to create sacred spaces in your work and home environment.

SEE ALSO:

→ Why detox? page 90

→ Everyday toxins, page 94

→ Massage, page 158

→ Aerobic exercise, page 224

→ Improve your breathing, page 240

→ Relaxation techniques, page 242

→ Meditation, page 244

→ Visualization, page 250

→ Yoga, page 252

→ Tranquil surroundings, page 264

→ Aromatherapy, page 278

→ Healing with herbs, page 288

5-minute unwind

So often we get home from work to be faced with yet more to do in the form of cooking and domestic chores – and in these circumstances, the last thing on our minds is how we can help ourselves to unwind. This easy bathroom routine can be fitted into the busiest schedule. All you need is a standard bath towel.

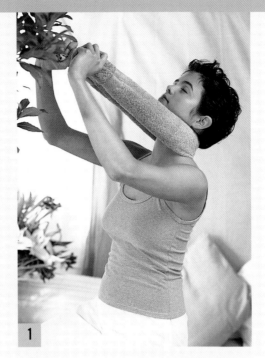

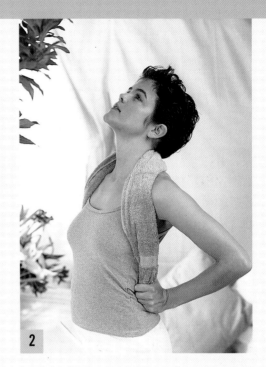

1 **Stretching the neck** Cradle your neck in a warmed, rolled towel. Arch the head back and hold for two or three breaths.

2 **Stretching the neck and shoulders** Pull the ends of the towel down and wrap it around your shoulders. Press your fists into the small of the back, pinching the elbows back to increase the pressure and expand the chest. Hold for two or three breaths. *Repeat Steps 1 and 2 six times.*

3 **Pressing the body** Sitting on the floor, hold the rolled towel down your spine. Tuck one end under your buttocks and hold the other end extended over your head. Slowly ease your body down on to the floor on top of the towel, centring your spine over the end. Release the top end of the towel, bend your knees and place your hands on your hips. Rest and relax, allowing the muscles on either side of the

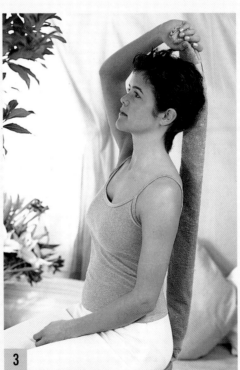

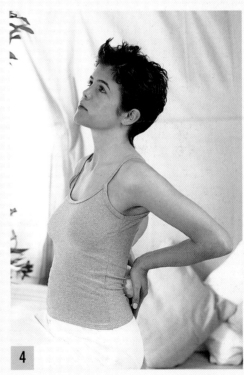

rolled towel to open and relax with the pull of gravity. Stay in this position for a few minutes. Any physical pain and tiredness can be dispelled in just a few minutes by just lying in this position.

4 **Releasing the pressure** Put two tennis or soft balls into a sock and knot the top. Press the balls into the tight muscles on either side of the spine at the base of your back and hold for two or three breaths.

Stress in the workplace

Stress and work are two words that unfortunately seem to go together. Increasingly, if you ask someone how their life is going they will reply that they are stressed by their work. It is not surprising then that work stress is thought to be the primary cause of physical and mental illness in Western society.

Most of us work for practical reasons and to feel fulfilled through using our individual abilities, but work should not make us sick. Certain workplace factors can be controlled only by the employer, but employees can also take steps to control their own response to stress.

Warning signs

A host of physical and mental signals indicate stress (see box below). The most common signs of stress at work are persistent fatigue, irritability and poor concentration. Psychologically, the symptoms are a tendency to worry, feelings of apprehension, being rude and irritable, and losing interest in hobbies outside work and in the job itself. When you recognize these signs and, most importantly, accept that you are not the only one suffering in this way, you can start taking steps to solve the problem.

Remedies

There are simple remedies, some already covered in this section, and activities that you can do at work. A relaxing visualization exercise (see page 250) need take only a few minutes and can be done at your desk or at lunchtime. Physical exercises to relieve the strain of using a keyboard are also unobtrusive. Chi kung (see page 294) is one therapy that has a lot to offer in terms of work stress relief, providing mental relaxation and preventing the physical problems caused by working at a computer for long periods and using poorly designed office furniture.

Practical steps

Consider the following simple suggestions to make your work life physically and mentally more comfortable and enjoyable.

Working environment If you work in an office, you should have an appropriate style of office chair, a proper desk and workspace and a screen for your computer monitor, if you use one, to cut out the glare from the screen. Try to make your workspace as attractive as possible within the allowed limits. Plants, in particular, are good for this as they radiate energy. If you like crystals, you could place one or two on your computer as they are thought to reduce the amount of electromagnetic radiation from the computer.

Make sure that your workspace is well lit and, if possible, do not face a wall or have your back to the office door. The best position is to be near a window, with plenty of natural light.

Correct sitting posture Sit upright at your desk, with your knees and

Signs of stress

- headaches
- muscle tension in the neck and shoulders
- palpitations
- excessive sweating
- dizziness
- increased smoking
- increased drinking

Massage for eye tension

1 Lace the fingers of both hands together and press your thumbs inside the corners of your eyes, either side of the bridge of your nose. Hold for 2–3 seconds, release slightly and *repeat six times*. If you prefer, lean on your elbows to give more pressure to the action, but do avoid any contact with the eyeball itself.

2 Pinch the top of the nasal bone (between the eyebrow and eye socket) with your index finger and thumb. Hold the fleshy area for two or three breaths, release slightly and *repeat six times*.

3 Rub your palms together until they feel really warm, then lightly cup them over your eyes. Hold in place for a few breaths. *Repeat whenever you need a boost.*

Massage for neck tension

1 Cradle the back of your head in your hands and circle your thumbs around the soft, fleshy area at the base of the skull.

2 Slide your fingers up from the base of the hairline at the back of the neck and over the crown. Gather your hair at the roots and tug gently from side to side, keeping your knuckles close to the scalp. Now slide your fingers through your hair from the temples to the sides of the head. Gather your hair and pull gently from side to side.

Repeat both steps two or three times. Finish by smoothing through the hair.

feet shoulder-width apart. Make sure your chair is at the right height so that you can sit with both your feet comfortably on the floor. Avoid sitting for long periods with your legs crossed.

Taking a break When you are sitting at your desk, take a complete break from your computer by switching it off if you can. The constant noise it makes, the screen glare and the electromagnetic radiation are all irritants, even when you are not working on the computer. Do this whenever possible, particularly if you have lunch at your desk.

Releasing tension Rest your wrists on your desk or on your knees. As you breathe out, stretch your fingers away from you. Keep stretching them and visualize all toxins and blockages in your circulatory system leaving your body on every out-breath.

This is an exercise that you can practise frequently throughout the day when you feel stressed. This tension-releasing exercise is particularly good for people who drive for long periods of time. You can do the exercise while at traffic lights or when you are stuck in a traffic jam. Stretching the fingers away from you releases all the 'fight or flight' in your muscles.

Relieving tension headaches and eyestrain Working to deadlines is a pressure that builds up and sometimes just won't go away. The end results are tension headaches, eyestrain and lack of mental focus which, if left unchecked, can greatly impair productivity. Taking a few minutes off every once in a while to do the self-help pressure-release techniques above will prevent and relieve stress.

SEE ALSO:

→ Self-help hair and head massage, page 147

→ Sparkling eyes, page 140

→ Relaxation techniques, page 242

→ Meditation, page 244

→ Visualization, page 250

→ Tranquil surroundings, page 264

→ Chi kung, page 294

Peaceful slumber

Is there any state more natural than sleep? Newborn babies do it for anything up to 23 hours a day and older people find it impossible to resist in the middle of the afternoon. Yet many of us lose that innate ability to drop off anywhere in the intervening decades.

This is as much to do with our lifestyles as any physiological changes, so we can change it. Experts have observed that, as the 24-hour society has become established, we are getting less sleep. By one estimate, our available sleeping time fell by 25 minutes over just five years in the 1990s. That deprivation shows more than anywhere in our faces – in bags or dark circles under the eyes, in saggy eyelids or a drained and pallid complexion.

The number of people seeking help for sleep problems has never been higher. The trend has led to a new branch of 'sleep medicine' and the establishment of specialized sleep clinics. What these seek to do is monitor a sufferer's sleep pattern and diagnose the problems, from heavy snoring to an inability to switch off. But

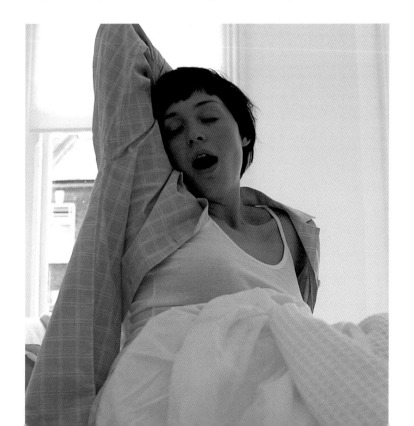

unless your problem is acute, you would do well first to adopt a code now known as 'sleep hygiene'. Only if your condition has not improved after a fortnight need you seek professional help.

Sleep allows the body to relax and regenerate damaged and tired cells, so adhere to the following rules to increase your quota:

- Go to bed and get up at roughly the same time each day.
- Avoid artificial stimulants – alcohol, smoking and caffeinated drinks – before you go to bed.
- Keep all work-related papers or books out of the bedroom.
- Make sure that the room is well ventilated.
- Allow yourself time to unwind before you get into bed.
- Burn a sedative essential oil in your room.
- Avoid very heavy meals in the evening.
- If you cannot sleep, sit up and read until your eyelids begin to droop. Then, when you lie down, adopt the basic yoga relaxation pose (see Corpse pose, page 261) to help you drop off again.

Aromatherapy

If you tend to have trouble sleeping, there are several things you can try. An aromatherapy bath is a good way of slowing down the mind and relaxing the body at the end of the day (see page 282). Similarly, two or three drops of the Sweet dreams oil (see page 269) on a tissue, placed on your pillow, may help you to unwind if your mind is spinning. If you still feel tense, give yourself a facial massage (see opposite), which you should find particularly relaxing. Alternatively, use undiluted lavender or neroli oil in a burner and put the burner in the bedroom about half an hour before you go to bed. (Be sure to extinguish the burner before climbing into bed.) Other essences with sleep-inducing aromas include rose, frankincense and camomile.

5-minute self-massage for sleep

This self-massage will take you about five to ten minutes, depending on how slowly you make the strokes. You can do it after a bath or even when you are already in bed, although you would need a large pillow to support your back. Take your time and leave the oil on all night. If you don't mind having oily hair until you shower in the morning, you can also massage the oil into your scalp.

To begin, mix half of the Sweet dreams oil (see page 269) with 25 ml (1 fl oz) of almond oil, grapeseed oil or any cold-pressed vegetable oil. Shake well and apply the oil mixture to your face and neck.

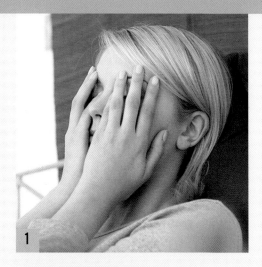

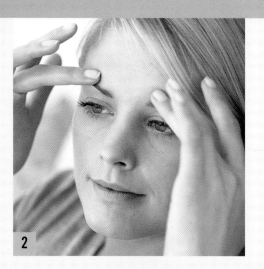

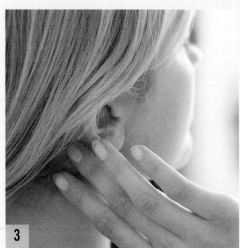

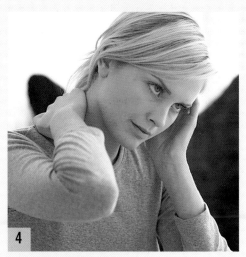

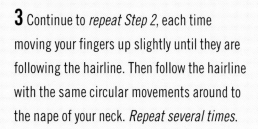

1 Rest your three central fingers of each hand on each eyebrow. Close your eyes lightly and remain in that position for a moment, taking a few deep breaths.

2 Place the middle finger of each hand either side of, and immediately above, the bridge of your nose, between your eyebrows. Now, following the line of the brows, make small circles with your fingers along the length of your brows as far as your temples. When you reach your temples, hold your fingers over them for a moment with a slightly increased pressure. Return to the centre of the forehead, this time with your fingers placed very slightly higher, and trace another line out towards your temples in the same way.

3 Continue to *repeat Step 2*, each time moving your fingers up slightly until they are following the hairline. Then follow the hairline with the same circular movements around to the nape of your neck. *Repeat several times*.

4 Make the same circular movements from the neck hairline down your neck, with your fingers either side of (but not on) your spine. You may want to use more pressure here.

5 Use the same movements from the centre of your forehead back across your scalp to the nape of your neck. Finally, using the whole hand, cover the whole of your head, as if you are kneading your scalp.

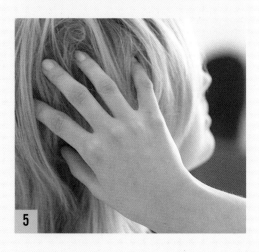

SEE ALSO:

→ Yoga, page 252

→ Aromatherapy, page 278

→ Aromatherapy bath, page 282

Improve your breathing

Breathing is something we do automatically – we simply don't think about it. Of course, it would be very difficult to think about our breathing all the time, but it is useful to spend a few minutes each day doing full, healthy breathing. Most of us breathe too shallowly, using only the upper chest and about one-third of our lung capacity, so that only a small proportion of the oxygen that should be reaching our bloodstream is inhaled. This means the body's cells do not receive sufficient oxygen to reproduce at their optimum rate. And, as the lungs fail to fill properly over the years, they lose their elasticity and so cannot reach full capacity.

This poor breathing may be merely a habit and is often related to stress. The more tense we feel, the shallower our breathing is likely to become. And, just as tension and shallow breathing often bring with them thoughts galloping out of control, slow, deep breathing calms the mind.

Breathing exercises have a very relaxing effect and slow the body down considerably. In the deep breathing exercise and the alternate nostril breathing exercises demonstrated here, focus your attention on your breath and try to observe its progress through your body.

Breathing and exercise

One of the great benefits of aerobic exercise (see page 224) is that it improves the way we use oxygen. However, many of us do not breathe correctly when we exercise and this undoes all the benefits. Most of us tend to hold our breath whenever we do anything strenuous, but this actually makes whatever we are doing more difficult and encourages the accumulation of tensions in the body. By breathing correctly during exercise, we can actually rid the body of those tensions.

Rather than holding the breath or gasping it in, breathe out as you make an effort and in as you release it. This helps you to perform any exercise better, aids your concentration and revitalizes your energy levels.

Deep breathing

This exercise helps establish a slower, deeper breathing rhythm, which in turn slows the heart rate and the pulse and aids relaxation. It is designed to be used on a regular, preferably twice-daily basis, morning and evening, but it can also come in handy when you're in a stressful situation – you don't always have to lie down.

1 Lie on the floor, placing your hands on your abdomen, fingertips touching. **Take a long, slow breath in through your nose**, counting to five. Your lungs and abdomen will expand, making your fingertips part.

Hold the deep breath for the count of five. Then, very slowly, this time on a count of 10, **exhale through your mouth**. Feel your fingertips touch again and keep on going, trying to empty your body completely of air. *Repeat the whole sequence 10 times.*

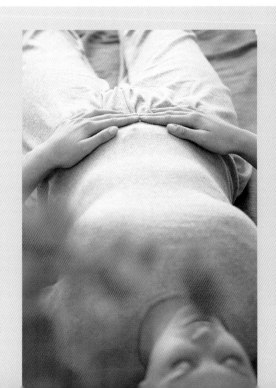

Yoga and breathing

In yoga, ill health is regarded as the product of imbalances and blockages in the flow of energy, or *prana*, through the body. The practice of *pranayama* takes the form of breathing exercises. Unlike circulation or digestion, we can consciously control our breathing, and this acts as a link between the conscious and unconscious parts of our bodies.

Besides improving oxygen intake, purification and circulation of the blood and lymph, and thereby increasing the flow of oxygen to every cell in the body, *pranayama* exercises are also believed to improve mental alertness, concentration and creativity, as well as being a form of deep relaxation, producing a sense of calm and serenity. Used at times of stress, when breathing typically becomes fast and shallow, they can dispel tension.

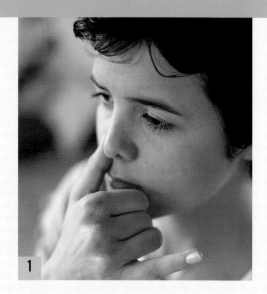

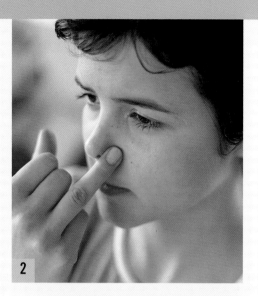

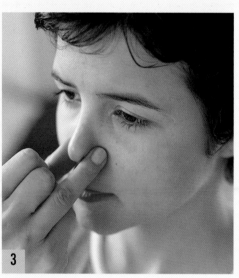

Alternate nostril breathing

Alternate nostril breathing is central to yogic meditation and is proven to be effective in dealing with stress. The techniques given here are adapted from classical yoga and are best performed while you sit comfortably on the floor, legs crossed, keeping your spine straight. Alternatively, kneel on the floor, sitting back on your heels, or sit on a chair (see Postures and positions, page 247). Choose whichever position is most comfortable for you.

1 Keeping the three main fingers of your right hand closed, extend your thumb and little finger. With the right nostril blocked by your thumb, **breathe deeply**, **inhale** for five seconds and **exhale** for five seconds through the left nostril.

2 Bring your fourth or your little finger across to block your left nostril, then release your thumb.

3 **Inhale** for five seconds and **exhale** for five seconds through the right nostril. *Repeat the exercise 10 times on the right nostril* and *10 times on the left.* Next, try **inhaling** for five seconds, holding for three seconds and **exhaling** for five seconds. *Repeat 10 times on each nostril.*

SEE ALSO:

→ Aerobic exercise, page 224

→ Living with stress, page 230

→ Yoga, page 252

Relaxation techniques

Even 10 minutes of relaxation a day will make a very big difference to your stress levels, your ability to cope and your overall health. The following exercise is very loosely based on the yoga *nidra* or relaxation technique, and you lie on the floor in what is known as the Corpse pose (see page 261). *Nidra* means 'yogic sleep', but you are, in fact, very much aware, and carry your awareness around your body, focusing on each area in turn. Bearing this in mind, it is important not to fall asleep – so make sure the room is warm but not stuffy before you start. Once you are able to achieve a deep rest using this basic pose, you may wish to introduce some meditation (see page 244).

Preparing for relaxation

Many people find it helpful to record the instructions on tape (see box, below) and play it while they do the relaxation exercise. If you do use a tape, place the player within easy reach so you don't have to get up to switch it on after the preparation.

Your body temperature will drop somewhat during relaxation, so make sure you have something, such as a blanket or towel, to cover yourself with. A pair of socks is also a good idea, as the feet can feel cold. Most importantly, endeavour to make sure you will not be disturbed, which would stop the whole relaxation in its tracks, defeating the object of the exercise.

Recording a relaxation tape

When making a relaxation tape, remember that your mind and body slow down during relaxation so you must speak very slowly and calmly. Repeating the instructions several times helps you to focus your mind during the exercise. Pause between each instruction – it is a good idea to take at least one long, deep breath between each sentence, with a longer pause between each individual instruction. In some places, for example where you have to repeat a series of procedures, you will have to leave enough of a pause for these on the tape.

You may not be able to focus on one part of your body immediately, and it is important to give yourself plenty of time. Don't put any modulation into your voice; it may sound boring to you as you record it, but you don't want any surprises or excitement during relaxation!

The tape of the exercise provided here, with pauses, should take 30–40 minutes, but you can take longer if you wish.

Some people like music in the background, but this can be a distraction. You might start listening to the music instead of focusing on your body. There are tapes available featuring music designed for relaxation and, when you have practised the technique for a while, one of these may make an interesting change.

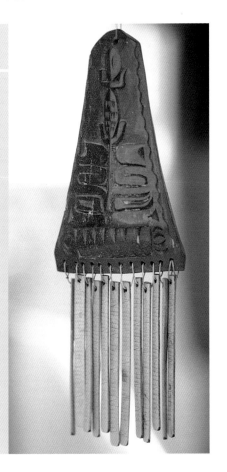

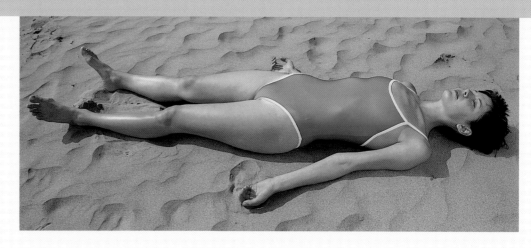

Relaxation exercise

1 Lie on the floor with your feet about 45 cm (18 in) apart, your legs rolling outwards slightly. Make sure your back is comfortable with your shoulders lowered, not tensed. Hold your arms straight but relaxed, your hands about 30 cm (12 in) away from your body with the palms facing upwards. It may seem more comfortable palms down, but when they are uppermost, the upper back and shoulders are more relaxed. **Close your eyes**. Feel your whole body heavy on the floor.

2 Take three long, slow, deep breaths, concentrating on the exhalation so that your body feels quite empty before you breathe in again. Starting at your toes, and working up through your legs and body, tense each group of muscles in turn, then relax them and move on to the next. Do not expect your muscles to relax completely at this stage, simply become aware of them. Move some parts of your body, such as your shoulders and your head, by rolling or rotating very slightly, rather than tensing. When you have become aware of all parts of your body, simply lie still for a few moments, still with legs slightly apart and hands by your sides, and then begin step 3.

3 Starting at your toes, **begin to feel the relaxation spreading** through your body,

moving upwards like a wave. Put all your concentration into each area in turn, first the toes, then the feet and ankles. **Feel the wave spreading up into your legs,** through the shins and calves, the knees and into the thighs. Let your legs roll outwards from the hips. Let the hips and buttocks go – a surprising amount of tension is often stored here. **The whole body is softening** and the effect now reaches the abdomen, which drops down further against the back, while the lower spine relaxes further into the floor.

4 The stomach, waist and ribs all expand and soften. The **breathing is now quite light**. As the relaxing wave flows through the torso and into the back, they fall deeper into the floor. The relaxation comes into the shoulders and neck and out along the arms to the very fingertips. The back of the neck is almost touching the floor, the scalp softens, almost loose against the skull, and the whole face – jaw, chin, throat, cheeks – melts away. The lips part and the tongue rests gently behind the lower teeth. The eyes sink gently back into the head; temples and forehead smooth out.

5 The whole body is at rest. **Enjoy this sensation**, be aware of it. As thoughts come into your mind, watch them and see them float away like clouds. Float any doubts or worries away in the same way. Stay in this place for three to five minutes. Now see the sun in your sky and feel its life-giving light and warmth. Feel the air around you and, as you take a **deep breath in**, feel that you are drinking in from the sun's vast source of energy, making you calmer and stronger.

6 **Deepen your breathing**, letting the ribs expand and the lungs fill. After three breaths, begin to feel your toes and fingers coming to life. Wriggle them. Still with your eyes closed, lift your arms above your head and stretch your arms and legs away from each other. When you are ready, roll on to your side and open your eyes. Take a few moments before you get up, and take things easy for a while.

SEE ALSO:

→ Living with stress, page 230

→ Yoga, page 252

→ Autogenic training, page 262

Meditation

Meditation is not just daydreaming or relaxation; it works to train the conscious mind to a state of stillness and tranquillity and brings both physiological and psychological benefits. Many people feel that the Eastern or religious trappings associated with meditation mean that it is not for them. In fact, meditation takes on many forms and philosophies and no religious bias is necessary – you can take from it whatever it is you need. Primarily, it is a discipline for training your mind to a point of both deep concentration and relaxation.

Its early beginnings were, of course, religious, though it would be a mistake to imagine they were only Eastern – the early Christians meditated, too. The most common forms of meditation we know today do come from the East and have been perfected over the centuries by such religions as Buddhism, Hinduism, Taoism and Islamic Sufism. Within this context, the aim of meditation is to help reach a point of spiritual enlightenment. However, for many people in the West today it is basically a practical self-help technique for coping with the high levels of stress found in our daily lives.

Why meditate?

Methods of meditation may differ, but they all have in common the aim of producing a state of deep relaxation which, it is claimed, rejuvenates both mind and body. People who meditate regularly say it gives them a new zest for life, with increased energy, improved concentration and an inner peace that leads to better relationships. Sportsmen and women even claim it improves their performance.

When you see someone meditate, it looks as if very little is happening. You may notice that his or her breathing has slowed down, but otherwise he or she remains quite still, eyes closed. The work is all taking place on the inside. Most of the meditation techniques that are used these days are really concentration techniques. Their effect on the mind might be compared with the effect of exercise on the muscles of the body. They aim to tone up the capacity for memory, analysis, perception, inference, concentration, recognition and recall. By developing in these daily sessions the mind's strength and flexibility, it is able to perform much more efficiently and effectively the rest of the time. In essence, it gives you the ability to stay focused on whatever you happen to be doing.

Learning to meditate

You can learn to meditate at home on your own simply by following the basic guidelines below. There are numerous audio tapes available, too, to draw you through what is usually known as a 'guided meditation'. This may take the form of a journey or visualizing a series of images in your mind. There are also tapes that simply play 'meditational' music. However, unless you are meditating solely on that sound, these may prove to be more of a distraction than a help.

There have, of course, been many great teachers of meditation over the millennia. The most famous in recent times is the Maharishi Mahesh Yogi, who taught the Beatles and other pop stars to meditate and attracted countless Western devotees in the 1960s. He then went on to establish his Centres of Transcendental Meditation, now found worldwide, which use the technique of a repeated word or mantra. Many people do find it much more effective to have a teacher to guide them, especially when they are first starting to learn to meditate. Having other learners around can be helpful, too, making it easier to discuss difficulties.

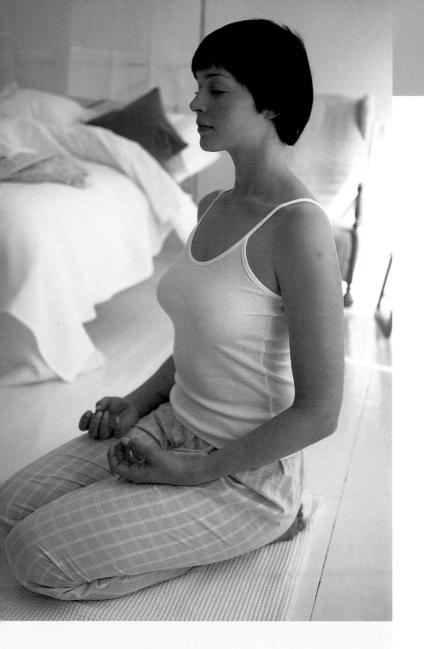

What is meditation?

It is a common misconception that meditation and conventional forms of relaxation are the same thing. However, meditation is not the passive act that it appears, and when practised regularly it has the potential to bring far greater benefits than simple relaxation. While relaxation offers temporary relief from stress, meditation aims to achieve both relaxation of the body and a heightened state of awareness. Regular meditation can bring greater control over restless thoughts and emotions, leading to a sense of wellbeing. The practice of meditation has a cumulative effect and the benefits can be felt almost immediately – a sense of detachment from life's pressures and lasting peace of mind.

Allow yourself time to succeed

The main thing to remember when learning to meditate is that the intrusion of thoughts is inevitable. Meditation is a technique that may take years to do with ease and this is only natural – you would not start learning tennis and expect to be playing at Wimbledon that week. Do not try too hard – you are not supposed to be forcing your mind into concentrating on a particular image. In fact, you are trying to release yourself from conscious thought. When anything enters your mind – thoughts, worries, ideas, lists of what you have to do when you stop meditating – observe its presence gently, make no judgement about the thought itself and, above all, do not become irritated with yourself for having it! Having recognized the thought, let it go, as if it floats away of its own accord, and attempt to draw your focus back to your breath, or the word or image on which you are meditating. Eventually conscious thoughts will be released, leading to a physical release.

Your shoulders or jaw are often the first to drop. After some practice, you should feel a lot of tension dropping out of your face. You may also find that some parts of your body become numb. If it is helpful to you, introduce some visualization (see page 250). Think of, for example, a quiet stream into which your worries trickle, of a warm pink glow suffusing your body or of your tension floating away in a cloud above your head – or indeed any graphic image that helps you, personally, to imagine your own particular stresses being absorbed and removed far away.

SEE ALSO:
→ Living with stress, page 230

→ Relaxation techniques, page 242

→ Visualization, page 250

→ Yoga, page 252

→ Autogenic training, page 262

How meditation works

Nobody knows for sure how meditation works, although it is evident that in time we become more able to control our thoughts and emotions in everyday life (not just when we are meditating), rather than being at the mercy of our emotions. Most people who meditate regularly find that they have greater clarity in all their thought processes, better memory and concentration and an ability to stay calm, by observing the thoughts and emotions that enter their minds and discarding those that will not be useful.

Clinical research shows that a number of changes take place in the brain during meditation. Electroencephalograph (EEG) tests show that electrical waves produced during meditation are different from those we produce at other times, whether asleep or awake. Electrical activity takes on a slow rhythm, with regular, even waves recorded from different parts of the brain and, with sustained practice, this evenness and regularity continues after meditation, too.

This change in brain wave pattern is called alpha rhythm and is associated with feelings of peace and tranquillity. Common beneficial side-effects reported by meditators include reduced stress levels, improvement in insomnia and quality of sleep, and a reduction in any tendency towards addiction (cigarettes, alcohol, drugs or food). Medical research has shown that meditation has marked physiological effects, many of which are beneficial for stress-related conditions. Specific effects include:

- Lowering the blood pressure
- Slowing the pulse rate
- Slowing the respiratory rate, but with the same levels of oxygen in the blood
- Reduction of activity of the autonomic nervous system
- Improvement in circulation
- Reduction of harmful lactic acid in the body.

Research is still ongoing into whether meditation can have any effect on cancer. Certain types of cancer are thought to appear at times of great stress because stress can damage the function of the immune system, which is needed to destroy cancer cells. Diminishing stress by meditation is therefore thought by some practitioners to have a place in cancer treatment though, as yet, there has not been sufficient research to judge.

Preparing for meditation

In some respects meditation is no different from physical exercise. Both require a certain amount of self-discipline if the habit is to be established. It is a good idea to meditate at the same time every day, even if it is only for 10 minutes, so encourage yourself by making that time of the day a special time. Create an inviting atmosphere with candles, incense and a small vase of lightly scented fresh flowers.

You need to be comfortable but alert to meditate. Do not try to meditate while you are very tired – you will probably just fall asleep – or when you have recently eaten or drunk alcohol. You should also avoid being disturbed – take the phone off the hook, if necessary. Find a quiet spot, wear loose, comfortable clothing and take off your shoes.

You do not have to sit in a yogic posture to meditate – although if you are used to a lotus or half-lotus, either can be a very comfortable way of holding a position for 20 minutes. You can sit cross-legged on the floor or in a straight-backed chair. The important thing is to be able to sit with a straight back and stay still for the session, so find a position you know your body can take without strain (see opposite).

Before you begin, take a few moments to focus on your body. Take some slow, deep breaths and try to let go of any areas of tension. Finally, scan your mind for immediate thoughts and worries. Observe them and simply leave them on one side for later, so your mind is clear to meditate.

Postures and positions

When you first start meditating, it is important to try to establish good habits early on, specifically those concerning correct posture and breath control. Both of these are useful for aiding concentration when your thoughts wander, as they will do in the early stages of meditation. Do not become too preoccupied with details, but aim to ease yourself into meditation so that relaxation and serenity soon come as readily as sleep.

If using a chair, choose a straight-backed chair to sit in so that you get support and do not cramp your diaphragm. Your feet should be flat on the floor and slightly apart in line with your shoulders. Place your hands on your knees, palms down. Your chin should be slightly inclined towards your chest, but do not let it sink right into your chest as this will restrict your breathing. Look straight ahead.

The classical postures to adopt for meditation are full-lotus position, half-lotus position and Egyptian position. The traditional cross-legged postures used in yoga and Buddhism (full- and half-lotus) require a degree of suppleness that does not come easily to Westerners. However, you can train yourself to adopt these positions which you may feel enhances the meditation experience.

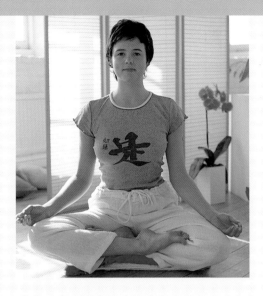

Full-lotus position For the full-lotus position, place your right foot on your left thigh and your left foot on your right thigh. Rest the backs of your hands on your knees to ensure circulation of energy around the body.

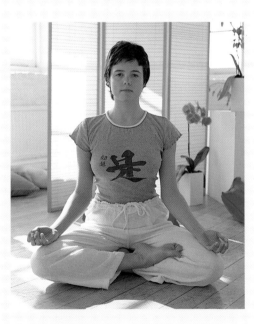

Half-lotus position For the less demanding half-lotus position, the right foot rests on the left thigh while the left foot lies under the right thigh, or vice versa. Palms can be turned upwards in a receptive gesture or cupped around the knees.

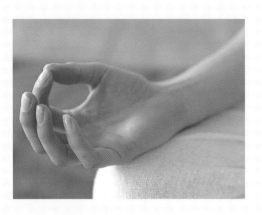

Position of your hands Closing the thumb and index finger symbolizes the completion of the energy cycle and wholeness.

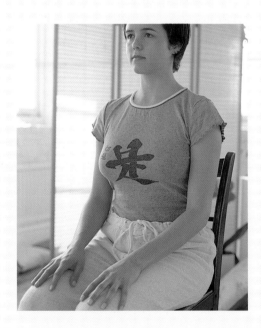

Egyptian position This traditional posture is ideal for the beginner as it is simple and easy to sustain over a long period.

Meditation techniques

It does not really matter which meditation technique you use. Generally, people find that one suits them better than another. However, it is important to give each one a good try – say, 10 days – before you decide whether to try another. When you have found a method you like, you should practise it regularly. Start with one or, preferably, two 10-minute sessions a day and build up to 20 minutes for each. Try to make your meditation session the same time of day in the same place. When you become adept, you will be able to meditate at any time and in all kinds of places – even when there is noise or other people around.

Breathing meditations There are several different forms. Start with the easiest, which is to close your eyes and count each breath. Inhale on one, exhale on two, inhale on three and so on. The breath should be even and you can focus the counting on either the sensation of the air entering through the nose or the rise and fall of the abdomen. If you lose count, start again at one.

The second form of counted breathing counts only the exhalations – this is harder because the gaps between counting are longer. Next, try counting only the inhalations. On the inbreath, the mind is inclined to wander more easily, making this slightly more difficult again. Finally, simply follow the breath without counting. Observe the natural flow of your breath, the movement of the abdomen, as you would watch the gentle breath of a sleeping child.

Visualization This is a form of meditation that can take several forms (see page 250). Focusing involves closing your eyes and becoming aware of your own physical body lying on the floor or sitting on the chair and the everyday noises around you. A more concentrated form is to focus upon a particular object. In colour visualization you choose any colour and, closing your eyes, try to fill your mind with it to the exclusion of everything else. Mental visualization can take the form of a place or an object, real or imagined, that you look at with your mind's eye.

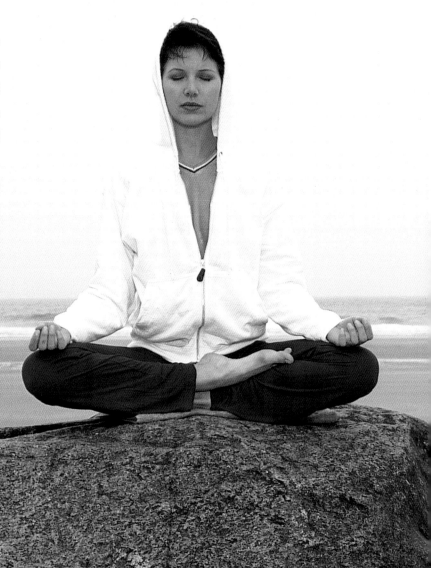

Mantra A mantra can be any word repeated aloud or silently on which the mind focuses. You can choose any word or sound you like; it can be a word with significance for you, like 'peace', or one that has a resonant sound – the best-known being the 'om' mantra (pronounced 'aum'). The most effective mantras tend to be mono- or duo-syllabic words with an emphasis on vowel sounds. Try 'one'/ 'one-O' or 'I'/'I-ing'. The idea is to repeat the word or sound until it has pushed all other conscious thoughts from your head.

After meditation

After 10–20 minutes, allow the focus of your meditation to fade gently away and bring your mind back to the present. Take some long, deep breaths and let your focus take in your body and how it is feeling, gradually becoming aware of your surroundings and the noises around you. Open your eyes and do a little gentle stretching. You are now refreshed for the rest of the day.

Remember, meditation can seem quite difficult to many people because their minds are full of thoughts and apparently unable to focus for any time at all on any of the techniques. This is quite normal. Do not feel that you are 'failing' to meditate; it is all part of the process of stilling the mind. If you try one of the above methods and find it does not suit you, try another. In any case, with time and practice, the ability to quieten the mind improves and these thoughts will bother you less.

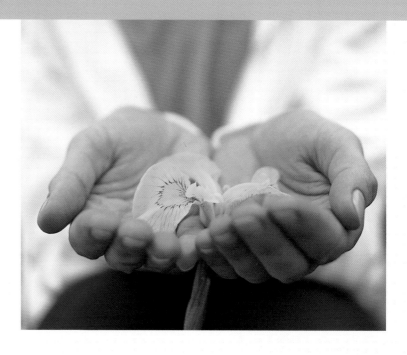

Spiritual meditation

Many people who meditate find not only a sense of deep personal inner peace, but also of connectedness with those around them and an inner store of wisdom and strength which is available to them to tap into whenever they need it. This often encourages them to explore the more spiritual and religious aspects of meditation. There are many Buddhist centres around for those who are interested, as well as a wealth of books on such subjects. More advanced methods of meditation should certainly be learned under the guidance of an experienced teacher and will inevitably have a moral and spiritual element, though not necessarily a religious one.

SEE ALSO:

→ Visualization, page 250   → Yoga, page 252

→ Improve your breathing, page 240

Visualization

A form of meditation that helps to calm and focus the mind, visualization can take several forms, three of which are covered here. Focusing on an object is a good introduction to meditation, as you can remind yourself of what you are doing every time your eye wanders from the object. Mental visualization skips the real object and goes straight to the mental image. Colour visualization appeals to many people, as they find a colour much easier to concentrate on than a more complex image.

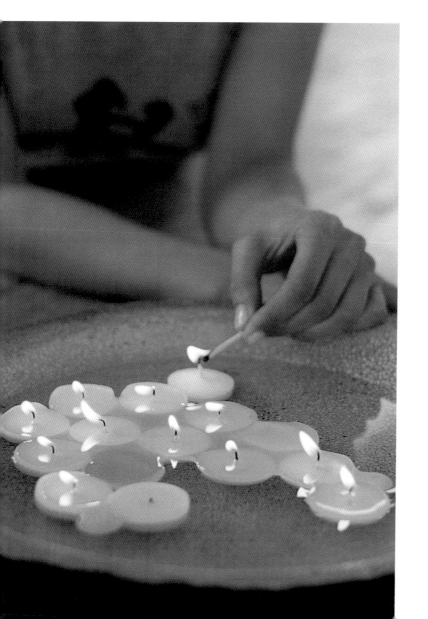

Preparing for visualization

Just as with meditating, when you are in a visualization session, you need to be free from distractions. So unplug the phone and, if there are other people about, ask them to be as quiet as possible and to keep out of the room. However, having someone else with whom to do the visualization exercise can often prove beneficial, adding to the focused atmosphere. Wear loose, comfortable clothing, make sure the room is warm but not stuffy, and sit in a position you can hold for up to 20 minutes. You can sit on the floor with your legs crossed or sit in a chair; the most important considerations are to be comfortable and not to have to move during the session.

Before you begin, take a few minutes to settle yourself both physically and mentally. Make sure you are sitting comfortably, and then focus on your mind. There will probably be plenty of thoughts whizzing around in your head, but just watch them, don't get caught up with them. Then place them on one side to deal with when you have finished.

Ideally, a visualization session should last for 20 minutes. If, however, you find this too difficult at first, begin with 10 minutes and try to extend the session a little each time. When the session is finished, remain seated for a few minutes, breathing slowly, and try to retain the tranquillity for a while afterwards.

Mental visualization

Close your eyes and picture a place or an object, that you see solely with your mind's eye; this place can be real or imagined. Observe this place or object in the greatest detail, focusing on it completely. A place of great tranquillity, such as a deserted beach, has a particularly calming influence.

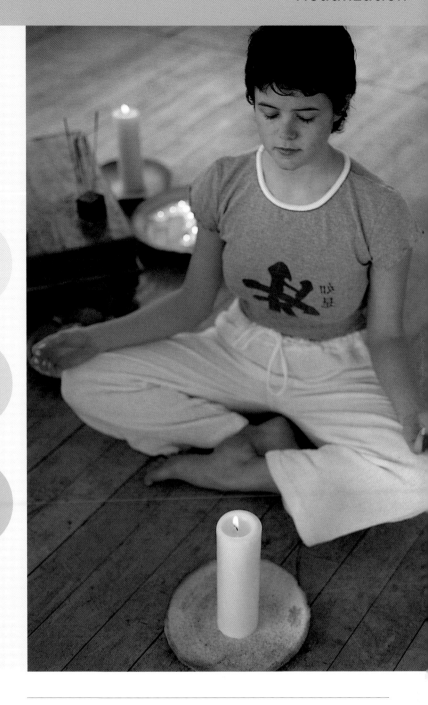

Focusing

1 Choose an object – something small and static, such as a flower, a stone or a candle flame. Place this in front of you, preferably about 1 m (3 ft) away and at eye level.

2 Close your eyes and become aware of your body on the floor or chair. Become aware too of the noises around you – cars going by, dogs barking, babies crying. Simply observe these sounds and then let them go.

3 Open your eyes. Look, without blinking, at your chosen object for a minute, or as long as you can. Then close your eyes and look at the image it has left in your mind's eye. When the image fades, open your eyes and look again. Continue in this way, alternating looking at the real object with the mental image, until the end of the session.

Colour visualization

Choose a colour on which to focus and, closing your eyes, try to fill your mind with the colour to the exclusion of everything else. It may be helpful to start by giving the colour a picture – the blue sea, a snow scene or a field of golden corn, for example. Then gradually try to go in closer and closer on the image so that you can no longer see the outlines of your mental picture, just the colour of it. Continue until only the colour floods your mind.

SEE ALSO:

→ Stress in the workplace, page 236

→ Relaxation techniques, page 242

→ Meditation, page 244

Yoga

Yoga is often portrayed as a mystical Eastern relaxation system that involves intricate postures that only the most supple and double-jointed people would dare to attempt. However, the movements can also be so simple that most people can benefit from yoga. The details of the origins of yoga are indistinct but it is known that it was practised by Indian philosophers, or *yogis*, who lived hermetic lives of meditation. Today the benefits of yoga have spread internationally and it is now practised in non-religious, non-cultural-based classes all over the Western world.

What is yoga?

Yoga is a gentle exercise system that benefits both body and spirit. The word yoga comes from the Sanskrit word for union. Practising the discipline is believed to encourage union of mind, body and spirit, thereby restoring the whole person to balance. Yoga benefits the body by relaxing muscles and improving suppleness, fitness and physical function. It also relaxes the mind and teaches us how to control stress, destructive emotions and unhealthy habits. A relaxed mind encourages the concentration and serenity that allows spiritual development.

The three aspects of the code on which yoga concentrates most are breathing (*Pranayama*), postures (*Asanas*) and meditation (*Dhyana*).

How it works

Harmony between body, mind and spirit is achieved through correct breathing, postural exercises and meditation. Breathing correctly is considered by yoga practitioners as a way of controlling all mental and bodily functions and essential for relaxation and meditation. Most of us tend to breathe incorrectly: anxiety and

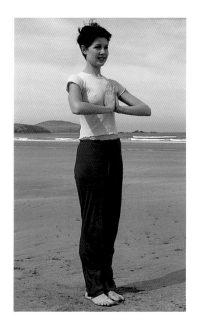

tension cause us to take short breaths that are centred in the upper chest, while lack of energy can cause weak breathing lower down in the diaphragm. Yoga breathing on the other hand encourages us to make full use of our lungs, so we strengthen them, increase our energy and vitality, and improve our circulation. The yoga postures exercise the body muscles and encourage relaxation and meditation. They must be practised regularly to be beneficial. The famous cross-legged lotus position (see page 247) represents self-awareness and is the pose most often adopted by experienced meditators. Some of the postures, for example the Cobra (see page 258), are based on the naturally relaxed and graceful movements of animals. These movements stretch the muscles to release pent-up tension and encourage strength and flexibility in the limbs and spine. Postures are often performed in a particular sequence, designed to exercise all the major muscle groups in the correct order, to encourage good circulation and to flush toxins out of the body (see Chapter 2). Meditation (see page 244) is a form of deep relaxation used to calm or focus the mind. It is an important but, particularly with beginners, not essential part of yoga. Meditation is often regarded as a natural progression from becoming competent at performing the postures and breathing exercises.

Who should practise yoga?

Yoga is safe for people of all ages and levels of fitness. Even pregnant women and people with chronic health problems can practise yoga under the guidance of a qualified instructor. Sufferers of any type of stress-related problem such as anxiety, high blood pressure, circulation and heart problems, backache, asthma, fatigue, arthritis and depression will all benefit from practising yoga regularly, especially since it can be practised to the level you are comfortable, and fit enough, for.

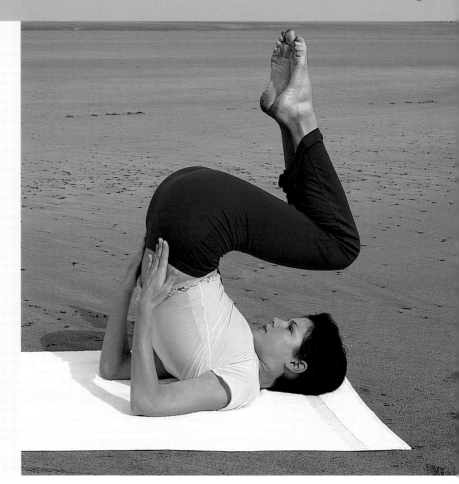

Performing yoga

To carry out the postures with ease and comfort you should work barefoot and wear clothes that allow movement. You will need a rubber mat on which to work and a room that is warm, quiet and well ventilated. It takes time to master the postures completely so do not push yourself too hard or become disillusioned. Perform them slowly and smoothly and hold each one only for as long as is comfortable, concentrating on your breathing throughout. Early morning sessions are recommended, but you can practise yoga at any time of day, providing you only do so at least two hours after eating your last meal.

Like any other exercise or relaxation system, yoga needs to be practised regularly to have a lasting effect. It should become part of your everyday lifestyle. However, even after only one session, most people will feel more relaxed and many people find they start to sleep better immediately.

Initial sessions

For your first session of yoga, try the **Salute to the sun** (see pages 254–6) two or three times. When you have finished, take five minutes to relax in either the **Child** or the **Corpse pose** (see page 261). When you are a little more experienced, begin each yoga session by running through the **Salute to the sun** between three and ten times, followed by the remaining postures illustrated on pages 257–260, carried out in the order in which they are shown (**Triangle**, **Cobra**, **Shoulder stand and plough**, **Fish**). These postures have the effect of stretching, stimulating and bringing into balance various parts of the body. Again, end the session by relaxing in either the **Child** or the **Corpse pose**.

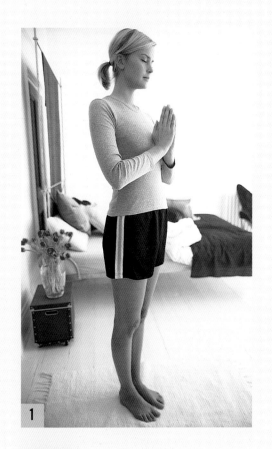

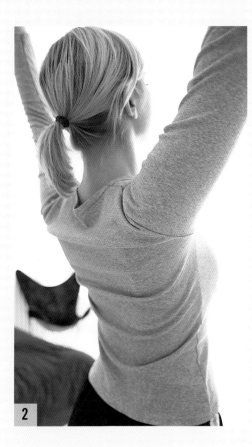

Salute to the sun

This is one of the best-known — and best — yoga postures. It stretches your whole body, as well as giving an internal massage to various organs.

1 Stand up straight, looking straight ahead, palms together in the prayer position just in front of your breastbone. Check that you are balanced equally on both feet and you are not tensing any area of your body. Take a few long, **deep breaths**.

2 Breathe in deeply and stretch your arms up to the ceiling. Continue the movement so that your arms move slightly backwards, taking your body with them in a curve. Don't force this position any more than feels comfortable.

3 Return to the erect position, still with your arms raised above you and, as you **breathe out**, bend forwards from your hips, keeping your back straight.

4 Place your hands on the floor, keeping your legs straight. If this isn't possible, hold the backs of your calves or ankles and gently stretch the backs of your legs.

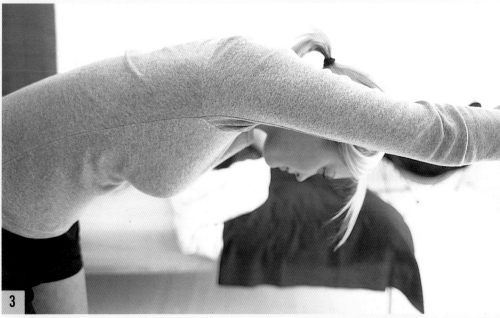

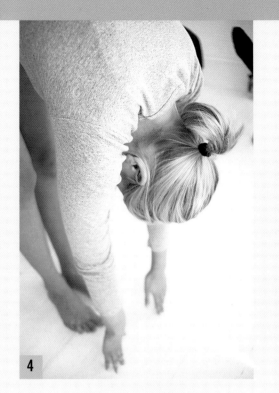

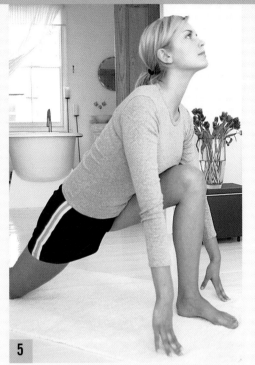

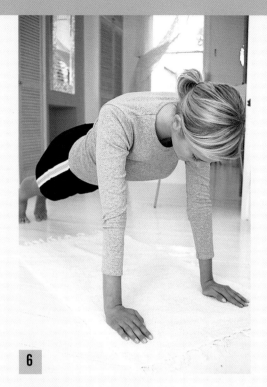

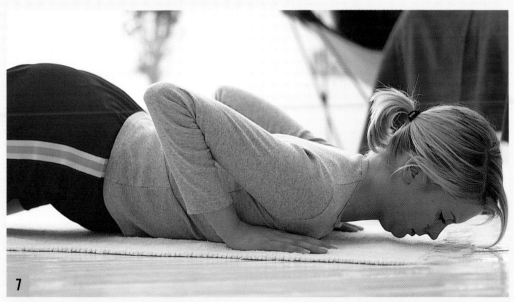

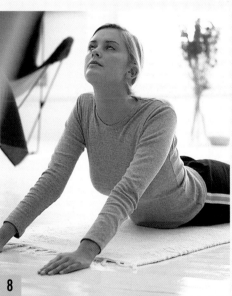

5 Take a deep breath in and bend your left knee, at the same time stretching your right leg out behind you and placing your hands on the floor. Look up to the ceiling.

6 Breathing out, take your left leg back so that you are supported on your hands and feet and your body is in a long straight line.

7 Breathe in and drop your knees and chest to the floor as you **breathe out**. Keep your hips raised off the floor.

8 As you **breathe in**, drop your hips to the ground and in a long, snake-like movement, push your upper body through your arms as far as it will go until your back is arched and you are looking at the ceiling.

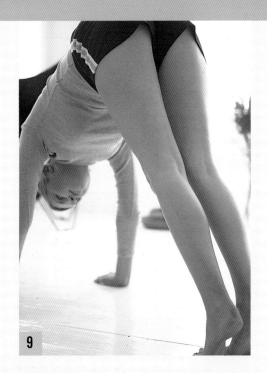

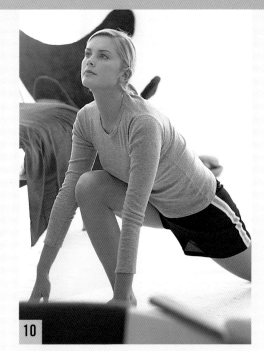

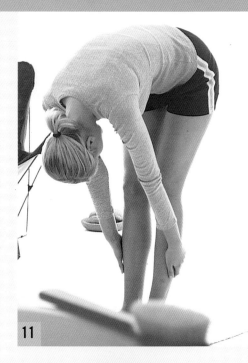

9 As you **breathe out**, push up to lift your hips up to the ceiling and drop your head so that you make a triangle.

10 Breathe in, bringing your right knee forwards, leaving your left leg stretched out behind you. **Breathe out** and look up towards the ceiling.

11 Breathe in and, as you **breathe out**, bring your left leg up to meet your right and stretch your legs, your hands flat on the floor or holding the backs of your calves. Keep your head dropped towards the floor. Only stretch as far as feels comfortable and, unless you are very supple, keep your knees bent.

12 Breathe in and very slowly start to lift your body from the waist, arms stretched out in front of you. Go past the upright position so that you lean back, arms behind you.

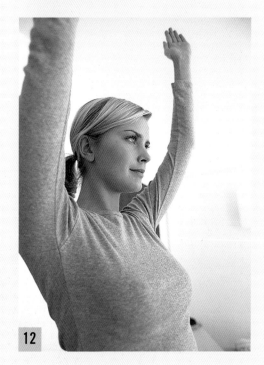

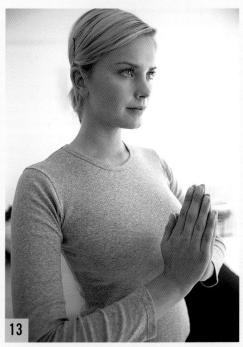

13 Return to standing and bring your palms together in the prayer position. *You can repeat this whole sequence a few times*. Those who are **experienced** at yoga may do so up to *10 times*. However, **if you are a beginner**, you should do it no more than *two or three times*

at first. You will find that you can stretch a little further each time you do it.

You may also find it helpful to take one sequence very slowly, holding each of the 12 positions for a few moments and taking a **few breaths** to relax into them.

The triangle

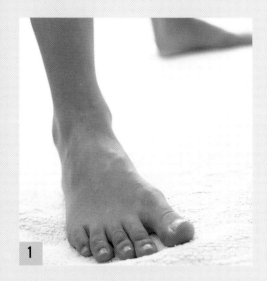

This posture involves a sideways bend that is beneficial to the spine and balances muscle groups.

1 Stand with your feet together, keeping your back stretched, and looking straight ahead. Your body should feel alert yet relaxed. Place your feet 60–90 cm (24–36 in) apart, then turn your right foot so that it points outwards at a right angle to your body. Your left foot should point slightly to your right.

Breathe in deeply and raise your arms to shoulder height, parallel to the floor. As you **breathe out**, bend to the right, placing your right hand on your right thigh, and sliding it down your calf as far as you can towards the floor. Do not twist your body as you slide down; your hips should be facing directly forwards.

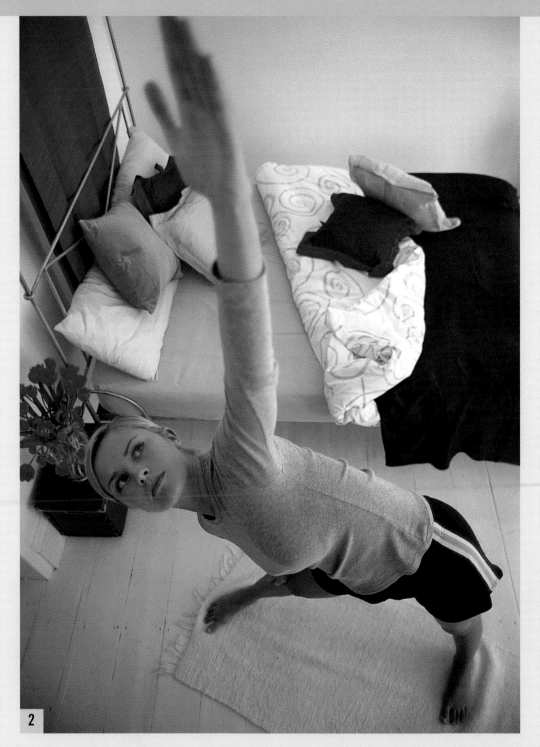

2 Raise your left arm so that your fingers point to the ceiling and your palm faces forwards. Turn your head so you are looking up at your hand. Feel a long stretch down your left side and between your right and left hands. Take at least **three long breaths** in this position, ten if you can. **Breathing in**, slide your right arm back up, dropping your left arm until you are facing forwards again. *Repeat on the left. Do three stretches on each side.*

The cobra

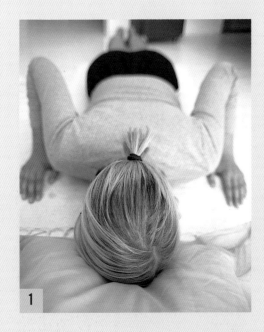

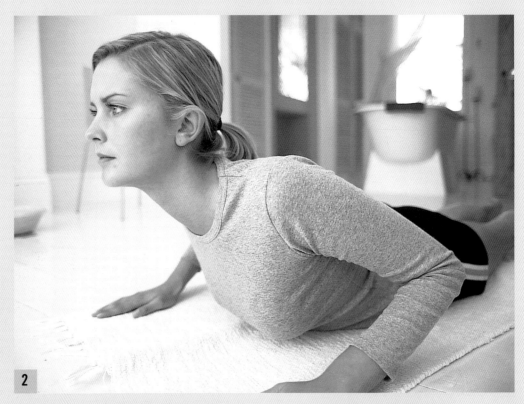

This posture stretches the front of the body and compresses the spine. The whole movement should be done slowly, with controlled movements, both while raising the body off the floor and when coming down again.

1 Lie face down on the floor, legs together, toes pointing away from you. Place your hands flat on the floor, parallel with your chest. Your forehead should be touching the floor.

2 Breathe in deeply and slowly start to raise your head, feeling a stretch through the back of your neck. Look at the floor to avoid tension in your neck. **Breathe out**.

3 Breathe in again and continue to lift your head. As you do so your chest should come up from the floor. Bring your arms in front of you and use them to support your body as you lift the whole ribcage off the floor. Look directly in front of you. When you have lifted as high as you can without undue strain, press down on your hands, **breathe out** and, if you can, hold this position for several breaths.

Breathe in deeply and return to the starting position, going through all the stages you did on the way up. Rest for a moment and *repeat the sequence once more if you feel you can*.

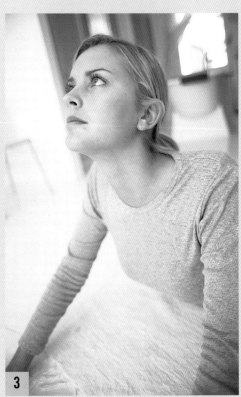

Shoulder stand and plough

The Shoulder stand increases energy flow, improves the circulation and stimulates the thyroid gland. It also promotes body awareness. The Plough is another inverted posture that calms the mind but also stimulates the body.

CAUTION: Do not do the Shoulder stand or Plough if you are menstruating or have back problems. If you suffer from hypertension (high blood pressure) or neck problems, check with your doctor before trying these postures.

1 Lie on your back, arms by your sides, and **breathe in** as you bend your knees to your chest. **Breathe out** and straighten your legs as far as comfortable, taking them further back so your hips start to come off the floor.

2 Use your hands to support your back and push yourself a little higher. The aim is to straighten your legs so that they are completely perpendicular, while resting on your shoulders.

3 If you are able to get your legs into a vertical position, hold this position, **breathing slowly**, for one to three minutes. You can stretch and flex your feet in this

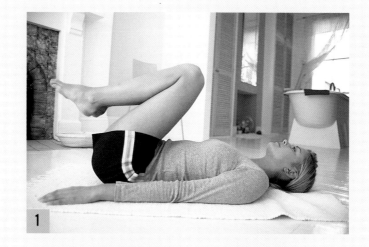

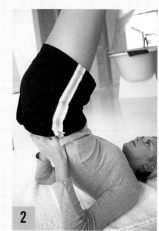

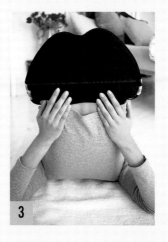

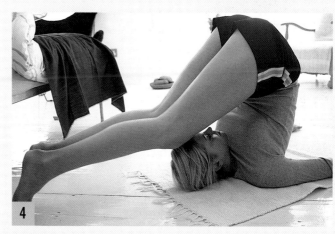

position to help your legs relax. However, you may find this difficult at first and it may be more comfortable to leave them at a 45° angle to your body. If so, go on to Step 4.

4 Take your legs over your head and, if you can, place your feet on the floor behind you, toes curled under and legs straight. This is the Plough position. When you are secure in

this position, place your arms behind you, flat on the floor. Take several **deep breaths** in this position.

You can return to the Shoulder stand and go back to the floor by reversing the first two steps, continuing very slowly. Alternatively, roll your spine down slowly back to the floor from the Plough position.

The fish

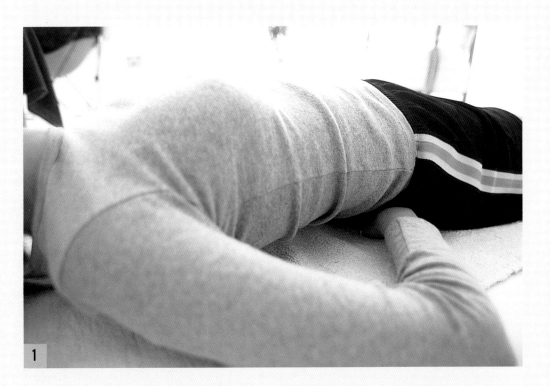

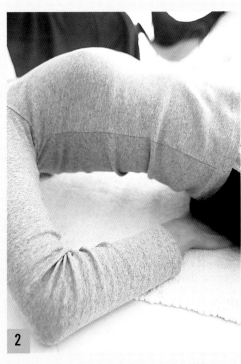

This posture opens the chest and compresses the vertebrae in the spine, so it acts as a counter position to the Shoulder stand.

CAUTION: Do not do this exercise if you have neck problems. If you suffer from hypertension, avoid putting your head on the floor in Step 2, as there is a vital pressure point at the top of the head. As an alternative, you can bend your head back until it is about 2.5 cm (1 in) from the floor.

1 Lie on your back with your legs held together in front of you and your toes stretching away. Raise your back off the ground.

2 Arch your back, supporting yourself on your elbows with your lower arms flat on the floor, palms facing down. Lower the top of your head to the floor. Hold the position and take several **deep breaths**. Slide the back of your head and then your neck back down to the floor. Relax for a few moments.

Child pose

This traditional yoga pose is good for both stretching and relaxing at the end of a yoga session.

1 Sit on your heels, back straight. Place your hands on the soles of your feet. **Breathe in** and bend gently backwards, looking up. **Breathe out** and bend slowly forwards until you can place your forehead on the floor. You will have to let go of your feet, and your bottom may come up a little. You may place your cheek on the floor for comfort, and lie your arms by your sides. **Breathe deeply and slowly**, eyes closed. After a minute or two, allow your breathing to become shallower, but keep your eyes closed. When you are ready, come up very slowly.

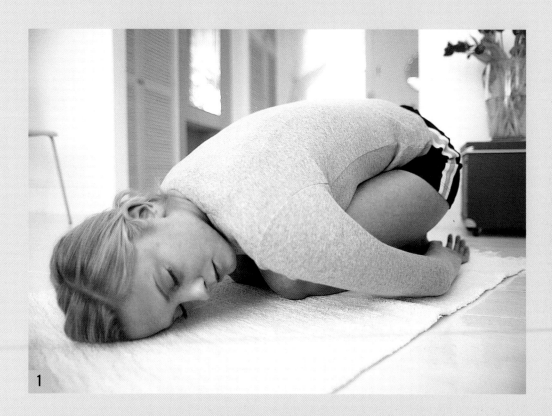

Corpse pose

This is so relaxing that you might even fall asleep. Make sure you have something to cover yourself with in this position as otherwise you may begin to feel cold.

1 Lie on your back with your arms slightly out from your sides with the palms facing the ceiling. Your legs should be slightly apart with relaxed feet. Close your eyes.
Breathe slowly and deeply for one or two minutes, concentrating on the breath itself and the sensation of your lungs filling with air. Then breathe naturally for a few more minutes before getting up.

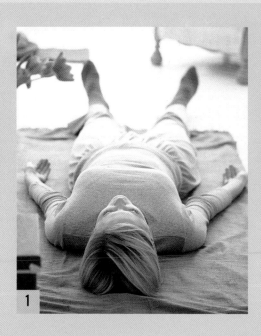

Autogenic training

Stress undermines the immune system as much as pollution or bad diet. Autogenic training (AT), a quick and easy form of relaxation that verges on meditation, can be used as a long-term relaxation therapy and as a quick defuser of stressful situations.

Ideally, AT should be learned with a therapist, who will take you through the stages over a period of weeks. Unfortunately there are still relatively few AT teachers, so the bones of the technique are described here. If you feel that you are falling into a relaxed state very quickly at the start of each session, try proceeding to the next stage. It isn't a race, and it doesn't matter how long it takes you to progress.

Each session takes a matter of minutes, becoming slightly longer at each stage. The best times for AT are first thing in the morning, mid-morning, just before lunch, mid-afternoon, just before supper and last thing at night in bed. AT is a very effective way of inducing a deep sleep.

Stage 1

Close your eyes and repeat these phrases slowly, silently to yourself three times each, pausing before each repetition, and focusing on the relevant body part. Pause for longer before the next phrase, so that your mind has time to refocus. At the right speed, it will take a minimum of three minutes, closer to five.

- My right arm is heavy
- My left arm is heavy
- Both my arms are heavy
- My right leg is heavy
- My left leg is heavy
- Both my legs are heavy
- My arms and legs are heavy

Stage 2

When you find yourself relaxing very easily in **Stage 1**, you may go on to **Stage 2**, but wait until you feel completely relaxed and then the next stage will give you more benefit.
In **Stage 2**, you lengthen the session a little by adding one further step. Repeat each phrase slowly, with pauses, as before.

- My right arm is heavy
- My left arm is heavy
- Both my arms are heavy
- My right leg is heavy
- My left leg is heavy
- Both my legs are heavy
- My arms and legs are heavy
- My neck and shoulders are heavy

Stage 3

In **Stage 3**, a third centre for your focus is added – **the breathing**. This is not a particularly deep breath but, as you can see from the phrase '**My body breathes me**', you become aware of how the breath is affecting your entire body. Again, you repeat all of the phrases from the previous stages first.

- My right arm is heavy
- My left arm is heavy
- Both my arms are heavy
- My right leg is heavy
- My left leg is heavy
- Both my legs are heavy
- My arms and legs are heavy
- My neck and shoulders are heavy
- My body breathes me

Basic guidelines

You can sit or lie down during autogenic training. While you are learning the technique, it is a good idea to find a quiet room where you will not be disturbed, but once you become more adept, you can use it anywhere for instant stress relief – in the office, on the train or before an interview.

As with all forms of meditation and relaxation, focus your mind quietly, without worrying if you find your mind drifting. Just bring it gently back to where it is supposed to be. AT focuses on parts of the body in turn and the sense of physical relaxation induces a mental relaxation. Don't worry if you don't feel heaviness initially – this will come, or if you feel other physical sensations, such as numbness or floating. This is perfectly normal.

When you practise the technique in bed or on the floor, lie on your back with your arms at your sides, allowing your limbs to fall naturally. If you are seated, sit up straight with your back well supported, your feet flat on the floor and your hands on your thighs. Begin with a few quiet moments breathing slowly and deeply. When you have finished, sit quietly with your eyes closed for a few moments, gently focusing back on your surroundings.

Stage 4

Adding the breathing – **Stage 3** – usually takes quite a long time to focus on. Make sure you can really feel the focus of the first three stages before you attempt **Stage 4** – here you focus on your face: try to feel the sensation of coolness. When you feel ready, progress with the same speed, pauses and repetitions.

- My right arm is heavy
- My left arm is heavy
- Both my arms are heavy
- My right leg is heavy
- My left leg is heavy
- Both my legs are heavy
- My arms and legs are heavy
- My neck and shoulders are heavy
- My body breathes me
- My forehead is cool and relaxed

Stage 5

Again, don't rush into this stage. Here, you take your focus from outside to inside to become aware of your heartbeat.

- My right arm is heavy
- My left arm is heavy
- Both my arms are heavy
- My right leg is heavy
- My left leg is heavy
- Both my legs are heavy
- My arms and legs are heavy
- My neck and shoulders are heavy
- My body breathes me
- My forehead is cool and relaxed
- My heartbeat is calm and regular

Stage 6

Finally, you take your focus to the mind itself.

- My right arm is heavy
- My left arm is heavy
- Both my arms are heavy
- My right leg is heavy
- My left leg is heavy
- Both my legs are heavy
- My arms and legs are heavy
- My neck and shoulders are heavy
- My body breathes me
- My forehead is cool and relaxed
- My heartbeat is calm and regular
- My mind is calm and serene

Tranquil surroundings

Tranquility and emotional balance are not just about massage techniques and relaxation exercises, however helpful these may be. To achieve a sense of inner peace you have to have a place where you can escape from the stresses and strains of modern life. Your home has to become a stress-free zone. This may sound like a major undertaking but, in fact, there are lots of simple things you can do to improve your home environment, whether it's your living room, your bathroom, even your garden.

Colour

When it comes to decorating your home, the colours most likely to help you to relax are the neutrals and pastels. Creams, blues, lilacs, pinks and greens are all ideal background colours that lower the environmental temperature and help you unwind. This is not to say that you should never use bold or dark colours, but they can be rather oppressive if you are exposed to them long term. Dramatic reds and purples or dark greens and blues are best saved for rooms, such as dining rooms and hallways, where they look very effective but where you don't spend a lot of time.

Some strong, bright colours, however, lift your mood, such as sunshine yellow or duck egg blue. These work particularly well in busy rooms, such as kitchens, where they share wall space with cupboards. Splashes of bright or dark colours, say on pictures or cushions, also add interest to neutral rooms which may otherwise feel a little bland.

These colour rules work in the garden, too. Lighter pastels and plenty of green will make a tranquil setting in an area where you often sit, and can be used to create a relaxing oasis. Save the flamboyant reds, yellows and oranges for an impressive entrance or a pathway in a different part of the garden.

Water

Both the sight and the sound of water are profoundly relaxing. Just think of the sound of the sea as it breaks on the shore or a stream running over stones. While few of us are lucky enough to have a stream or the sea at the bottom of the garden, even a tiny patio will have a corner for a small pond or fountain. A barrel or ceramic bowl with aquatic plants or a simple fountain where the water splashes on to stones can have a surprisingly soothing effect. If you have room for a bigger pond, watching your fish glide through the water can be very relaxing at the end of a stressful day.

You don't need to have a garden in order to have a simple fountain. It can work equally well in a bathroom where the rhythmic splashing and gurgling of water is the perfect background music for a relaxing bath.

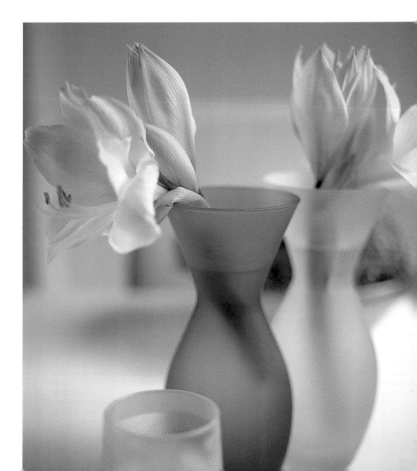

Plants and flowers

Plants and flowers bring the natural world into the house and along with them a calmer atmosphere. Our living rooms are very hard edged nowadays. We have more and more hi-tech equipment – televisions, DVDs, computers, music systems – all enclosed by the inevitably geometric lines of walls and ceilings. Contemporary life can be fun and futuristic but it is a long way from nature where you never see a straight line. The softer shapes, colours and scents of flowers and plants break up hard contours and can transform a room. For a breath of the countryside, simply fill a bowl with the heady scent and delicate petals of roses, lilies or sweet peas.

Lighting and fragrance

Central ceiling lights are rarely relaxing. A more subtle version, using strategically placed lamps, will give attractive pools of light that are both more flattering to your décor as well as being easier on your eyes. Candles, too, give a very pretty, soft light that is particularly relaxing. They are ideal on the dining table, or when you are listening to music, and make the perfect background lighting for a massage. Always remember, though, to check that the flames are completely doused before you go to sleep.

There are many scented candles available now, too, often with an aromatherapy oil such as rose or lavender that has particularly soothing qualities. Aromatherapy oils can be used in incense burners or simply put a few drops into a bowl of water and place it on top of a radiator. Research has shown that we respond to smell on an emotional level more strongly than to the other senses. It's not

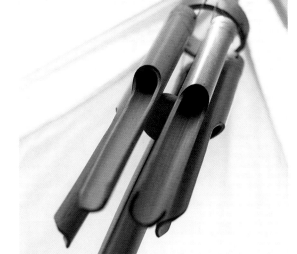

surprising that oils such as lavender, rose, neroli, geranium and jasmine can balance out our emotions, relieving anxiety, depression, mental fatigue and insomnia.

Pets

Another important, often under-used, sense is touch. Touch is the first form of communication and a young child needs stroking and skin contact almost as much as food and warmth. This need for touching does not stop in infancy and this is one of the reasons that pets have been found to be so effective in reducing stress. Dogs and cats love being stroked and petted and as you touch them, you relax too. Physical contact may not even be necessary. Watching fish or listening to a bird sing has much the same effect.

Creating an oasis

Noise, as we all now know, can be extremely stressful. Traffic noise and loud music have a unique ability to invade our sense of privacy and space. We need to create our own oasis of tranquil sound in which to feel at peace. The sound you choose depends very much on personal preference but, generally, quiet music is more relaxing than loud. Besides listening to music, there are also tapes of relaxing sounds. These include sounds from nature, such as birdsong and whale music, new age music and chanting. Wind chimes are popular, too, placed near a window, and are an important device in *feng shui*, the Chinese art of creating a perfect environment. *Feng shui* also stresses the relationship between a cluttered room and a cluttered mind. You can't avoid feeling stressed if you're surrounded by mess. So, clear a space, create an oasis of calm and relax.

Weekend home health spa

Some short-term stress is not a bad thing; it can actually motivate us. In the long term, however, it can cause many physical and emotional ailments. This relaxing weekend programme is for those who are experiencing prolonged stress, which can manifest itself in the form of anxiety, headaches, digestive problems, depression, skin eruptions – or simply feeling unable to cope. By the end of the weekend, you should have brought both the physical and emotional symptoms of stress under control and be feeling rested and calm.

The first thing to do is create an oasis of time. Choose a weekend, and clear all arrangements. Unplug the phone for the whole weekend and switch off the rest of the world. If you have children, ask your partner or your mother to take them for the weekend. Alternatively, try and arrange a reciprocal weekend with another parent, who will have a free weekend when you take their children.

You do not have to spend the whole time in isolation at home. The weekend includes a visit to a professional therapist for a massage. Apart from this, you should make sure you get out for a breath of fresh air every day. Take a walk, go cycling or do some gardening. Ask a friend to follow the weekend programme with you. You can compare notes on how you are feeling as you progress. However you decide to spend it, the most important thing is to relax and enjoy yourself, and not feel guilty about spending time on what you are doing.

Look through the recipes for the weekend and make a list of the food and drink you need to buy in advance. It is a good idea to prepare as much as you can beforehand so you have as few chores as possible during the weekend itself. There may be other preparations, too – you might want to make a relaxation tape for the weekend (see page 242). If you decide to go out for a professional massage on Saturday, book your appointment well in advance, and most importantly, tell everyone you are unavailable that weekend.

Weekend Schedule

Friday
7.00 pm
Meditation
8.00 pm
Evening meal
9.00 pm
Aromatherapy bath
10.00 pm
Self-massage for sleep

Saturday
8.00 am
Yoga
9.00 am
Breakfast
10.00 am
Relaxation and meditation
12.00 pm
Lunch
2.00 pm
Massage
4.00 pm
Facial massage
6.00 pm
Evening meal

8.00 pm
Breathing techniques
and meditation
10.00 pm
Bed

Sunday
8.00 am
Yoga, relaxation and
meditation
9.00 am
Breakfast
11.00 am
Acupressure
1.00 pm
Lunch
3.00 pm
Aromatherapy facial
4.00 pm
Meditation
6.00 pm
Evening meal
8.00 pm
Aromatherapy bath
10.00 pm
Bed

Friday

7.00 pm
Meditation
8.00 pm
Evening meal
9.00 pm
Aromatherapy
bath
10.00 pm
Self-massage for
sleep

Many of us feel severely overstretched, trying to balance work, family commitments and a social life. You are so busy coping, you forget to, or are unable to, relax. The point of the programme for this weekend is to reverse this trend. Not only will you give yourself time and several pampering treats, but you will also learn a number of techniques that help to combat stress. Ideally, these should be incorporated into your everyday life. Tonight's meditation session and aromatherapy bath are the first items on the agenda to get your relaxing weekend off to a good start.

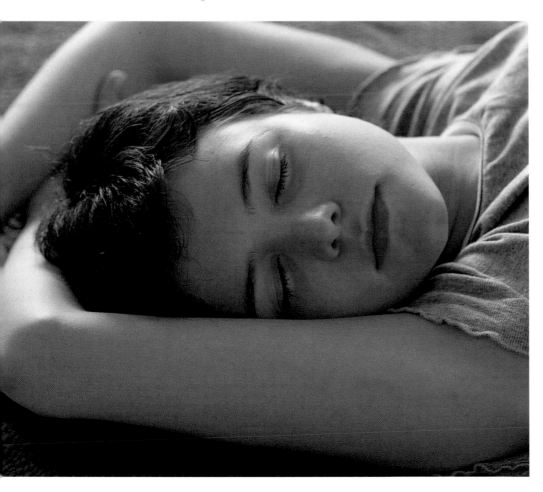

7.00 pm Meditation

There are numerous relaxation techniques that can overcome the immediate stresses and strains of contemporary life. However, a period of prolonged stress is another matter, manifesting itself in many different ways. To overcome these problems, a quite different form of deep relaxation is needed to disperse severe stress of body and mind.

Regular meditation has emerged as the most effective way of achieving deep relaxation. A considerable body of clinical research, focusing mainly on the most dramatic and measurable manifestations of stress, such as heart disease, has shown that meditation results in substantial reductions in blood pressure and cholesterol levels. Other clinical tests have shown that the risk of much of the physical and mental deterioration associated with ageing is reduced considerably by regular meditation. Meditation is not, however, merely a prophylaxis. Some of its other benefits include:

- Physical relaxation
- Improved concentration
- Increased tranquillity and ability to deal with stress
- Improved awareness
- Improved creativity and memory

Friday

Primarily, meditation (see page 244) is a discipline for training your mind to a point of both deep concentration and relaxation. During this weekend, you can only hope to achieve an idea of what meditation is like. The first session may seem a little strange, but if you get into a regular rhythm of meditation during the course of these three days, you may well find that its benefits make it something you want to continue.

There are various meditation techniques you can use. Two options are breathing and the mantra (see pages 248 and 249). Over the course of the weekend, you may want to try both to see if one seems more suitable than the other. When you have found one you like, you should practise it regularly, preferably at the same time of day in the same place. After the allotted time, allow the focus of your meditation to fade away gently and bring your mind back to the present. Take some long, deep breaths and become aware of your body and its sensations, gradually becoming aware, too, of your surroundings and the noises around you. Finally, open your eyes, but remain still for a few more minutes.

You can establish a meditation routine for the future during the course of the weekend – in the morning and in the evening. It will be particularly beneficial if you meditate after gentle exercise, but avoid practising for at least an hour after a meal. If you find your sessions immediately beneficial, you can add an extra one during the course of the day.

8.00 pm Evening meal

There are several techniques and treatments that will aid relaxation of body and mind, and diet has an important part to play in this. While weight loss is not the purpose of this weekend, if your body is working overtime to digest rich food, it is going to be more difficult to slow down generally. Therefore, your diet for the weekend should be light, nutritious and easy to digest. Your evening meal each night is a nourishing soup and the main meal of the day is eaten at lunchtime, when the body's digestive system is working most efficiently. If you don't think one bowl of soup is enough, have a second serving, or eat a slice of wholemeal bread with it.

If you want a deep, restful night's sleep, you should eat neither too much nor too late in the evening. Don't be tempted to drink alcohol; although it makes you feel sleepy initially, it is a stimulant and may well break your sleep in the middle of the night. Tea and coffee are also stimulants, so avoid these as well. Instead, drink plenty of bottled or filtered water throughout the evening.

Try to eat no later than 8.00 pm and eat slowly, concentrating on your food while you eat – don't watch television or listen to the radio at the same time. This will give your body the chance to slow down.

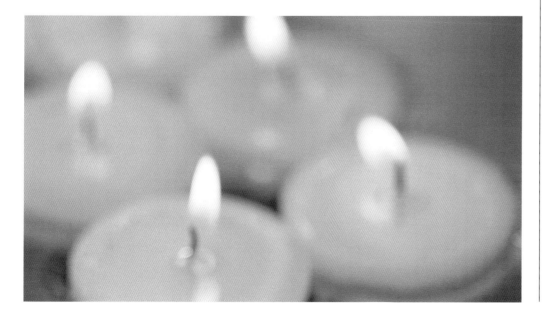

9.00 pm Aromatherapy bath

The very fact you feel in need of this relaxing weekend plan means you are likely to be stressed. As a result, you may well be having trouble sleeping. One of the aims of this weekend is to have three deep, restful nights of sleep without recourse to medication and its unwanted side-effects. Aromatherapy is a very pleasant alternative to sleeping pills, and doesn't leave you feeling drowsy the next day.

You need to take time to wind down at the end of the day, which is why this first evening is so carefully planned, starting with the meditation. Eating a light meal fairly early in the evening also helps. If you feel thirsty later, have a cup of herbal tea to drink before bed. Camomile with honey and lemon is ideal. If you have a tendency to indigestion, try drinking peppermint.

An aromatherapy bath is the next step and is a very good way of slowing down the mind and relaxing the body at the end of the day. This bath has little to do with washing; it is all about pleasure and relaxation. Prepare the room in advance to make it as tranquil as possible. The bathroom and towels should be warm. Lighting is also important; keep it as low as possible. Candlelight has a calming effect, and candles scented with relaxing oils are widely available.

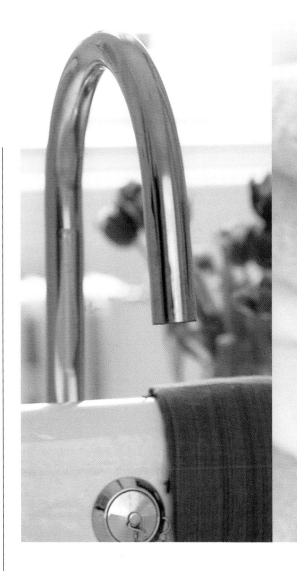

Sweet dreams oil

12 drops lavender essential oil
8 drops neroli essential oil
5 drops rose essential oil

Mix the ingredients and store in a glass bottle until use.

Fill the bath with water. It should not be too hot or the essential oils will simply evaporate. Add 5-10 drops of Sweet dreams oil (see box, above) to the water and mix it in well. Alternatively, add 4 drops each of lavender and sandalwood essential oils to the water. The lavender will help reduce anxiety and depression, while the sandalwood will help overcome the risk of insomnia by gently quietening the brain.

Relax in the bath for at least 20 minutes. If you have difficulty unwinding, listen to soft, tranquil music. After your bath, wrap yourself in a big, warm towel and pat yourself gently with the towel or just wrap yourself in it until it absorbs the water on your body, so that a little of the oil remains on your skin.

10.00 pm Bed

There are various techniques for inducing sleep after your bath. These include burning aromatherapy essential oils in the bedroom (don't forget to extinguish the candle) and self-massage for sleep (see page 239).

Saturday

8.00 am Yoga	**12.00 pm** Lunch	**8.00 pm** Breathing
9.00 am Breakfast	**2.00 pm** Massage	techniques and meditation
10.00 am Relaxation and meditation	**4.00 pm** Facial massage **6.00 pm** Evening meal	**10.00 pm** Bed

Today begins with a yoga session before breakfast. Yoga, the ancient Indian 'science of life', deals with physical, mental and spiritual health in its three disciplines of postures (*asanas*), breathing exercises (*pranayama*), and meditation (*dhyana*). During the course of this relaxation weekend, you will try all of these aspects of yoga, which together aim to bring the mind, body and spirit into balance.

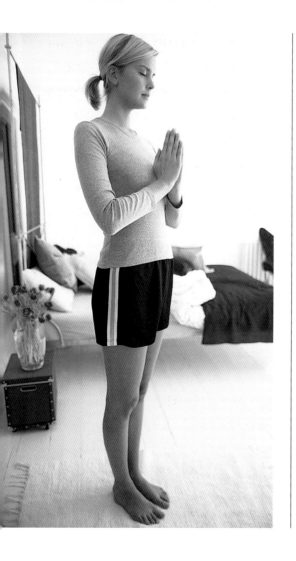

8.00 am Yoga

Yoga is a systematic, gradual process of relaxation, and is therefore a perfect technique for this weekend. The physical relaxation that results from the practice of yoga postures (see pages 254–261) and breathing exercises (see page 240) brings with it the release of old stored tensions, often emotional in origin. The body becomes much more supple, and the muscles become stretched and toned without increasing their bulk. Ailments connected with tension and contracted muscles are therefore often considerably relieved by yoga. These include chronic back pain, headaches and migraine. The effect of loosening immobile joints makes yoga particularly helpful for anyone who suffers from arthritis or rheumatism.

Start the day with the yoga exercise, Salute to the sun (see page 254), which is traditionally performed in the morning – before you breakfast or shower. Even if you are not at your best first thing in the morning, this exercise will wake up your body and help to focus your mind. It also works as a massage for the internal organs. Wear loose clothing and make sure the room is warm before you start exercising – cold is not beneficial to stretching muscles. Repeat the exercise a few times then take five minutes to relax in either the Child pose or the Corpse pose (see page 261).

9.00 am Breakfast

It is best to have breakfast after you have had your yoga session – exercise on a full stomach is not recommended. If you can, drink a herbal infusion rather than ordinary tea or coffee, but if you really can't do without these, try decaffeinated versions – you will sense the benefit when you do your relaxation session later in the morning, and when you

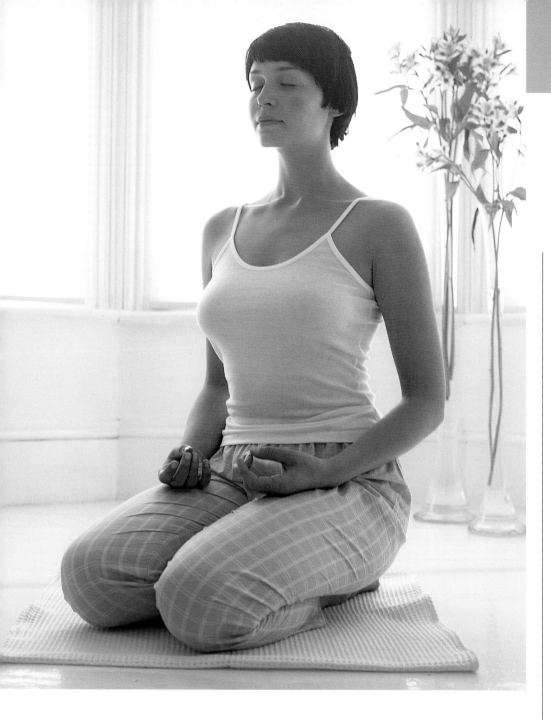

go to bed at night. Drink plenty of filtered or bottled water or more herbal teas throughout the day and, if you want a snack, have a piece of fruit or some dried fruit and nuts.

Keep breakfast simple – perhaps a piece of wholemeal toast or a non-sugary cereal with some fruit and a herbal tea. Have a large glass of fruit juice as well – you could try making your own fresh juice mix (see page 42 for recipes).

10.00 am Relaxation and meditation

After breakfast, you can slowly begin to prepare yourself for the rest of the day, allowing yourself time to digest breakfast before you think about your next session.

Dress for the relaxation exercises in clothes that are loose and comfortable. Bear in mind that, during relaxation, your body temperature will drop, so make sure that you are going to be warm enough. Socks are a good idea and put a blanket or sweater nearby in case you begin to feel cold as the session progresses.

There are no secrets to relaxation, and when you try the exercises you may be surprised to find how closely the mind and body track each other. Where one leads, the other will follow; therefore by relaxing one, the other must also relax. However, you have to give yourself the chance to relax – free from interruption. Take the phone off the hook or put on the answer machine and, if anyone is likely to come in and disturb you, put a 'keep out' notice on the door.

There are two ways of completing the relaxation process. You can either read through the instructions on page 243 and remember them, saying them to yourself in your mind, or you can record the whole sequence in advance (see box, page 242). This allows you to focus entirely on your body.

If you get up too soon at the end of the exercise, you may feel dizzy. Instead, lie on the floor for at least five minutes, gradually coming back to your normal consciousness. You may want to lie on the bed for a while afterwards or even take a short nap. Do whatever you feel instinctively and spend the time until lunch as quietly as possible.

Saturday

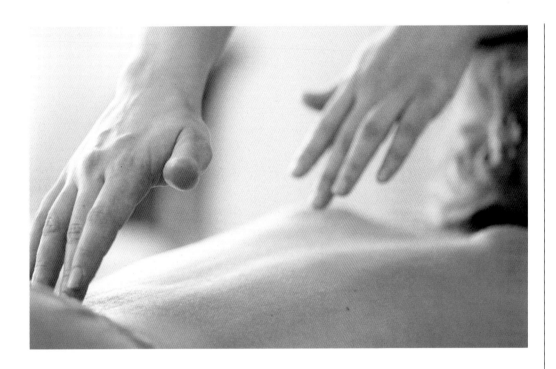

8.00 pm Breathing techniques and meditation

See pages 240–1 for the two breathing exercises you need to do. In both exercises, focus your attention on your breath and try to observe its progress through your body.

The breathing exercises are very relaxing and slow the body down considerably. This puts you in the ideal state for meditation. So, as soon as you are ready, do your second meditation session, choosing either the breath or the mantra method (see page 248).

12.00 pm Lunch

Lunch will be the main meal of the day for the weekend, so do enjoy it. Have a salad such as tuna, prawn or bean salad (see pages 62–65), followed by fruit and frozen yogurt. Give yourself plenty of time to savour the food and eat slowly.

2.00 pm Massage

Delay the massage until you have had a chance to digest your lunch. The ultimate treat is to have a professional massage – and it is particularly relaxing if aromatherapy oils are used. Look for a qualified therapist at your local gym, swimming pool or sports centre, and make sure you book your appointment well in advance. Some therapists will even come to you. This is the best possible option, as after you have had your massage you can simply relax in the comfort of your own home.

4.00 pm Facial massage

A lot of tension is stored in the muscles of the face. A facial massage (see page 126) releases this tension and leaves your face looking relaxed, and therefore younger. Also, because the massage stimulates circulation to the face, your complexion should be toned and glowing by the end of this session.

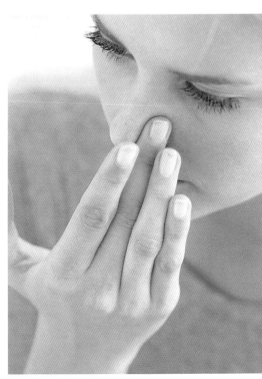

Sunday

8.00 am	**3.00 pm**
Yoga,	Aromatherapy
relaxation and	facial
meditation	**4.00 pm**
9.00 am	Meditation
Breakfast	**6.00 pm**
11.00 am	Evening meal
Acupressure	**8.00 pm**
1.00 pm	Aromatherapy
Lunch	bath
	10.00 pm
	Bed

You should be feeling much more relaxed and well rested today than you did when you woke up on Saturday. As yesterday, the day starts with a yoga session.

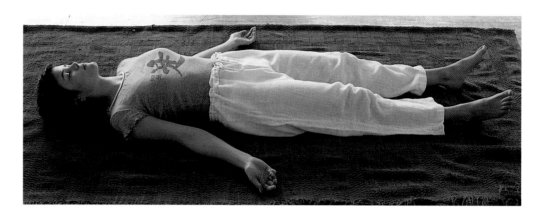

8.00 am Yoga, relaxation and meditation

Begin with Salute to the sun (see page 254), repeating this between three and ten times, depending on how experienced you are and how fit and supple you feel. Then proceed to the Triangle, Cobra, Shoulder stand and plough, and Fish postures (see pages 257–260). As with all yoga exercises, do them slowly and do not put any unnecessary strain on your body. If you feel uncomfortable or have any pain, come out of the posture, rest and then move on to something else.

At the end of this longer yoga session, spend at least 5 minutes in one of the relaxation poses, either the Corpse or the Child pose (see page 261). You will now be in an ideal frame of mind for meditation.

Meditate (see page 248) for up to 20 minutes and, if you wish, do the relaxation techniques session (see page 243).

The remainder of the day...

Try a session of acupressure (see page 286) at 11.00 am. This is similar to acupuncture, but has the big advantage that you can do it yourself and no needles are involved. It is particularly useful for relieving stress.

After lunch, treat yourself to an aromatherapy facial and hair treatment (see page 116), followed by another session of meditation (see pages 248–249).

After a light evening meal, take an aromatherapy bath (see page 282) to prepare for a night of peaceful sleep, ready to face the week ahead feeling relaxed and rejuvenated.

SEE ALSO:

→ Making juices, page 40

→ Everyday toxins, page 94

→ Aromatherapy facial, page 116

→ Massage, page 158

→ Aerobic exercise, page 224

→ Improve your breathing, page 240

→ Relaxation techniques, page 242

→ Meditation, page 244

→ Visualization, page 250

→ Yoga, page 252

→ Aromatherapy, page 278

→ Acupressure, page 286

Therapies and treatments

7

There are plenty of therapies and treatments to help you improve and maintain your physical, mental and emotional wellbeing. Intended to energize, revitalize and balance body and mind, many have already been introduced earlier in this book and range from exercise regimes and detox programmes, to pampering beauty treatments and de-stressing relaxation routines. Many are self-help applications and programmes easily managed at home, while others are treatments best received from professionals. Those disciplines not yet dealt with elsewhere are covered here.

Choosing a therapy

The therapies and treatments in this chapter can improve all aspects of wellbeing. Many complementary therapies recognize the value of healing the whole person, so they are not just designed to deal with physical symptoms, though many are effective when used in this capacity. They are often better than orthodox medicine at addressing mental and physical problems brought about by tension, stress and emotional issues. Some are now subject to scientific testing and results are encouraging. Orthodox doctors are also becoming more aware of their benefits.

You don't have to be ill to gain from one of these therapies – often their greatest benefit is the sense of wellbeing they engender. This makes them ideal for relaxation and stress-busting. While they can be very effective for specific physical symptoms, they should not be used instead of orthodox medicine. Consult your doctor to make sure the therapy will complement your existing treatment.

Aromatherapy uses oils from plants, either inhaled or absorbed through the skin by massage or in baths. Different oils have different properties, affecting both physical and emotional states.

Reflexology is based on the idea that there are reflex points on the feet which correspond to every organ in the body. Energy flows between all parts of the body via channels. When these channels are blocked, illness occurs. Applying pressure to the reflex points on the feet unblocks the channels and restores balance throughout the body.

Acupressure is similar to reflexology in that it recognizes channels of energy flowing through the body. If there are any blockages, pressure is applied to points along the channels (anywhere on the body) to restore the flow of energy and the overall health of the patient.

Herbal treatments Mankind has exploited the curative properties of plants since ancient times. Many ready-made herbal remedies are available, or you can make your own teas, tinctures and infusions.

Chi kung is a series of meditation exercises designed to harness the body's own vital energy, having an energizing effect on both physical and mental health. A few simple exercises can be done at home, but it is better to be taught properly in a class.

Reiki is a form of healing where the practitioner channels healing energy through his or her hands to the patient, usually without actual contact. The energy activates the body's natural ability to heal itself.

Using a therapist

Some therapies like aromatherapy and chi kung can be done yourself at home. However, they will be more effective carried out by a professional practitioner as the treatment can be tailored more closely to your needs.

Choose a therapist with care. For most therapies, practitioners don't have to be registered, so contact the regulatory body and ask them to recommend one in your area. Ask questions before you commit yourself, and discuss what you hope to gain from the treatment. Ask about the cost of sessions and how many are needed. Trust your instincts and avoid anyone who makes unreasonable promises, or with whom you feel uncomfortable.

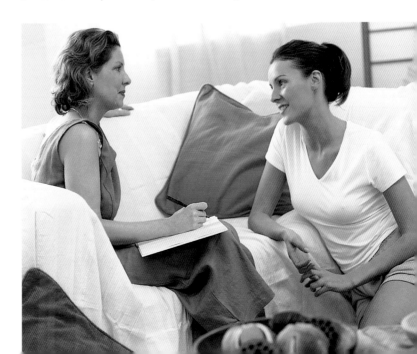

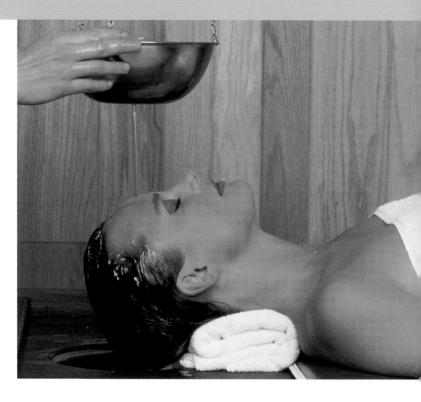

Professional pampering

Many home treatments are effective, but nothing is more relaxing than letting yourself go in someone else's trusted hands. As well as the therapies covered more fully, these can also promote wellbeing:

Ayurvedic massage The ancient Indian healing tradition of Ayurveda is designed to restore harmony and vitality to the whole body.

Ayurvedic medicine incorporates many natural disciplines, such as herbalism, detoxification, diet, yoga and meditation. Three life forces flow through the body and are the basis for diagnosis and treatment: *vata*, *pitta* and *kapha* (loosely translated as wind, fire and mucus). The practitioner evaluates your constitution and current state to assess the balance of the three forces in your overall constitution.

Treatment may include massage with appropriate oils and herbal preparations, and is effective for acute or short-term skin problems.

Indian head massage This is a specialized form of Ayurvedic scalp massage. Practitioners attribute the increasing incidence of premature greyness and baldness to tension in the head. The head massage aims to relieve this tension. Its effect on the face is equally marked, as tension in the scalp muscles is transmitted to the facial muscles.

The Ayurvedic practitioner massages shoulders and head using a warmed oil suited to the patient's constitutional type. If you carry a lot of tension in your scalp, you may get a headache afterwards, but the visible softening of your facial contours and the deep sleep that typically follows, should soon bring a smile back to your face.

Colonic irrigation A soft, pliable tube is inserted into the anus and warm water is passed up it into the large intestine, dislodging and diluting waste material. The outflow of water takes with it faeces, wind, mucus and bacteria. Devotees report feeling instantly lighter and cleaner and see a greatly improved complexion within a day or so.

Cranial osteopathy Cranial osteopathy aims to release twisted connective tissue beneath the skin by restoring the body's natural, internal rhythms. In adults it is useful for headache, migraine, dental problems, poor circulation and inefficient elimination. It also treats poor sleep, restlessness and infections, all of which can affect the skin.

To rebalance the cranial rhythms, the practitioner places her hands gently on the skull and other parts of the skeletal system to identify the areas of tension and to follow the subtle internal twists of the craniosacral system until points of resistance are released.

Aromatherapy

Aromatherapy encompasses the use of plants in their most natural forms. By capturing the essence of the oil from various different parts of the plant their beautiful, healing and mood-altering characteristics can be unleashed in various ways to improve the mind, body and spirit.

The therapeutic benefits of plants have been known for many, many centuries – evidence shows that as far back as 7000BC, Neolithic man combined olive and sesame oils with plant fragrances to produce ointments – and recent decades have seen a tremendous resurgence of interest in our ability to harness these benefits through the essential oils the plants yield.

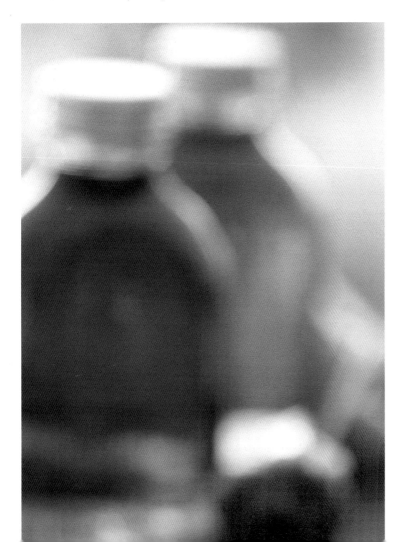

René Gattefosse first coined the term 'aromatherapy' in the 1920s while studying the powers and properties of essential oils. Gattefosse's work was put to the test when he accidentally burnt his hand one day in his laboratory. Plunging it into a container of pure lavender oil to cool the burn, he discovered that the burn quickly lost its redness and swiftly began to heal.

Essential oils

An essential oil, or essence, is a concentrated, aromatic, volatile liquid made up of tiny oil-like molecules that blend easily with vegetable or nut oil. Essential oils do not contain any fatty substances, so do not stain. The 'oil' comes from the small cavities in the cellular structure of plants or peel of fruits and is extracted by various methods such as distillation or cold pressing, which concentrates them into powerful substances. Essential oils extracted from plant species that contain little oil or that require complicated extraction are usually the most expensive – for example it takes 100 kg (220 lb) of rose petals to produce 20 ml (¾ fl oz) of rose oil. However, their potency means they are used in a very dilute form. If mixed with a carrier oil, a dilution of 1–2 per cent is enough; in a bath, five to eight drops is sufficient.

Using essences

Although essential oils are applied externally, they are able to penetrate to the body's organs and systems via the nose and the skin. The oils exert their unique properties by influencing both physical and emotional states. Many oils have antiviral, antibacterial, antiseptic, immunity-boosting, anti-inflammatory and pain-killing properties. Some essential oils tranquillize and calm, some uplift, enliven or clear the brain. Others are reputed to impart sensual aphrodisiac-like effects, probably by stimulating or suppressing certain hormones.

Ways to inhale or absorb essential oils

- **Aromatherapy massage** (see page 282)
- **Bathing:** add essential oils to bath water (see pages 282–3), or to a natural bland shower gel
- **Room freshening:** add essences to a plastic plant spray of water for a natural air freshener, or sprinkle pot pourri with essential oils
- **Vaporizing:** use essential oils in burners or add to molten candle wax (take care as essential oils are flammable)
- **Household cleaning:** add essential oils to a plant spray of water to make an effective cleaning spray
- **Beauty applications:** see pages 116 and 146 for face and hair treatments
- **Scented drawer sachets** (see page 283)
- **Diffusing:** add a drop or two of essence to a light bulb ring or an electric plug-in diffuser, or a bowl of water set over a radiator. When heated, the oil molecules are released into the atmosphere
- **Steam inhalation:** add drops of essence to a bowl of hot water, lean over the bowl and place a towel over your head to make a tent of steam. Stay there for five minutes, breathing deeply. Inhalations are good for treating respiratory disorders but should not be used by asthma sufferers

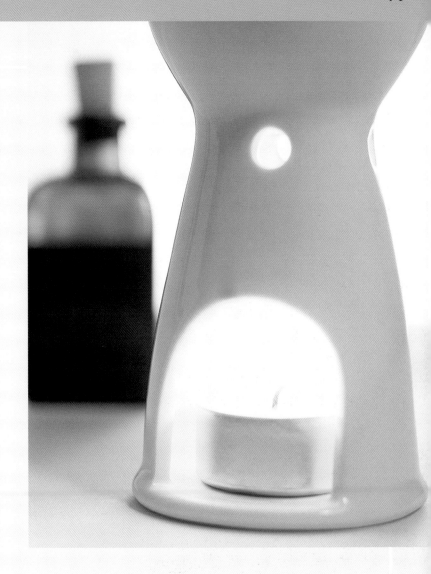

- **Sleeping aid:** drip a relaxing essence such as lavender on to balls of cotton wool or a tissue and place inside your pillowcase at night

• **Absorption** The essential oils are absorbed by the skin through the tiny hair follicles covering the body. The oil joins and mixes with the sebum at each follicle base and then diffuses into the bloodstream or is carried by the lymphatic system or the intestinal fluids.

When massaged into the skin the oil stimulates the circulation and gets the blood pumping around the body more effectively, allowing the oil to exert its pain-relieving properties. Aromatherapy massage is therefore the best technique for muscular disorders, menstrual and abdominal pains and circulatory disorders.

• **Inhalation** An essential oil that is inhaled, particularly via steam inhalation, is absorbed into the bloodstream much faster than one absorbed through the skin. The inhaled oil enters the nose, moves to the lung linings and is absorbed into the bloodstream. Inhalation is the best way of treating any respiratory, bacterial or viral ailments.

Buying and storing essential oils

Always buy good-quality oils from a noted manufacturer to ensure that the method of extraction has been carried out well and the quality of the plant that produced the harvest was good. The best essential oils will be the most expensive, but a little goes a long way.

Essential oils are volatile substances and require care to ensure that their properties remain active. The undiluted oils are easily corrupted by light (which is why they are stored in dark glass bottles), temperature extremes and exposure to air. Buy oils in small quantities and store them, tightly capped, in a cool dark cupboard or drawer.

Stored correctly and unopened, essential oils will last for many years, some such as patchouli even becoming more potent with age. However, citrus-based oils such as orange, lemon and lime have a shorter shelf life. Once you start using the oils they become exposed to the air each time you remove the cap but, with careful usage, the oils will remain at their peak for about a year.

Once an essential oil has been diluted in a carrier oil its shelf life is reduced considerably. It is therefore advisable to dilute only what you are going to use within the next two to four months.

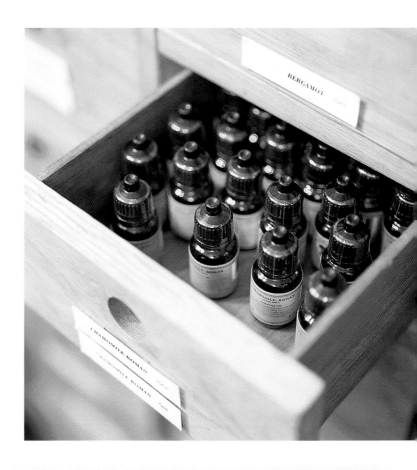

Aromatherapy care

- Be sure to use essential oils with care. Very few oils can be used in their undiluted form. Always dilute them unless instructed to use them neat.
- Before using an essential oil, check that it is safe for you to use. If you have a pre-existing medical condition, are receiving medical treatment, taking homoeopathic remedies, are pregnant or breastfeeding, or have sensitive skin or a skin condition, do not use the oils until you have checked with your medical adviser and a fully trained aromatherapist.
- Always carry out a patch test first to check that your skin does not react adversely to the oil. Place a diluted drop on the skin and leave on for 24 hours. If there is any adverse reaction such as reddening, scaling or other disturbance of the skin texture, do not use.

ESSENTIAL OIL	PROPERTIES	BLENDS WELL WITH	CONTRAINDICATIONS
Bergamot	Calms and helps prevent inflammation, limits bacterial growth. Good for infected skin. Digestive stimulant. Helps grief, depression and anxiety	Geranium, lavender, neroli sandalwood, ylang ylang	
Camomile, Roman	Calms and helps prevent inflammation and bacterial infection. Good for dry, sensitive skin and thread veins. Good stress reliever	Lavender, rosewood, sandalwood	Avoid in early pregnancy
Cypress	Aids blood and lymphatic flow, has antiseptic and decongestant properties. Useful for stress	Citrus oils, geranium, ylang ylang	Avoid if pregnant and if suffering high blood pressure or cancer
Frankincense	Tones and firms, boosts immunity. Antiseptic, calming and soothing	Citrus oils, geranium, lavender, sandalwood	
Geranium	Tones, firms, stimulates blood. Diuretic, astringent. Mood uplifter	Lavender, bergamot, rose, neroli, sandalwood	Increases sensitivity to UV rays
Lavender	Aids regeneration of damaged skin, calms inflammation. Soothes headaches. Antidepressant	Bergamot, geranium, palmarosa, rosewood, sandalwood	
Lemon	Increases circulation, strong antibacterial, antiseptic agent. Helps promote clarity of thought	Bergamot & other citrus oils, rose otto, ylang ylang	Increases reaction to sunlight. Irritates sensitive skin
Neroli	Firms, aids cell regeneration, helps with thread veins, stretch marks and scars. Immunity booster and decongestant. Has stress-relieving effects and helps stress-related symptoms. Powerful antidepressant	Bergamot, geranium, lavender, sandalwood, ylang ylang	Not for very sensitive skins
Peppermint	Strong brain stimulant. Invigorating and soothing. Good for stomach upsets	Eucalyptus, geranium, lemon, rosemary, tea tree	Avoid during pregnancy and when breastfeeding
Rose	Helps many skin conditions. Is sedative and aids digestion, easing nausea and stomach upsets. Good for menstrual and menopausal complaints	Frankincense, geranium, lavender, neroli, sandalwood	Do not use during the first four months of pregnancy
Rosemary	Strong mental and circulatory stimulant. Digestive aid. Antidepressant	Citrus & resinous essences	Avoid if pregnant, and if suffering epilepsy or high blood pressure
Sandalwood	Destroys bacteria, soothes dry, sensitive and irritated skins. Digestive aid. Antidepressant, aphrodisiac	Bergamot, geranium, lavender, neroli, palmarosa, rose	Not for sensitive or irritated skin
Tea tree	Strongly antiseptic, antiviral, anti-inflammatory and immunity boosting. Can be applied neat in tiny doses to spots, stings and cuts	Eucalyptus, lavender, lemon, rosemary, ylang ylang	
Ylang ylang	Powerful aphrodisiac, sedative effect, balances extreme emotions	Citrus & light floral oils, cypress, geranium, lavender, palmarosa	

Aromatherapy massage

Massage is an essential part of aromatherapy, relaxing both mind and body, as well as acting therapeutically to treat all manner of minor ailments. Essential oils for massage need to be diluted in a carrier oil. This can be any odourless vegetable oil, but those such as almond, apricot kernel, peach or grapeseed oils are preferable as these are rich in vitamins A, D and E, which are fat soluble and so more easily absorbed by the skin. Oils such as coconut, walnut, sesame and olive have their own unique aromas and their own therapeutic properties and, provided these are sympathetic to your essential oil, they can also be used successfully.

Always use a dropper to measure as this will enable you to count the number of drops more easily – but remember to use a clean dropper for each essential oil in order to avoid cross-contamination between oils.

For a body massage, two or three drops of essential oil should be diluted in 5 ml (1 teaspoon) of base carrier oil. This should be sufficient for one massage – you do not need to be lavish with the oil. If you are using a mix of more than one type of essential oil, the proportion of drops to the 5 ml (1 teaspoon) of carrier oil should be maintained. Reduce the essential oil by half if you are going to use it on your face (see page 116).

Choice of oils For oils with uplifting and relaxing qualities, choose from lavender, rose, neroli, ylang ylang, geranium, jasmine or the citrus oils and make sure you dilute them properly. One recipe for a relaxing massage oil is to place 10 drops each of lavender and geranium essence with five drops of jasmine essence in 50 ml (2 fl oz) of

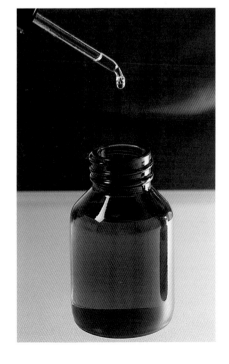

carrier oil, such as almond or grapeseed. Mix well and store in a tightly sealed dark glass bottle, ready for use.

For essential oils that can help increase circulation and detoxify choose from cedarwood, cypress, black pepper and rosemary. These all have the effect of widening the capillaries beneath the skin into which they are rubbed.

Aromatherapy baths

Aromatherapy baths are wonderfully relaxing at the end of the day. You should give yourself at least 20 minutes to allow the essential oils to be absorbed and try to make your surroundings as relaxing as possible, too. Light candles instead of turning on the light and listen to soft music. For a relaxing bath at the end of the day, try five to ten drops of one or two of the following essential oils, mixed in well with the water before you get in:

- **Lavender** is one of the gentlest essential oils. It is safe to use directly on the skin, even for children. It has strong calming and sedative qualities and so is very effective for problems such as insomnia or any sort of tension. You can also put a few drops on your pillow to ensure a good night's sleep.
- **Rose** has a lovely scent which both relaxes and rejuvenates. It is also very helpful for detox side-effects such as headaches.
- **Sandalwood** is both calming and an antidepressant, so use it if you are feeling low and this is causing sleeplessness. It is of particular benefit to dry skin and has a lovely, woody, warm fragrance.

Tips and tricks

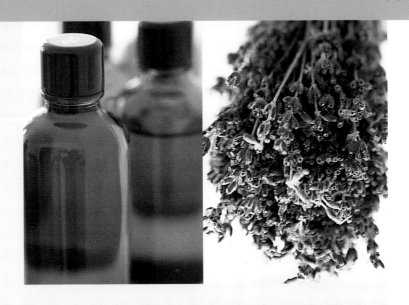

- Essential oils are inhaled and absorbed into the bloodstream. Most oils cannot be applied neat and require diluting in oil, cream or water.

- Aromatherapy massage increases blood flow to the skin manually and helps the absorption of essential oils by creating heat.

- Experiment with different essential oils and in different combinations, but don't try blending more than three oils at a time as you may find that you 'confuse' the oils and negate their therapeutic benefits.

- Individuals differ in their preferences for certain oils. Despite the therapeutic benefits of an essential oil, if you dislike its smell it will be of little value to you.

- Adding essential oils is the simplest, safest and most beneficial way to perfume a vegetable or nut oil.

- Colds and flu symptoms often make the sinuses congested. Make a steam inhalation by adding a couple of drops each of eucalyptus and tea tree essential oil to a bowl of hot water. Place your face over the steam, make a tent over the bowl and your head with a towel and stay there for five minutes, breathing deeply.

- Kickstart your day by adding to your bath three drops of basil (to help perk up the brain) and three drops of lemon, cypress, neroli or bergamot, all of which have a fresh, lively aroma.

- Whenever the weather has made you wet and miserable, a blend of spicy and warming ginger (three drops), patchouli (one drop) and frankincense (two drops) will get the circulation flowing, warm up hands and feet, and impart a relaxing, warming glow to both mind and body. Add the essential oils to a carrier lotion to apply as a warming massage, or to the water of a hot bath.

- Scented drawer sachets keep clothes smelling sweet and fresh. Make a small cushion and stuff it with lavender sprigs. As the smell of the sprigs gradually fades, freshen it by adding a few drops of lavender oil. Alternatively, stuff the sachet with cotton wool and add any essential oil you like.

• **Neroli** is made from orange blossom and has a delicious, heady, floral scent. It is very uplifting as well as calming. It particularly suits dry or mature skin.

For a bath at the beginning of the day, you need stimulating rather than relaxing essential oils. Try basil, peppermint, pine, cypress, juniper, rosewood or any of the zesty citrus oils such as grapefruit, bergamot, orange or lemon.

SEE ALSO:

→ The detox process, page 92

→ Weekend home health spa, page 102

→ Aromatherapy facial, page 116

→ Facial massage, page 126

→ Healthy hair naturally, page 146

→ Massage, page 158

→ Peaceful slumber, page 238

→ Weekend home health spa, page 266

→ Healing with herbs, page 288

Reflexology and acupressure

Both reflexology and acupressure are pressure point practices and are ideal self-help techniques. Practical, hands-on therapies with down-to-earth applications in everyday life, they both rely on using the body's energy centres. They can ease both long-term conditions and sudden crises, and are suitable as a supporting complementary back-up to orthodox medical treatment.

WARNING: Reflexology and acupressure should not be considered as replacements for professional medical treatment. A doctor should be consulted in all matters relating to health, and especially in relation to any symptoms that may require diagnosis or medical attention. Care should be taken during pregnancy in the use of pressure points.

Reflexology

The underlying principle of reflexology (sometimes known as reflex zone therapy) is that there are reflex points on the feet (and the hands) that correspond to every organ and function in the body. The theory is that by treating the feet, you treat the whole person.

According to reflexologists, all parts of the body are connected by subtle energy, which flows from the head to the feet through 10 zones (also called channels or vessels). When there is illness or discomfort the channels become blocked and the flow of energy is disturbed. Working on the hands and/or feet unblocks the channels, allows energy to flow and restores the balance, relaxing the body, enhancing the circulation and relieving uncomfortable symptoms.

Relief can be almost immediate, but long-standing conditions may take time, as the healing begins on a deep level. Reflexologists believe the body heals itself from the inside out. If symptoms have been suppressed by medical treatment they may return briefly in the order in which they were suppressed, which is why symptoms sometimes become worse for a while after the first few treatments.

• **Foot charts** The feet are extraordinary. Each of our feet contains 26 bones (together the feet hold one-quarter of all the bones in our bodies), plus 7200 nerve endings and 107 ligaments. All of these structures provide exceptional strength and range of movement.

Our feet are among the most sensitive parts of our bodies, making them the best place for reflexology treatments. Our hands, treated with a lot more respect, are actually much less sensitive than our feet.

• **The treatment** Since the purpose of reflexology is to treat the whole person, rather than a single symptom, a reflexologist normally starts by working on the entire foot to treat the whole person, before homing in on an area that requires extra help. A full reflexology treatment includes each of the body system routines and each section is begun and finished with long smooth strokes down the foot, towards the ankle. The same is done after working on any sensitive areas, to ease discomfort and draw excess energy out of the area.

Reflexology enhances circulation and the nerve supply to all organs, so there is a balancing effect – which reflexologists call restoration of 'homeostasis', the body's equilibrium. Treatment may stimulate the body to release any stored toxins, which could cause headaches or nausea. You should drink plenty of water after a treatment to help the kidneys work efficiently to flush waste products out of the body.

• **Soothing pain** Anxiety and stress respond very well to reflexology treatment, as do back pain, headache, migraine, blocked sinuses and circulatory problems. Opposite are just two examples of the various types of pain that you can ease yourself with reflexology. For more advanced care, you may choose to have professional treatment from a qualified reflexologist. Always consult a doctor if you have symptoms that won't go away, even if they seem trivial.

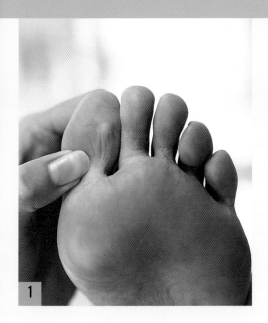

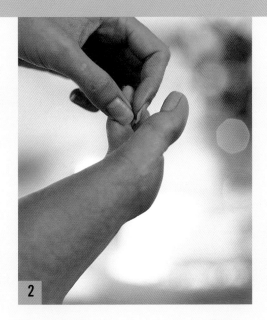

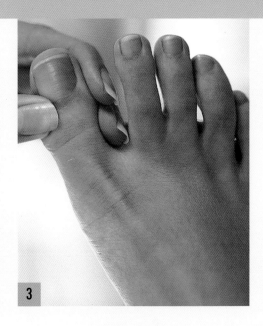

Headaches

If the work you are busy doing causes a headache, go for a walk and get some fresh air – if headaches are frequent, try to do this in time to defuse them. Check your posture; if your shoulders are hunched or if

you are straining your eyes, headaches will be inevitable. Try to visualize breathing out pain as you carry out the following self-help treatment.

1 Thumb- or finger-walk all over the pad of the big toe – this movement is also said to stimulate the brain.

2 If a headache is caused by sinuses, squeeze the sides and back of each toe.

3 A headache across the forehead brought on by tiredness can be eased by pressing just below the big toenail.

Aching shoulders

Aching shoulders are almost always caused by strain, and can in most cases be relieved by improving your posture (see page 182).

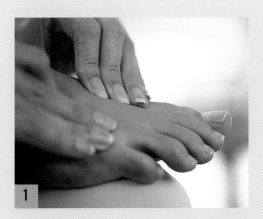

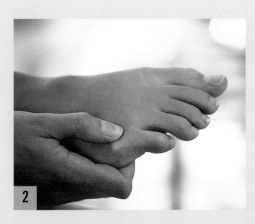

1 Knead and massage your way across both the top and the sole of the foot, about 2.5 cm (1 in) from the toes.

2 Pinch, press and gently hold for a count of five on the shoulder point, which is located on the foot between the bases of the fourth and fifth toes.

Acupressure

Acupressure provides many of the benefits of acupuncture, with the great advantage that you can do it yourself, and no needles are involved. As with all forms of Chinese medicine, the underlying principle is that the smooth flow of the body's energy, or *chi*, is vital to health and wellbeing. It travels around the body along invisible energy channels known as meridians. Dotted along these, like stations along a railway line, are 'acupoints'. If there is a blockage in a point as a result of physical or emotional disturbances, energy cannot flow. If the energy flow is blocked, the body is thrown off balance. By stimulating and restoring the flow of *chi* through these points via pressure from the fingers (or punctures with needles), health is restored.

Stress is all too likely to affect the flow of *chi*. It can result in many symptoms and ailments, including headaches, digestive upsets and insomnia.

The correct pressure You can use your thumb or fingertip to apply pressure on a particular acupressure point. Use a firm, constant pressure with the finger or thumb held straight on the point. Keep the pressure even for two minutes.

General stress relief

There are two main pressure points for general stress relief, both of which are easy to locate yourself.

1 **The foot pressure point** is on the top of the foot, about halfway up. It is the point where the bones between the first and second toes meet. This pressure point is also good for the relief of headaches.

2 **The hand pressure point** is located in the web between the thumb and forefinger on the back of the hand.

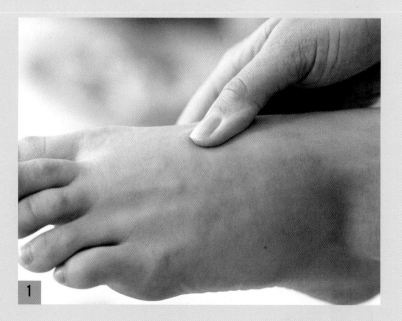

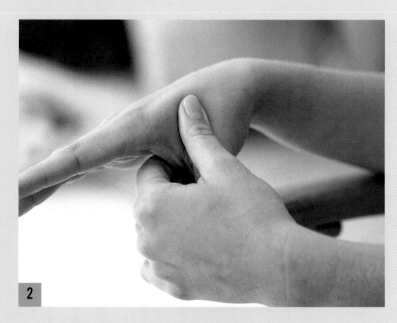

Insomnia

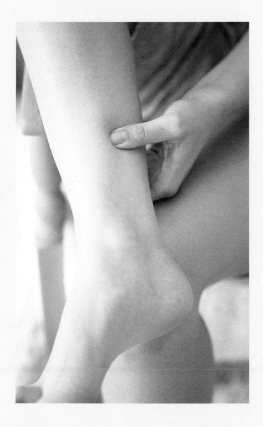

The pressure point for insomnia is located four finger widths above the ankle bone, on the inside of the leg, close to the tibia.

Caution: Never put pressure on this point during pregnancy.

Indigestion

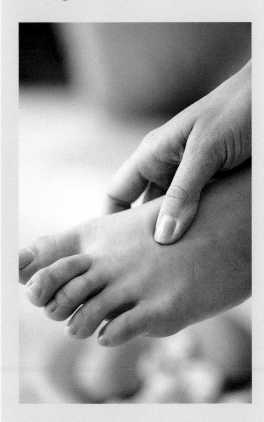

Find the point between the second and third toes, where the bones meet on the top of the foot. This pressure point will help relieve heartburn and nausea.

Headache

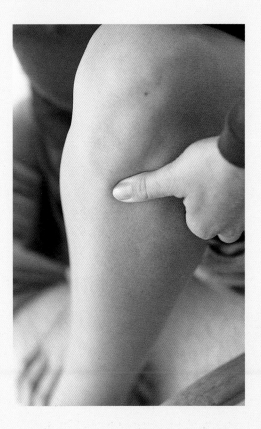

The foot pressure point for general stress relief is good for headaches as well as stress. Another point is located four finger widths below the knee, outside the tibia.

SEE ALSO:

→ Footcare, page 176

→ Posture, page 182

→ Pilates, page 184

→ Professional pampering, page 277

→ Chi kung, page 294

→ Reiki, page 298

Healing with herbs

Herbs have been used for healing since ancient times, and herbs and their derivatives form the basis of many modern medicines. For example, willow bark has been chemically reproduced as aspirin. Modern herbal medicine is a combination of tradition and modern science. The wide range of over-the-counter and self-help herbal remedies constitute a growing multimillion-dollar business. 'Natural' medicines are increasingly sought to replace potent, synthesized drugs prescribed by orthodox practitioners, a trend fuelled by concerns over side-effects and a preference for the less invasive and more intuitive approach of herbalism.

Consulting a herbalist

While herbs can be ideal for self-help use at home (see pages 290–3), professional advice is sometimes needed. There is a growing choice of qualified professional medical herbalists who use Western herbs, as well as those trained in the related disciplines of Ayurvedic (see page 277) and Chinese herbal medicine.

Herbalists can treat a wide range of ailments: aches and pains, high blood pressure and digestive problems, and chronic conditions like rheumatoid arthritis, chronic fatigue syndrome (ME) and asthma.

A consultation with a herbal practitioner will probably last 30 minutes to an hour. It will involve a review of the current illness, conventional diagnostic techniques such as feeling pulses and looking at tongues and a full medical history and lifestyle analysis. At the end of the consultation, the medical herbalist will most probably make and dispense his or her own remedies.

As well as a combination of herbs tailored to suit, the patient may be given a list of dietary suggestions or foods to avoid or eat more of, relaxation routines to follow or Bach Flower Remedies (see opposite) to help specific emotional factors that affect physical wellbeing.

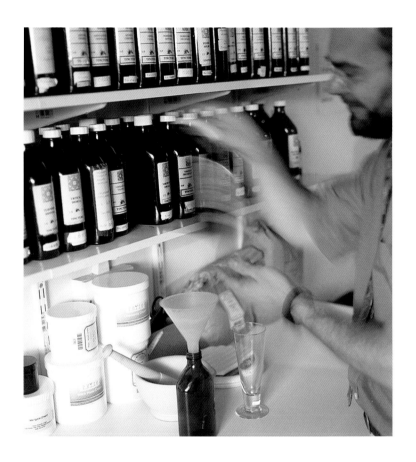

The Bach Flower Remedies

These remedies provide support for any condition involving emotional issues and help counteract the effects of stress. They are derived from 38 healing flower extracts identified by Dr Edward Bach in the 1930s, which are still widely used today, although more exotic essences – such as gem extracts and Australian bush plant derivatives – have also joined the repertoire. The Bach Flower Remedies are plant extracts preserved with brandy and are ready-to-use preparations that are dropped on your tongue or mixed in water. They are not addictive; they do not interfere with any other medication and are suitable during pregnancy and for all ages.

The Bach Flower Remedies

REMEDY	DR BACH'S SUGGESTED USE
Agrimony	For those who suffer mental torture behind a 'brave face'
Aspen	For vague fears of an unknown origin
Beech	For critical intolerance of others
Centaury	For the weak willed
Cerato	For those who dither, doubt their own judgement and seek advice of others
Cherry Plum	For irrational thoughts and fears of mental collapse
Chestnut Bud	For a refusal to learn from past mistakes
Chicory	For possessiveness and selfishness
Clematis	For the inattentive and dreamy escapist
Crab Apple	A cleansing remedy for those who feel unclean or ashamed
Elm	For those temporarily overcome by feelings of inadequacy
Gentian	For the eternal pessimist, ever despondent and easily discouraged
Gorse	For hopelessness and despair
Heather	For the self-centred, obsessed with their own woes
Holly	For those who are jealous, angry, envious or who feel hatred for others
Honeysuckle	For homesickness and nostalgia
Hornbeam	For 'Monday morning feelings' and procrastination
Impatiens	For the impatient
Larch	For those with ability but who lack confidence
Mimulus	For feelings of self-consciousness and fear of known things

REMEDY	DR BACH'S SUGGESTED USE
Mustard	For deep gloom and severe depression
Oak	For those who struggle on against adversity to the extent of overdoing things and losing strength
Olive	For complete exhaustion
Pine	For feelings of guilt and self-blame
Red Chestnut	For excessive fear for others, especially loved ones
Rock Rose	For extreme terror and panic
Rock Water	For the self-repressed who overwork and deny themselves any relaxation
Scleranthus	For uncertainty and indecision
Star of Bethlehem	For shock
Sweet Chestnut	For extreme anguish; the limit of endurance
Vervain	For tenseness, overenthusiasm and overeffort
Vine	For the dominating and inflexible
Walnut	Provides protection at times of change such as the menopause or during other major life-stage transitions
Water Violet	For the proud, reserved and isolated
White Chestnut	For mental anguish and persistent nagging worries
Wild Oat	For uncertainty about which path to take; an aid to decision-taking
Wild Rose	For the apathetic who lack ambition
Willow	For the resentful and bitter who wallow in self-pity and who are fond of saying 'not fair'
Rescue Remedy	A widely used remedy, made up of some of the above. Helpful for emergencies, calming nerves and relieving anxiety

Treating ailments

Herbs can be used at home safely for a very wide range of ailments – from colds and period pains to chronic conditions such as arthritis or irritable bowel syndrome, see pages 292–3 for just a small selection of the many ailments that can be treated with herbs. They can also provide supportive self-help in more serious conditions. However, remember to tell your doctor if you are taking herbal remedies; similarly, tell your herbalist about any current orthodox medication.

Herbal remedies can be taken internally or applied to the skin. Chewing fresh herbs may be the simplest way of taking a remedy, but it is rarely palatable or convenient. The most common forms of remedies are infusions, decoctions, tinctures, tablets and capsules; others include washes, macerations, inhalations, syrups, creams, ointments, infused oils for use in the bath, compresses and poultices.

• **Herbal infusions** Herbal infusions, sometimes called tisanes, are made in a similar way to ordinary tea, except that the usual medicinal dose is 25 g (1 oz) of dried herb, or 75 g (3 oz) of fresh herb, to 600 ml (1 pint) of water that is just off the boil. Infuse for 10 minutes, then strain and drink the infusion in three equal wine glass or cup doses during the day. Infusions are made with the flowers, leaves or stems of plants. If making individual cups, then you will need about 1–2 teaspoons of dried herb per cup. The infusion should be stored in a covered jug or teapot in a cool place and used within 24 hours.

• **Decoctions** Decoctions are similar to infusions but are made from the roots, barks, nuts and seeds or the twiggy parts of plants. A decoction is usually made with 25 g (1 oz) of plant material per 750 ml (1¼ pints) of cold water, brought to the boil and then simmered until reduced by about one-third. Strain and drink three wine glass or cup doses during the day. For individual doses, use 1–2 teaspoons of herb per 1½ cups of water.

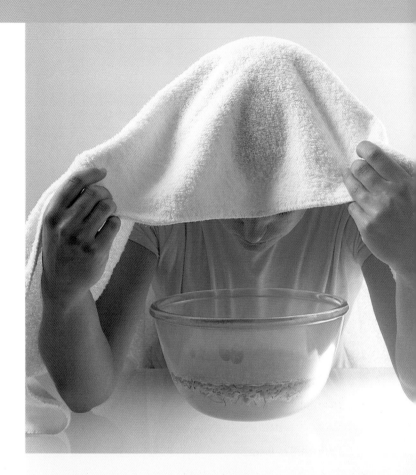

Herbal medicine safety

Although herbal medicines have a better safety record than pharmaceutical drugs, they should still be treated with care. Do not take herbal remedies unnecessarily, in greater doses or for longer than you need. Some herbs are toxic when taken in large doses and many are unsuitable for use if you suffer from particular medical conditions. Consult both your doctor and a herbalist for advice.

In China decoctions, often called 'soups', are always used instead of infusions with as much as 125 g (4 oz) or more of dried herbs per 600 ml–1 litre (1–1¾ pints) of water. The decoction can be reduced to 300–600 ml (½–1 pint) by simmering, and then this concentrated mix can be given in drop dosages, either neat or diluted in water or fruit juice. Strong decoctions can be extremely bitter and

Home herbal medicine chest

- **Bergamot essential oil:** nature's antidepressant – add five or six drops to a bath.
- **Calendula cream:** a wonderful antiseptic for cuts, scrapes and minor skin irritations.
- **Camomile tea:** soothes digestive upsets and helps teething and colicky babies.
- **Comfrey ointment:** a useful remedy for bruises and sprains.
- **Echinacea tablets:** wonderful for fighting infection and warding off colds, flu and sore throats.
- **Elderflower tea:** excellent for coughs, colds, flu, fevers and hay fever symptoms. Combine with peppermint for relief of catarrhal problems.
- **Garlic:** raw or in capsule form, is best used as a preventive for coughs, colds and to reduce blood cholesterol. Its antiseptic and antifungal properties make it invaluable for chest infections and fungal infections such as thrush.
- **Ginger:** good for indigestion and wind, circulation, arthritis, morning sickness and travel sickness. Chew on fresh ginger root, make it into a tea or take it in capsule form. Ginger in the form of drops of dilute tincture, ginger wine, crystallized ginger, ginger ale or ginger biscuits can also help to alleviate general feelings of nausea.

- **Lavender essential oil:** relieves stress and promotes relaxation – add five or six drops to a bath.
- **Lime blossom tea:** a relaxant, good for tension headaches or tension-related insomnia.
- **Lemon balm:** wonderful for relieving stress and stress-related digestive problems. Use the fresh leaves in a hot infusion.
- **Meadow sweet tea:** a gentle pain reliever, also good for acid indigestion.
- **Peppermint tea:** good for indigestion, flatulence, headaches and also colds.

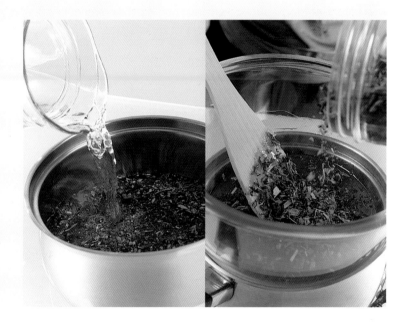

unpleasant to taste and diluting them can be a good way of persuading reluctant patients to drink them.

Strong decoctions can be stored in a refrigerator for up to about 48 hours, although they are better freshly prepared each day.

• **Other forms of remedy** A tincture is an alcoholic extract of the active ingredients in a herb made by soaking the chosen plant part in a mix of alcohol and water for two weeks, then straining the mix. Tinctures keep well, are easy to store and only a small amount is required at a time.

A compress is a cloth pad soaked in a liquid herbal extract and applied when hot to painful limbs, swellings and strains to help speed the healing process. A poultice is similar to a compress but involves the application of a herb paste directly to the affected area.

Herbal remedies for common ailments

THE COMMON COLD

Because colds are caused by a virus they cannot be treated by antibiotics, which are only good for tackling bacteria. Some herbs possess antiviral properties; the herbal approach also focuses on strengthening the body's immune system. Echinacea is one of the best herbs to take to strengthen the immune system and garlic is especially helpful if the cold develops into a chest infection. Anticatarrhals such as elderflower and yarrow can also ease the symptoms.

- **Make an infusion** using 1 teaspoon of dried **hemp agrimony** to a cup of boiling water. Add the juice of 1 lemon, 1 teaspoon of grated fresh ginger and 1 teaspoon of honey. Drink a cup three to four times daily.
- **Inhale steam** over a basin of boiling water (see page 279) to which you have added 10 drops of **eucalyptus** and five drops of **peppermint** essential oil.
- **At the first sign of symptoms** take up to 10 ml (2 teaspoons) of **echinacea tincture** in water or three 200 mg **echinacea capsules** three times daily for a period of up to five days.

BRUISES

Bruises are caused by blood escaping from damaged blood vessels underneath the skin following injury.

- **Apply arnica** or **comfrey creams** if the skin is unbroken. If the skin is broken use **marigold cream** instead.
- **Use a compress** soaked in a hot infusion of **arnica, comfrey, chickweed, hyssop, St John's wort, fenugreek** or **hemp agrimony.**
- Apply a **poultice** of mashed **cabbage leaves**.
- **To calm the sufferer and encourage more rapid healing** take homoeopathic **Arnica 6x** or **Bach Flower Rescue Remedy** (see page 289) internally .

EXHAUSTION AND FATIGUE

For a general lack of energy that falls short of clinical exhaustion, herbs can provide a longer-term energy boost.

- **Take up to 600 mg** daily of **Siberian ginseng, Dang Gui, ginseng,** or **withania capsules** for up to four weeks. (Dang Gui and Siberian ginseng tend to be more suitable for women.)
- **Drink an infusion** of **rosemary** and **gotu kola**, up to three cups daily .
- **Have a breakfast** of a bowl of oatmeal **porridge** each day.

LOSS OF LIBIDO

Stress, overwork, alcohol and excessive caffeine can contribute to loss of libido in both men and women. The menstrual cycle also plays its part in women, with libido often tending to rise mid-cycle, just prior to ovulation, and again before menstruation when pressure from the thick endometrium stimulates sexual activity. At other times it can be quite natural to feel less like sexual intercourse. Where low libido does become a problem, then there are many stimulating herbs to help.

- **Take 10–20 drops of chaste tree tincture** in water each morning.
- **Drink up to three cups daily of an infusion** containing equal amounts of **raspberry leaf, rosemary, motherwort** and **gotu kola**.
- **If tension and stress are contributing to loss of libido** drink a cup of **wood betony** and **vervain infusion** night and morning.
- **Take 10 drops of helonias tincture** in water three times a day.
- **Take up to 500 mg of evening primrose oil** and **600 mg of Siberian ginseng** daily.

CHILBLAINS

Herbal treatment for chilblains, usually caused by poor blood flow to remote parts of the body, combines warming circulatory stimulants such as ginger or cayenne pepper with ointments designed to give symptomatic relief.

- Apply a little arnica cream to chilblains to relieve symptoms, but only if the skin is unbroken. For chilblains where the skin is broken, use echinacea or camomile cream instead.
- Improve general circulation with stimulating herbs. Drink either two or three cups a day of a decoction of ginger or galangal to which is added a small pinch of powdered cayenne pepper, or a cup of rosemary infusion three times a day.
- Rub chilblains with lemon juice or a piece of raw onion.

HYPOGLYCAEMIA

Hypoglycaemia (low blood sugar) is caused by insulin overproduction. This occurs as a result of too many refined sugars in the diet, which overwork the pancreas, causing wide swings in blood sugar levels (see Carbohydrates, page 18). Symptoms include constant hunger, dizziness, headaches, fatigue, irritability, memory lapses and visual disturbances.

- To stimulate the digestion and help to normalize function put one or two drops of wormwood on the tongue.
- Drink infusions of white horehound, camomile or wood betony instead of caffeinated drinks during the day.
- Take up to 600 mg of ginseng or two 200 mg capsules of golden seal daily.
- Avoid alcohol, sugary snacks and refined carbohydrates, and eat small, regular meals throughout the day.
- Avoid sweets and chocolates and chew liquorice root instead.

PERIOD PAINS

The choice of herbs depends on whether the pain is congestive or spasmodic pain. Congestive pain builds up shortly before the period starts. It is associated with stagnation and congestion of the blood and can involve bloating and fluid retention. It eases once the period has begun. Spasmodic pain is due to uterine cramps; it begins once flow starts and can be linked to a prostaglandin imbalance and emotional tension. Motherwort and helonias will ease the stagnation sort of pain while black haw and black cohosh are better for cramps.

- For cramping pain dilute 20 ml (4 teaspoons) of black haw tincture in water. One dose is usually sufficient but it may be repeated after four hours if necessary.
- For stagnation pain take 40 drops of helonias tincture in water three times daily.

SUNBURN

Preventive measures such as large-brimmed hats, sunglasses, long-sleeved shirts and protective sunblock creams are the best solution, but if you do get burnt, herbal remedies can help.

- Pack a bottle containing 25 ml (5 teaspoons) of infused St John's wort essential oil with 25 drops of lavender essential oil when holidaying in hot climates. Apply liberally to damaged, sunburnt skin.
- Fresh aloe vera sap or aloe vera creams can also be effective.
- Drink an infusion of elderflower, yarrow and boneset to encourage sweating and cool the skin.
- Bathe the skin in a cooled infusion of marigold petals and common plantain leaves.
- To combat skin damage take supplements of beta-carotene, vitamins A and C and also zinc.

SEE ALSO:

→ Top foods for health, page 28

→ Herbal teas, page 44

→ Sun safety, page 154

→ Living with stress, page 230

→ Aromatherapy, page 278

→ Professional pampering, page 277

Chi kung

Chi kung (pronounced 'chee goong') is a form of moving meditation and a way of harnessing and releasing the body's own vital energy, or *chi*. It can have an extraordinarily beneficial effect on both physical and mental health and it is one of the most energizing forms of exercise.

There are many chi kung exercises. Some of them are for specific ailments, but the ones described here increase strength and energy, or *chi*. Given all of this, it is clearly a profound technique and one that cannot be covered in any depth in such a small amount of space. The best way to learn it is to find a good teacher, go to at least one class a week and practise at home in between. Here, however, are some basic chi kung exercises to serve as an introduction to this remarkable method. Dress in loose, comfortable clothing and soft shoes, socks or bare feet.

CAUTION: Do not do these exercises if you are pregnant.

Starting position

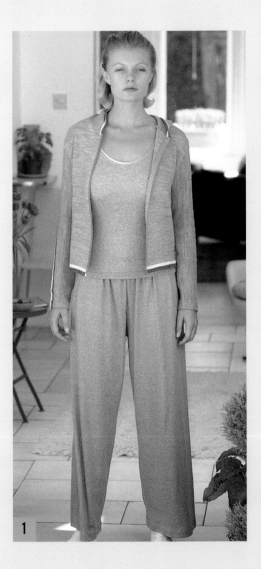

1 Begin in a **relaxed standing position**. Make sure there is no tension in your spine. Tilt your pelvis slightly forwards to iron out your back and neck, and let your hands hang loosely at your sides. Your neck should follow the line of your spine, so your gaze is straight ahead. Relax your knees.

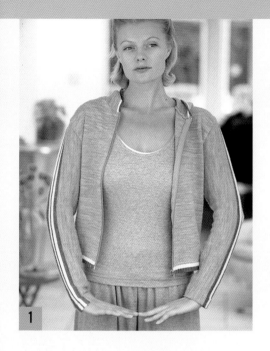

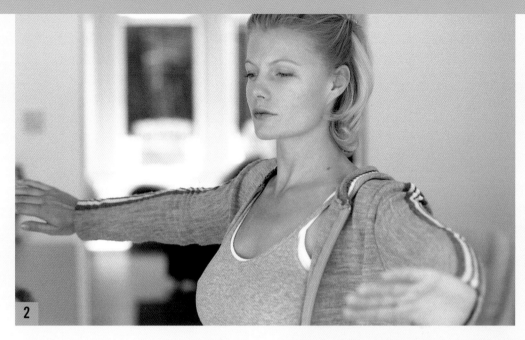

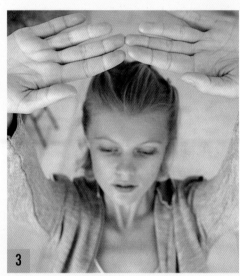

Lifting the sky

1 From the **starting position**, bring your arms in front of your body, fingertips touching and palms facing the floor.

2 Start to raise your arms out to the sides in a wide circle.

3 When your arms are level with the top of your head, turn the palms to face the ceiling and bring them directly overhead. As far as you can, straighten your arms, with your hands at right angles to your arms, fingertips slightly apart. Hold the stretch for a moment and then lower your arms until your hands are just above your head. Raise and lower in a continuous arc *up to 20 times*.

Embrace the tree

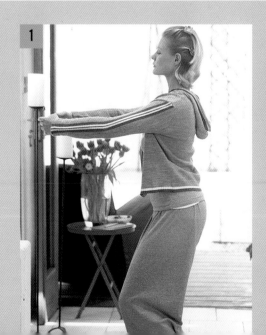

1 Stand in the **starting position**. Let your knees bend and feel your body's centre of gravity lower, but keep your spine straight.

Slowly raise your arms so that they make a wide open circle in front of you, with your palms facing your chest. **Stand in this position for one minute** and try to relax into it. With practice, you should be able to lengthen this to **five minutes**.

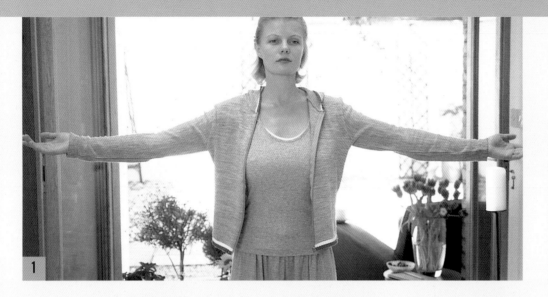

1

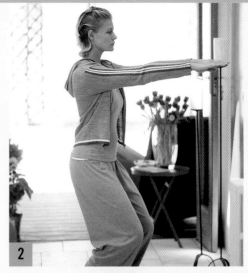

2

Low knee bend

1 Begin in the **starting position** and open your arms to your sides at shoulder height, palms facing upwards.

2 **Breathe in** and turn your palms so that they face downwards. Bring your arms round so they stretch straight out in front of you. Start to bend your knees.

3 **Breathe out** and bend your knees as if you were squatting or sitting on a beach ball. **Breathe in** and return to standing, with your arms still stretched in front of you.

4 Lower your arms to your sides, palms facing backwards. If you feel strong enough, *repeat the sequence at least four more times.*

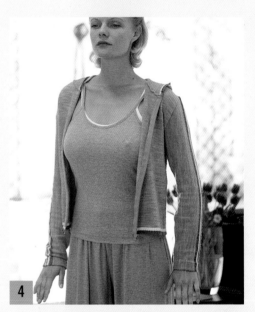

4

Pushing mountains

1 Stand in the **starting position.** Bend your arms at the elbows, palms facing forward, drawing your arms back.

2 Push forwards from the heels of the hands. Draw the arms back again and then *repeat up to 20 times.*

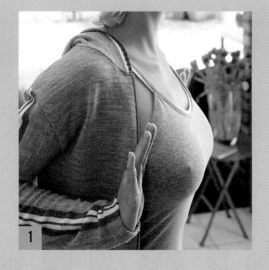

1

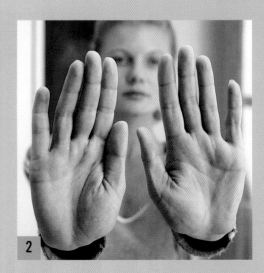

2

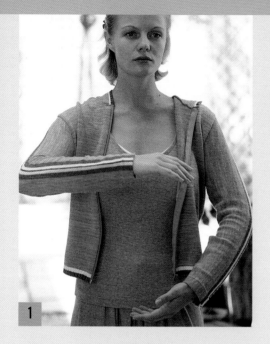

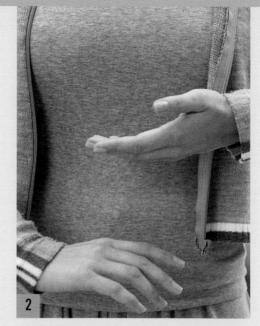

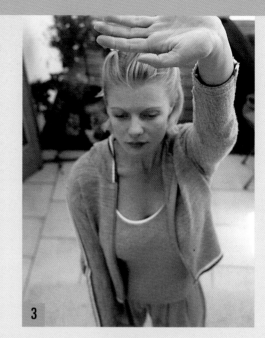

Plucking stars

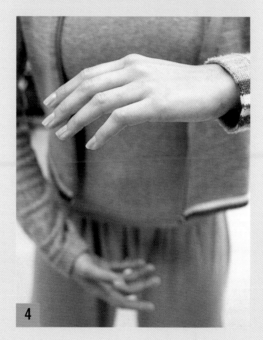

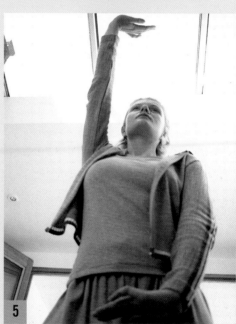

1 Stand in the **starting position**. Hold your arms out in front of you, elbows bent, your left arm level with your abdomen, and your right at chest level, as if you were gently holding a large beach ball.

2 Lift the left hand upwards, so the two hands pass by each other. When your left hand is level with your face, twist your arm round to allow the palm of your hand to continue to push towards the sky. The right hand should push simultaneously down towards the floor.

3 Push hard enough so that both arms straighten, fingers pointing inwards.

4 **Reverse the arms** to hold the ball again, this time with your left hand uppermost.

5 Lift the right hand upwards, turning your wrist up. Meanwhile bring your left hand down, to push towards the ground. This is the same position as Step 2, but **using the opposite arms.**

6 Straighten both arms as in Step 3. *Repeat up to 10 times.*

SEE ALSO:

→ Living with stress, page 230

→ Stress in the workplace, page 236

→ Improve your breathing, page 240

→ Relaxation techniques, page 242

→ Meditation, page 244

→ Yoga, page 252

Reiki

Reiki (pronounced 'ray-key') is a Japanese word that means 'universal life energy'. In all cultures and religions there is a name or concept which corresponds to the meaning of *Ki* in Reiki, for example *chi*, found in Chinese medicine, and *prana*, found in Hindu yoga.

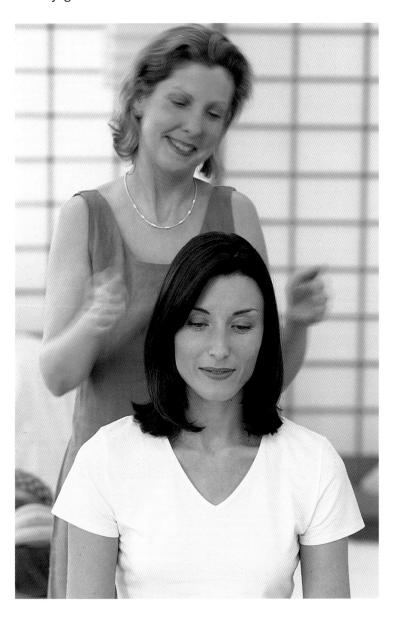

What is Reiki?

Reiki is primarily perceived as a practice for healing the body, but it is also a method for healing the mind and spirit. Reiki is healing energy in its truest sense. When the Reiki practitioner channels this life energy through their hands to the recipient, it activates the body's natural ability to heal itself. The energy goes to the deepest levels of a person's being, where illnesses have their origin. It works wherever the recipient needs it most, releasing blocked energies, cleansing the body of toxins and working to create a state of balance. It reinforces the recipient's ability to take responsibility for their life, and helps them to make the necessary changes in attitude and lifestyle to promote a happier and healthier life.

Reiki is a healing system that is a safe, natural and holistic way of treating many acute and chronic conditions and bringing about spiritual, mental and emotional wellbeing. These conditions include stress, sinusitis, menstrual problems, cystitis, migraine, asthma, chronic fatigue syndrome (ME), eczema, arthritis, menopausal problems, back pain, anxiety, tension, depression, insomnia and sciatica. Reiki is suitable for almost everyone (see box, opposite), including the very young and the elderly, pregnant women and those recovering from surgery. It is also a great tonic, and if you are in good health Reiki will help you to stay that way.

Reiki treatment complements and increases the effectiveness of most medications and other forms of treatment. However, as with all alternative healing, Reiki shouldn't be used as a substitute for orthodox medicine. No Reiki practitioner should advise any person receiving the therapy to stop taking prescribed medicines or not to see a doctor.

One of the best ways of learning more about Reiki first-hand is to visit an open evening. Here you can experience Reiki for yourself and meet people who practise Reiki both privately and professionally.

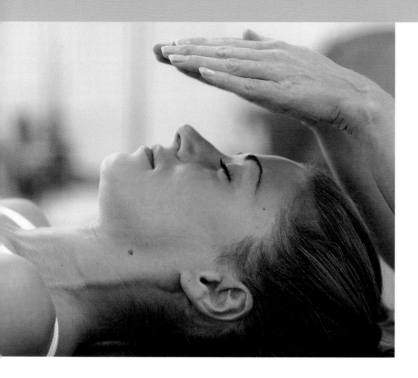

Contraindications

- People with pacemakers should be aware that the effect of Reiki energy on such a device can be very unpredictable. Reiki can also affect the levels of insulin required by the body, so diabetics treated with Reiki will need to monitor their insulin levels very closely.
- Reiki must not be applied to broken bones before the site of the break has been set in plaster. Otherwise there is a real chance that the bone may start to knit at an incorrect angle.

The treatment

Reiki is a simple, non-intrusive and powerful method of treatment. It requires no elaborate or difficult techniques, it does not require the recipient to remove their clothes and there is no pressure applied to the body. This makes it particularly useful for treating conditions where touching the body may be painful as in the case of someone who has been burnt or is recovering from surgery.

Reiki treatment aims to channel Reiki to all parts of the body. In this way the energy works to bring balance and healing to the whole person. One unique aspect of Reiki is that the energy has an intelligence of its own: attempts by the practitioner to direct the energy do not work. For example, if you have back pain and receive a Reiki treatment, the practitioner will treat your whole body and will give extra attention to your painful back. But the practitioner cannot direct the energy to go only into healing the back pain, so there is no guarantee that you will leave with your back cured. The energy will go first to where it is needed most in your body, and that may not be your back, even though it is the place where symptoms are apparent. This is why several treatments, each lasting 1–1½ hours, are usually needed and why the Reiki practitioner should not try to direct the energy during a treatment, but instead remain an open channel.

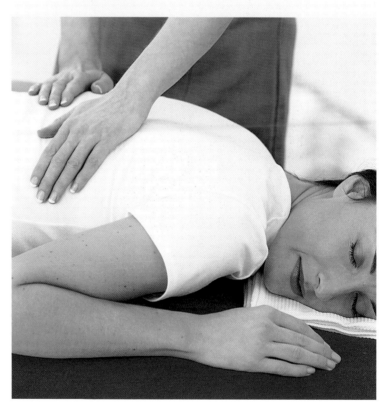

SEE ALSO:

→ Yoga, page 252

→ Reflexology and acupressure, page 284

→ Chi kung, page 294

Index

Index

Acknowledgements

Executive Editor Emily van Eesteren
Editors Sharon Ashman and Jo Lethaby
Executive Art Editor Rozelle Bentheim
Designer Lisa Tai
Picture Research Christine Junemann and Jennifer Veall
Production Louise Hall

ACKNOWLEDGEMENTS

GETTY IMAGES STONE/**Peter Cade** 12/**Peter Nicholson** 155
MAINSTREAM/**Ray Main** 265
OCTOPUS PUBLISHING GROUP LIMITED/**Colin Bowling** 3 bottom right, 232, 279, 280, 282, 288, 289, 290, 291 centre, 291 centre right, 292-293/**Peter Pugh Cook** 2 bottom centre left, 14, 25, 236/**Jeremy Hopley** 17 top left, 20 top right, 23, 26 bottom left, 27, 28 bottom left, 30, 31, 33, 35/**David Jordan** 38/**Sandra Lane** 24 left, 68, 74/**Gary Latham** front cover top right, front cover bottom left, front cover bottom right, 1, 40, 41 top centre, 41 top right, 90, 102, 104, 107, 183 centre left, 183 centre, 183 centre right, 183 bottom right, 185, 198 left, 198 right, 198 centre, 199 top, 199 bottom right, 199 bottom left, 200 top centre, 200 top right, 201 right, 201 top centre, 201 top left, 201 centre left, 201 centre, 201 bottom left, 201 bottom centre, 202 top right, 202 centre right, 203 top centre, 203 top right, 203 bottom right, 203 bottom left, 203 bottom centre left, 203 bottom centre right, 204 top left, 204 top right, 204 bottom right, 204 bottom left, 205 top, 205 bottom, 206 top, 206 bottom, 207 top left, 207 top right, 207 centre right, 207 bottom right, 207 centre right below, 208 top left, 208 bottom right, 208 bottom left, 209 top centre, 209 top right, 209 bottom right, 209 bottom centre, 210 bottom right, 210 bottom left, 210 bottom centre, 211 top right, 211 bottom right, 211 bottom left, 212 top left, 212 top right, 212 bottom right, 212 bottom left, 213 top, 213 centre, 213 bottom, 214 top left, 214 top right, 214 bottom right, 214 bottom left, 215 top, 215 bottom, 216 left, 216 right, 217 top left, 217 centre left, 217 top right, 217 centre right, 217 bottom right, 217 bottom left, 218 left, 218 right, 218 centre, 219 top left, 219 centre left, 219 top right, 219 bottom right, 219 bottom left, 220 top, 220 bottom right, 220 bottom left, 221 top left, 221 top right, 221 bottom right, 221 bottom centre, 222 left, 222 right, 222 centre, 223 left, 223 right, 223 centre, 224, 226, 243, 248, 249, 252, 253/**William Lingwood** 32, 37 top right/**David Loftus** 17 top right, 264/ **Neil Mersh** 18, 20 bottom left, 49, 50, 51, 53, 54, 55, 57, 58, 59, 60, 61, 63, 64, 65, 67, 69, 73, 75, 76, 78, 81, 82, 84, 85, 87/**Peter Myers** 83, 157, 182 top centre, 182 top right, 276, 298, 299 top left, 299 bottom right/**Sean Myers** 100 bottom right/**Emma Peios** 44, 45 /**William Reavell** front cover centre right, back cover top centre, back cover bottom centre, back cover bottom right, 2 bottom right, 2 bottom left, 2 bottom centre right, 3 bottom left, 6-7, 7 top left, 7 top right, 7 top centre right, 7 top centre left, 8 bottom right, 8 bottom left, 8 bottom centre left, 8 bottom centre right, 9 bottom centre right, 19, 24 right, 28 top centre, 28 top right, 34, 92, 93, 95, 96, 97 top right, 97 bottom left, 98, 99 top centre, 99 top right, 100 bottom left, 112, 114, 115 top right, 119 top, 119 bottom, 120 top centre, 120 top right, 121 main, 121 top right, 123 top centre, 123 top left, 123 top right, 123 bottom right, 123 bottom centre, 125, 126, 127 top centre, 127 top right, 128 top left, 128 top right, 128 bottom, 129 top centre, 129 top left, 129 top right, 129 bottom right, 129 bottom centre, 130 top centre, 130 top left, 130 centre, 130 top right, 130 centre right, 130 bottom right, 131 left, 131 right, 132 top left, 132 top right, 132 bottom, 133 top, 133 centre, 133 bottom, 135 left, 135 right, 136 left, 136 right, 136 centre, 137 top centre, 137 top left, 137 top right, 137 bottom right, 137 bottom left, 137 bottom centre, 138 top centre, 138 top left, 138 top right, 138 bottom right, 138 bottom left, 138 bottom centre, 139 top, 139 bottom right, 139 bottom left, 140, 143, 150, 151, 158 top right, 159 top right, 169 left, 169 right, 169 centre, 177 top centre, 177 top left, 230 top right, 230 bottom left, 233 top right, 238, 245, 263, 271, 283 top right/**Simon Smith** 15, 17 bottom right, 22, 42-43, 62, 66, 70, 71, 72, 77, 80, 86/**Richard Truscott** 158 bottom left, 160 top right, 160 bottom right, 160 bottom left, 160 bottom centre, 161 top centre, 161 top left, 161 top right/**Ian Wallace** back cover bottom left, 37 top centre, 52, 105, 106, 108 top left, 108 centre, 108 top right, 108 bottom, 109 top left, 109 centre left, 115 top centre, 116, 117 top left, 117 top right, 117 bottom right, 117 bottom left, 118, 141, 146, 152, 153 left, 153 right, 162 top, 162 bottom, 163 left, 163 right, 163 centre, 164 top left, 164 top right, 164 bottom right, 165 top left, 165 top right, 165 bottom right, 165 bottom left, 166 top right, 166 bottom left, 167 top left, 167 top right, 167 bottom right, 168, 170, 171 right, 171 top centre, 171 bottom left, 172, 173, 174 left, 174 right, 175, 177 centre right, 178 left, 178 right, 178 centre, 179 top centre, 179 top left, 179 top right, 179 bottom right, 179 bottom centre, 224 bottom left, 225, 233 bottom left, 234, 239 top left, 239 centre left, 239 top right, 239 centre right, 239 bottom right, 240, 242, 254 top left, 254 top right, 254 bottom, 255 top centre, 255 top left, 255 top right, 255 bottom right, 255 bottom left, 256 top centre, 256 top left, 256 top right, 256 bottom right, 256 bottom centre, 257 left, 257 right, 258 top left, 258 top right, 258 bottom right, 259 top left, 259 top right, 259 bottom right, 259 bottom left, 260 left, 260 right, 261 top, 261 bottom right, 269 left, 269 right, 270, 272 top left, 272 bottom right, 277, 278, 283 top centre, 285 top centre, 285 top left, 285 top right, 285 bottom right, 285 bottom centre, 286 left, 286 right, 287 left, 287 right, 287 centre, 294, 295 top left, 295 top right, 295 centre right, 295 bottom right, 296 top left, 296 top right, 296 centre right, 296 bottom right, 296 bottom left, 297 top centre, 297 top left, 297 top right, 297 bottom right, 297 bottom centre/**Philip Webb** 21, 56, 79/**Mark Winwood** 3 bottom centre left, 3 bottom centre right, 9 bottom centre left, 142, 159 bottom left, 176, 186 top right, 186 bottom left, 186 bottom centre, 187 top, 187 bottom right, 187 bottom centre, 188 top centre, 188 top right, 188 bottom, 189 top, 189 centre, 189 bottom, 190 top, 190 bottom, 191 top right, 191 bottom right, 191 bottom left, 192 top right, 192 centre right, 192 bottom, 193 top left, 193 top right, 193 bottom right, 194 centre, 194 top right, 194 bottom right, 195 top left, 195 top right, 195 centre right, 195 bottom left, 196 top, 196 bottom, 197 top, 197 bottom, 241 top left, 241 top right, 241 centre right, 247, 247 top right, 247 bottom right, 247 bottom left, 250, 251, 267, 268, 273/**Jacqui Wornell** 145, 147 left, 147 right, 147 centre, 235 top left, 235 top right, 235 bottom right, 235 bottom left **Photodisc**/26 top right, 227